PRACTICAL POINTS IN PEDIATRICS

PRACTICAL POINTS IN PEDIATRICS

FOURTH
EDITION

RAYMOND M. RUSSO, M.D., F.A.A.P.

VYMUTT J. GURURAJ, M.D., F.A.A.P.

PETER C. FREIS, JR., M.D., F.A.A.P., A.B.F.P.

MEDICAL EXAMINATION PUBLISHING CO.

Russo, Raymond M.
    Practical points in pediatrics.

    Includes bibliographies and index.
    1. Pediatrics—Handbooks, manual, etc. I. Gururaj,
Vymutt J. II. Freis, Peter C. III. Title. [DNLM:
1. Pediatrics. WS 100 R971p]
RJ48.R78   1985   618.92'0002'02   85-11588
ISBN 0-87488-618-X

This edition of

Practical Points in Pediatrics

is dedicated to our wives,

Joanne, Prema, and Kathleen

Contents

Preface

The purpose of *Practical Points in Pediatrics* has not changed since the first edition. From the start, it has been written with the intention of providing the student and the graduate child health provider with a practical, concise source of information. Enough subject matter has been included to assist the reader in diagnosing and managing the majority of common pediatric problems encountered in practice. The book was designed to be useful not only to the student and resident physician, but also to the pediatrician, the family physician, the nurse, and the physician assistant.

Standard textbooks of pediatrics as well as other pertinent literature have been reviewed in order to present a consensus regarding various aspects of infant and child health care. We have relied on our own clinical experience as well, especially in those sections entitled "Practical Points."

The purpose of the fourth edition is to incorporate the major changes in the diagnosis and management of pediatric illnesses occurring since 1981. The majority of the chapters have been extensively revised to keep apace with new information in these areas, and several newer subjects of increasing concern such as adolescent health, scoliosis, and accident prevention have been added.

We again want to emphasize that *Practical Points in Pediatrics* is intended only as a quick reference source, and wish to urge all readers of this book to delve deeper into the vast pediatric literature when time and opportunity permit.

We cannot sufficiently express our gratitude to the many readers of *Practical Points in Pediatrics* whose interest in the work has made a fourth edition possible.

We wish to acknowledge Dr. Peter Freis as a coauthor of *Practical Points in Pediatrics.* Dr. Freis brings an extensive experience in general pediatrics and adolescent medicine to the work.

We wish to thank Mrs. Lynn Funkhauser and Sannie Robinson for their invaluable assistance in the preparation of the manuscript.

notice

The author and the publisher of this book have made every effort to ensure that all therapeutic modalities that are recommended are in accordance with accepted standards at the time of publication.

The drugs specified within this book may not have specific approval by the Food and Drug Administration in regard to the indications and dosages that may be recommended by the authors. The manufacturer's package insert is the best source of current prescribing information.

Chapter 1

A PRACTICAL GUIDE
TO THE EXAMINATION OF THE CHILD

The physical examination of the pediatric patient differs in many respects from that of the adult. Techniques must be adapted to the degree of cooperation of the child. Interpretation of the physical findings is contingent upon a thorough knowledge of growth and development. In addition, the variation between normal and abnormal may be subtle, particularly in the infant. Regardless of the presenting complaint, a thorough physical examination should always be done with the child completely undressed. The feelings and modesty of the child should be respected. In certain age groups, the physician should examine last those body areas to which the patient will most often object in order to avoid excessive concern and resistance, i.e., ears and throat in the infant and the genitalia in the adolescent.

OBSERVATION

Considerable information can be gained by inspection or observation of the patient before proceeding with the actual examination. The information gained will be of great value in assessing the severity of the illness and will provide valuable clues in arriving at a diagnosis. Does he appear to be

well, acutely or chronically ill? Lethargic, alert? Does he
appear to be in pain? What is his state of nutrition? In the
older child, is the patient apprehensive?

POSITION OF THE CHILD

1. Head deviated to one side (congenital torticollis, which is
   most often accompanied by asymmetry of face and head,
   acute torticollis secondary to myositis, cerebellar tumors,
   dislocation of cervical vertebrae—congenital, traumatic,
   or secondary to disease pathology, e.g., rheumatoid arthritis, osteomyelitis, atlantooccipital dislocation,
   spasmus nutans, tilting of head secondary to ocular
   pathology)
2. Opisthotonos (central nervous infection, adverse reaction
   to phenothiazines, tetanus)
3. Head held in a retracted position (retropharyngeal abscess, tumor of the base of the tongue)
4. Patients with peritoneal inflammation (appendicitis or
   other inflammatory intraabdominal conditions) may lie
   on the unaffected side and keep the leg flexed at the hip
   and knee; patients who have pain due to an inflammatory
   process of the pleural cavity may lie on the affected side
   in order to splint this side to avoid pain with respiration;
   a patient with pericarditis may be more comfortable
   leaning forward in a sitting position

NATURE OF THE CRY

1. Weak (seriously ill infant or child); strong (often a good
   sign but may be indicative of pain); hoarseness (laryngitis,
   epiglottitis, foreign body in larynx, hypothyroidism)
2. High pitched (intracranial pathology)
3. Infrequent cry (mongolism, hypothyroidism, drug sedation)
4. Excessive cry (colic, parental anxiety, maladjustment)
5. Unusual cry (cri-du-chat syndrome)
6. Moaning (meningitis in infancy)
7. Grunting (respiratory distress-pulmonary or cardiac in
   origin or nasal obstruction, sometimes hypothermia)

FACIES

Facies is important, from the point of view of both severity of illness and various clinical entities. Are the eyes sunken? Is nystagmus present? Is there deviation of the eyes? What is the color of the skin – pale, cyanotic, icteric? (In black children pallor and cyanosis can best be determined by inspection of the mucous membranes and nailbeds. Icterus can be evaluated by inspection of the conjunctiva.) Is a rash present? If so, is it macular, papular, petechial, or vesicular? Are any unusual muscular movements present tremors; twitching of the facial muscles; tonic, clonic, choreiform, or athetoid movements of various muscles, exremity or truncal; absence of movement of one or more extremities?

MEASUREMENTS

The following eight measurements are essential parts of the physical examination, contingent upon age, presenting complaints, or periodic physical assessment.

TEMPERATURE
(Rectal, Axillary, or Oral)

Rectal temperature is indicated in the presence of suspected infection (up to 100°F may be considered normal). Axillary temperature may be taken in the newborn period or if the patient has diarrhea and is usually about 2°F lower than the rectal temperature. Oral temperature may be taken when the child is about 6 years of age or older and understands the nature of the procedure. If the patient is ill, temperature should be recorded at least every 4 hours.

PULSE

In young infants, apical or femoral; in older infants and children, radial. Rate, quality, and regularity are important. A thready pulse is weak and rapid and may be an indication of shock or circulatory failure. An irregular pulse may be due to sinus arrhythmia which may be judged by changes in rate with respiratory acceleration during inspiration and decrease during expiration. This may be considered as physiologic in childhood. An irregular pulse which appears clinically to be abnormal is an indication for an electrocardiogram. The diagnosis of an arrhythmia is solely by electrocardiography.

Pulse alternans is one strong beat followed by a weak beat; it is considered a sign of cardiac failure. Pulsus paradoxus is a marked decrease in amplitude of pulse beat on deep inspiration (greater than a drop of 10 mmHg with sphygomanometer); it is characteristic of an appreciable amount of pericardial fluid. Rapid pulse denotes excitement, fever (increase of about 10 beats/min for each degree Fahrenheit of temperature elevation); it implies cardiac disease and severe illness. Slow pulse may mean certain diseases (thyphoid fever), congenital cardiac disease, myocarditis due to exotoxin (diphtheria, scarlet fever), increased intracranial pressure, digitalis intoxication. Irregular pulse may be present with premature contractions, atrial fibrillation, digitalis, intoxication. Water hammer pulse (Corrigan pulse) is wide pulse pressure; it indicates aortic regurgitation or patent ductus arteriosus.

RESPIRATIONS

What is the character of the respirations? In assessing rate take into consideration age, fever, crying, depth, dyspnea (rapid flaring of nares, suprasternal and chest retractions, use of accessory muscles of respiration), and whether breathing is thoracic or abdominal in type.

BLOOD PRESSURE

Unfortunately, this procedure is too often not attempted or frequently not considered as an integral part of the examination. The size of the cuff is important. It should be about one-half to two-thirds the length of the humerus. The use of a cuff which is too small will result in an artificially elevated blood pressure; if too large, artificially low. In some instances, only the systolic pressure may be measured by palpation of the radial pulse. In infancy, the flush method may be mandatory. With ingenuity, an accurate blood pressure may be obtained by auscultation in the 2-3-year-old group. When indicated, blood pressure readings should be obtained in the upper extremities in both the erect and the reclining positions. In some instances (congenital heart disease), the blood pressure should be recorded in all four extremities. If taken by palpation, the first pulsation is about 10 mm below the true systolic pressure.

HEIGHT AND WEIGHT

See Appendices A-1-A-4.

HEAD CIRCUMFERENCE

Head circumference is best done by using a metallic tape measure and measuring circumference from the most prominent part of the occiput and just above the supraorbital ridges. (See Appendices B-1-B-2.)

CHEST CIRCUMFERENCE

Measure at the nipple line. Except for premature infants, in whom the head may appear unusually large, the head and chest circumferences are roughly equivalent until about 1 year of age. After this age, the chest grows much more rapidly than the head.

SITTING HEIGHT

To properly measure the sitting height, the infant must sit on a firm surface and the distance to the top of the head accurately determined. At birth, the ratio of the sitting height to total height is about 70%; age 3 years, 57%; girls at 13 years and boys at 15 years, 52%; thereafter, 1-2% increase. Until the age of 1 year, the head circumference is roughly equivalent to the crown-rump length (sitting height).

Height, weight, and head circumference should be plotted on the growth chart. (See Appendices A-1-B-2.)

Practical Points

1. One recording is of insignificant value. Changes in percentile as the child matures are important and efforts should be made to determine the reasons for these changes.

2. The Boston Children's Medical Center anthropometric charts were devised for "Caucasian infants and children of North European ancestry and living under normal conditions of health and home life in Boston, Mass." In many instances, these charts are not accurate for infants and children of other ethnic origins who live under less than the ideal conditions described above.

AUDIOVISUAL

EYES

1. Sclera: normal (black children may normally have a "muddy" color; newborns may have a bluish tinge because of a thin sclera), icteric, blue sclera (osteogenesis imperfecta, Ehlers-Danlos syndrome).
2. Extraocular movements: in cooperative children, the range of eye movements may be ascertained in all directions by having the patient follow a finger or small movable object. Inability of the globe to move in various directions may be due to pathology of ocular muscles or nerves. In the infant, extraocular motion is easily assessed by an induced nystagmus. The infant is held above the examiner facing him. The examiner rotates in a circle observing the normal horizontal nystagmus.
3. Strabismus: frequently present at birth but disappears before 6 months of age; subsequent to this, it may mean difficulties in visual acuity of various nature, deformities of the extraocular muscles, pathology of the nerves innervating these muscles, or central nervous system diseases.
4. Pseudostrabismus: secondary to epicanthal folds or position of the orbital fissure, tested by the following:
   a) Light shone into eyes - reflection of beam falls symmetrically on each pupil.
   b) Cover test for older, cooperative children—the eyes are made to focus on a light 2-3 feet from the patient's eyes. One eye is covered. No movement of uncovered eye should be noted. This is repeated by covering the opposite eye.

Evaluation of Vision

Does the child see? Infants blinking in response to a strong light indicates light perception. An infant who cannot see displays a constant searching movement of the eyes. A rough estimate of visual fields in older children is usually possible as is the use of standard Snellen eye charts or the Titmus vision tester.

EARS

1. Position: normally the epinna is slanted; however, an angle of slop exceeding 18° from perpendicular is associated with chromosomal aberrations and eponym syndromes; low-set ears (helix situated at a level below a horizontal plane) with corner of orbital fissure are a minor variant associated with chromosomal aberrations and renal anomalies.
2. Examination of the auditory canal and tympanic membrane with the otoscope. (See Figures 1-1 and 1-2.)
   a) Minimum restraint should be used - primarily the mother or assistant holding the child's wrists. The examiner should be able to control the patient's head.
   b) The largest size speculum that fits should be used, and it should be inserted a minimal distance to accomplish the examination.
   c) In infants the external auditory canal runs upwards. Thus, the pinna should be pulled downward to properly inspect the eardrum. In older children, the course of the external canal is downward and forward, and the pinna should be pulled upward and posteriorly to straighten the canal wall and thus obtain optimal visualization of the eardrum.
   d) The walls of the external canal should be carefully inspected for evidence of pathology - furuncles, vesicles, inflammation, seborrhea or eczema, sagging of the posterior canal wall (mastoiditis).
   e) Presence of discharge should be noted, as well as color, character, and odor. Discharge may be the result of external otitis or otitis media. Always inspect carefully for a foreign body.

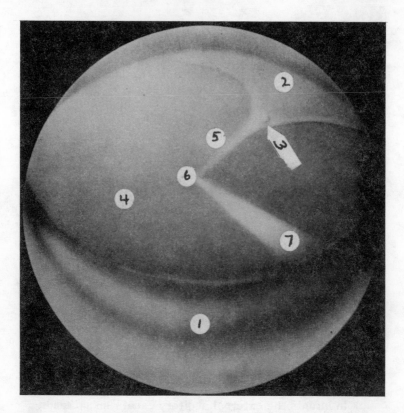

Figure 1-1 Right eardrum, infant. (1) Anulus tympanicus. (2) Pars flaccida, Shrapnell's membrane. (3) Short process, malleus. (4) Pars tensa. (5) Handle, malleus. (6) Umbo, malleus. (7) Light relex.

f) The abnormal eardrum:
    (1) Bilateral suffusion of the eardrums, with preservation of the normal landmarks, is frequently encountered as a result of crying. It is not indicative of a pathological process.
    (2) Early shortening of the light reflex with minimal injection of various portions of the eardrum, followed by obliteration of the light reflex and normal landmarks, with marked redness of the entire

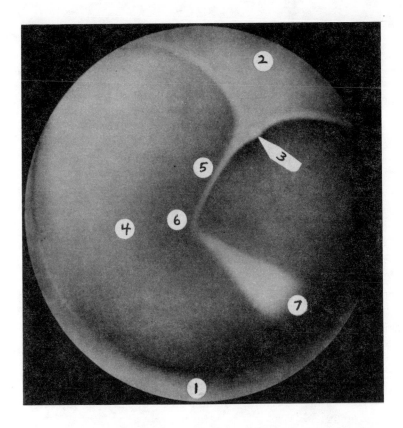

Figure 1-2   Right eardrum, child. (1) Anulus tympanicus.
(2) Pars flaccida, Shrapnell's membrane. (3) Short
process, malleus. (4) Pars tensa. (5) Handle, malleus.
(6) Umbo, malleus. (7) Light reflex.

eardrum and a bulging of the pars tensa, indicates
infection of the middle ear. This may be followed
by spontaneous perforation and the presence of a
purulent discharge, often pulsating in nature.
Otitis media is a dynamic process in which the
physical findings depend upon the duration and
severity of the infection.

(3) Serous otitis media—physical findings vary from the simple to the chronic form, from an opaque appearing eardrum having a yellowish or bluish light reflex to a grossly distorted eardrum showing presence of fluid and air, scarring, prominent but malpositioned landmarks (secondary to negative pressure and retraction of tympanic membrane), perforation of the drum (usually the pars flaccida) with presence of a cholesteatoma (a whitish appearing pseudotumor composed of shredded epithelial cells).

Evaluation of Hearing

1. The Newborn
   a) Reaction to loud noise—blinking or Moro reflex
   b) Reaction to stimulus using Neometer 70-80-90-100 decibels at a distance of 12 inches - same as (a)
2. The Infant
   a) Reaction to loud noise—contingent upon age
   b) Reaction to mother's voice—turning head toward her, cooing, smiling, transient cessation of activity, anticipation-contingent upon age
   c) Reaction to crinkling of paper—turning head toward source of sound, cessation of activity, excitement-age contingent
   d) Definitive testing—audiometry. Usually possible at age ≥ 4

After the above components have been accomplished, the examiner should continue his examination of the "whole" child in a thorough, systematic manner. It is to be emphasized, however, that the remainder of the examination should begin with that part of the body which appears from the chief complaint and the history to be the primary site of any possible pathological process. For example, the heart should be examined first if complaints relate to the cardiac system, the abdomen is to be examined first if there are abdominal complaints, etc. Throughout *Practical Points in Pediatrics,* various aspects of the history and physical examination are discussed.

Chapter 2

THE NEWBORN

EVALUATION OF THE NEWBORN

APGAR SCORE

Described by Virginia Apgar in 1950, the Apgar score is a
numerical score reflecting the status of the newborn at birth
and having a significant correlation to mortality and the
presence of neurological damage in the newborn period. Five
objective signs are scored on a scale of 0 to 2 at 1 minute
and at 5 minutes as shown in Table 2-1. The sum of these
scores constitutes the newborn's Apgar score. The 1-minute
score determines the need for resuscitation and the 5-minute
score is shown to be of greater value in predicting the survi-
vability of the infant in the immediate neonatal period as
well as the long-term prognosis for the infant. The assign-
ment of score can be done by anyone other than the one who
actually is delivering the infant and should commence exactly
at 1 minute and 5 minutes after the birth of the baby. A
total between 8 and 10 signifies a normal infant.

Table 2-1   Apgar Score

Sign	0	1	2
Heart rate	Absent	Slow	Over 100
Respiratory	Absent	Slow, irregular	Good crying
Muscle tone	Limp	Some flexion of extremities	Active motion
Reflect irritability	No response	Grimace	Cry
Color	Blue pale	Body pink Extremities blue	Completely pink

ASSESSMENT OF GESTATIONAL AGE

Until recently, the gestational age of the newborn was based principally on the obstetrical history (date of last menstrual period, time of onset of fetal movements, etc.) and clinical examination of the pregnant mother, (detection of fetal heart sounds, size of the uterus above the symphysis pubis). Uncertainties inherent in an obstetrical history and the occasional deviation of the obstetrical findings from the normal made accurate assessment of gestational age difficult.

When in doubt, gestational age can be accurately measured using real time or B-mode ultrasound. Measurement of the crown-rump (C-R) length to date a pregnancy is accurate within 1 day in the first trimester. Sonography performed at approximately 12-16 weeks gestation can be followed serially as indicated. Biparietal diameter of the fetal head is measured after 24 weeks gestation. Intrauterine growth retardation can, thereby, be diagnosed early and managed definitively.

Laboratory assessment of certain components of amniotic fluid provides additional data to determine gestational age. Amniotic fluid surface-active phospholipid levels reflect fetal lung maturity by indicating pulmonary surfactant production. Phosphatidylglycerol is present after 35 weeks gestation and correlates well with a mature lecithin-sphingomyelin ratio (L/S ratio) of 2.0 or more. An optical density of amniotic fluid at 650 nm of 0.15 is consistent with a mature L/S ratio.

It is now possible to estimate the postconceptual age with a good degree of accuracy by noting certain physical and neurological findings in the newborn (Figure 2-1). It has been demonstrated that weight gain and gestational age proceed in a predictable way. Gestational age accurately estimated at birth, when taken in conjunction with birth weight, can shed light on the deviations from the normal intrauterine growth. Using these two criteria, it is possible to classify newborn infants into three groups: (1) large for gestational age, (2) appropriate for gestational age, and (3) small for gestational age; each group with differing mortality risk (Figure 2-2). Such a classification helps one to anticipate, and more effectively manage, some of the special problems that may be associated with the two groups of children showing inappropriate weights for gestational age. Further, prediction as to the morbidity in these groups can be made, though to a limited extent, at the present time.

THE HIGH-RISK NEWBORN

Deviations from the normal length of gestation and from normal intrauterine growth can be classified as follows:

Shortened gestation - prematurity
Prolonged gestation - postmaturity
Small for gestational age babies
Large for gestational age babies

PREMATURITY: LOW BIRTH WEIGHT

Newborns born before 37 weeks of gestation (from the first day of the last menstrual period) are now classified as premature infants. Until recently, all children weighing less than 2500 g were classified as premature. This classification

Physical Findings (EST GA)	Findings across Weeks Gestation 24–44
VERNIX	APPEARS (24–25); COVERS BODY (26–37); DECREASES IN AMOUNT (38–40); NO VERNIX (41–44)
EXAM FIRST HOURS	
BREAST TISSUE / NIPPLES	NONE; BARELY VISIBLE; WELL DEFINED FLAT AREOLA; WELL DEFINED, RAISED AREOLA; 1–2 MM (36); 4 MM (38); 7 MM OR MORE (42)
SOLE CREASES	NONE; 1, ANTERIOR TRANSVERSE; 2, ANTERIOR TRANSVERSE; ANTERIOR 2/3 SOLE; CREASES INVOLVING HEEL
EAR CARTILAGE	PINNA SOFT, STAYS FOLDED; RETURNS SLOWLY FROM FOLDING; THIN CARTILAGE SPRINGS BACK FROM FOLDING; FIRM, REMAINS ERECT FROM HEAD
EAR FORM	FLAT, SHAPELESS; BEGINNING INCURVING OF PERIPHERY; PARTIAL INCURVING UPPER PINNA; WELL DEFINED INCURVING ALL OF UPPER PINNA
GENITALIA – TESTES & SCROTUM	UNDESCENDED; TESTES HIGH IN CANAL, FEW RUGAE; TESTES LOWER MORE RUGAE; TESTES DESCENDED, PENDULOUS SCROTUM, RUGAE COMPLETE
LABIA & CLITORIS	LABIA MAJORA WIDELY SEPARATED, PROMINENT CLITORIS; LABIA MAJORA NEARLY COVER LABIA MINORA; LABIA MINORA & CLITORIS COVERED
HAIR (APPEARS ON HEAD @ 20 WKS)	EYEBROWS & LASHES; FINE, WOOLLY HAIR; HAIR SILKY, SINGLE STRANDS
LANUGO (APPEARS @ 20 WKS)	LANUGO OVER ENTIRE BODY; VANISHES FROM FACE; SLIGHT LANUGO OVER SHOULDERS; NO LANUGO
SKIN TEXTURE	THIN; SMOOTH, MEDIUM THICKNESS; SKIN THICKENING, DESQUAMATION
SKIN COLOR & OPACITY	TRANSLUCENT, PLETHORIC, NUMEROUS VENULES (ABDOMEN); PINK, FEW LARGE VESSELS OVERALL; PALE PINK, NO VESSELS SEEN
SKULL FIRMNESS	SOFT TO 1 INCH FROM ANTERIOR FONTANELLE; SPRINGY AT EDGES OF FONTANELLE, CENTER FIRM; BONES HARD, SUTURES EASILY DISPLACED; BONES HARD, CANNOT BE DISPLACED
POSTURE – RESTING	LATERAL DECUBITUS; HYPOTONIA; SLIGHT INCREASE IN TONE, FROG-LIKE; SLIGHT, LOWER EXTREMITIES; TOTAL FLEXION
RECOIL	ABSENT; NONE UPPER EXT, GOOD LOWER EXT; SLOW UPPER EXT; GOOD UPPER EXT
LATER EXAM	
TONE – HEEL TO EAR	NO RESISTANCE; SLIGHT RESISTANCE; DIFFICULT; IMPOSSIBLE
SCARF MANEUVER	NO RESISTANCE; MINIMAL RESISTANCE; FAIR RESISTANCE; DIFFICULT
NECK EXTENSORS	ABSENT; SLIGHT; MINIMAL; GOOD; FAIR
NECK FLEXORS	ABSENT; NO ABDUCTION; COMPLETE WITH ABDUCTION
REFLEXES – MORO	BARELY APPARENT; COMPLETE, EXHAUSTIBLE; GOOD, COMPLETE
GRASP	FEEBLE; FAIR; SOLID, INVOLVES ARMS; MAY PICK INFANT UP
ROOTING	MINIMAL C REINFORCEMENT; GOOD C REINFORCEMENT; REACT
CROSSED EXTENSION	SLIGHT WITHDRAWAL; WITHDRAWAL; WITHDRAWAL & EXTENSION; WITHDRAWAL, EXTENSION & ADDUCTION
AUTOMATIC WALK	ABSENT; MINIMAL; FAIR TOES; GOOD, TOES; GOOD, HEELS
TRUNK ELEVATION	ABSENT; SLIGHT; GOOD
GLABELLAR TAP	ABSENT; APPEARS; PRESENT
HEAD TURNS TO LIGHT	ABSENT; APPEARS; PRESENT
Clinical estimate, GA	
Calculated GA	24 ... WEEKS GESTATION ... 44

Figure 2–1 A guide to the estimate of gestational age on the basis of physical and neurological findings. (From Lubchenco, L.O.: Assessment of Gestational Age and Development at Birth. Pediatr Clin North Am 17:125, 1970. Courtesy of W.B. Saunders Co., Philadelphia. PA.)

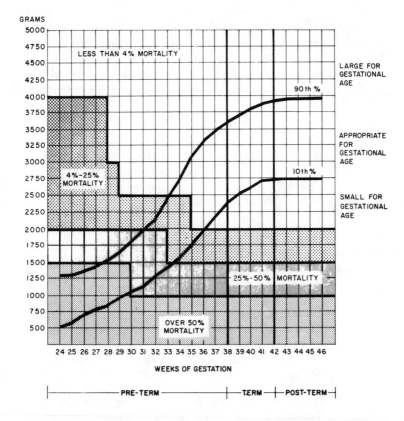

Figure 2-2   University of Colorado Medical Center classification of newborns by birth weight and gestational age and by neonatal mortality risk. (From Battaglia, F.C. and Lubchenco, L.O.: J Pediatr 71:161, 1967. Reproduced with permission of C.V. Mosby Co., St. Louis.)

included a number of children who were born at term but weighed less than 2500 g. Also, it excluded a small number of children who were, in fact, premature by gestational age but weighed more than 2500 g. At present, all newborns weighing less than 2500 g are simply termed low birth weight infants. A great majority of infants who are premature (gestational age less than 37 weeks) also belong to the low birth weight category (less than 2500 g).

Factors that cause premature birth of infants include abnormalities in the genital tract of the mother, complications of pregnancy such as toxemias, and a variety of chronic illnesses. Other circumstances that are generally associated with low birth weight infants are low socioeconomic status of the mother, history of frequent pregnancies, maternal age below 16 or above 35, and certain maternal habits such as cigarette smoking or narcotic addiction, inadequate maternal weight gain during pregnancy purposefully to meet societal demands or malnutrition. There is also a genetic factor that may influence the birth weight. It is known that black infants, on an average, weigh less than white infants and low birth weights are more common in the former.

Physical characteristics of infants born prematurely are consistent with their gestational ages. (See Figure 2-1). Generally, the head circumference of a premature infant will be less than 33 cm and the height less than 47 cm. These measurements are appropriate to gestational age.

Functional immaturity of different systems of the body explains some of the characteristics seen in premature infants. Inability to either concentrate or dilute the urine to the extent seen in full-term infants and a tendency to develop acidemia and edema reflect a state of immaturity of pulmonary and renal function. Limitation of digestive function is reflected in an inability to tolerate fat as well as the mature infant. Immunological immaturity accounts for the unusual susceptibility to infection; the predisposition of premature infants to develop idiopathic respiratory distress syndrome has been explained on the basis of immaturity of the lungs. The inability to maintain a stable normal body temperature is principally due to a lack of ability to compensate for the heat loss through their large body surface relative to their weight and minimal subcutaneous fat. The incidence of intracranial and pulmonary hemorrhage is high.

The immature cardiovascular system is not prepared for the placental transfusion at birth. Platelet dysfunction rather than hypoprothrombinemia results in capillary fragility. Hypercoagulability of blood, because of a deficiency of the anticoagulant antithrombin II, is prominent in preterm infants. Polycythemia is frequently present in term and preterm infants. This can result in cardiovascular or neurological sequelae as well as jaundice. Therapy with partial exchange transfusion is of benefit where indicated.

Hypoproteinemia and jaundice are common. The functional hepatic immaturity and enterohepatic recycling of bilirubin contribute to this problem.

Apnea, when present, is due to a lack of central nervous system (CNS) responsiveness to oxygen and carbon dioxide drives.

Management of the Premature Infant

Incubator Care

Temperature adjustment of the incubator air should be made to keep the axillary temperature of the infant between 36.5 and 37°C (Table 2-2). Relative humidity should be maintained between 40 and 60%.

Oxygen should be provided as indicated to provide adequate tissue oxygenation. An oxygen tension between 50 and 80 torr is satisfactory and will avoid excessive oxygen

Table 2-2 Guide for Incubator Temperature Setting for Neutral Thermal Conditions in Neonates

Weight (g)	Incubator Air Temperature (C)
Less than 1000	35-36
1000-1500	34-35
1501-2500	33-34
2501-3500	32-34
Over 3500	31-33

From Oliver, T.K., Jr.: Temperature Regulation and Heat Production in the Newborn. Pediatr Clin North Am 12:765, 1965. (Reproduced with permission of W.B. Saunders, Co., Philadelphia.)

administration and its complications such as retrolental fibroplasia. The mode of oxygen administration must be tailored to the individual infant's needs.

Endotracheal intubation, if indicated, should be performed promptly. Optimum positioning of an endotracheal tube at midtrachea can be calculated as follows:

$$\text{nares} - \text{midtrachea distance} = 0.21$$
$$\text{x crown-heel length}$$

Consultation with a neonatologist or transfer to a neonatal intensive unit must be coordinated by the pediatrician.

Feeding

The preterm infant may be unable to suck well and require intravenous, gavage tube feeding. In a term infant, intravenous fluid is offered as 10% glucose at 70 ml/kg/day initially. This is increased at 3 days of age to 80, then 90 ml/kg/day on day 4. At 1 week, the baby requires 120 ml/kg/day. Sodium and potassium 2-3 mEq/kg/day are added on day 2 or 3 of life. The preterm infant has a higher insensible water loss and requires slightly increased maintenance fluid. If possible, early po feeding, about 4-8 hours after birth, is recommended to minimize the dangers of hyperbilirubinemia and hypoglycemia. The amount and route of feeding should depend on the condition of the infant. Initially, start with sterile water. Feedings may be changed to a standard formula after two feedings. The amount is increased at each feeding by 1-2 ml/feeding depending on the individual infant's ability to take more, until a total of about 150-160 ml/kg/day is reached which will provide between 120 and 150 cal/kg/day.

Frequently, an infant can tolerate only 100 ml/kg/day of po fluids. This is adequate if the neonate gains 15 g of weight each day. Most preterm and term neonates have sufficient growth on 120 cal/kg/day. However, these physiologic requirements can be increased to 160-185 cal/kg/day by disease and activity. Feedings should be supplemented with vitamins A, C, D, and E. Administration of iron (10-15 mg of elemental iron/day) is indicated in these rapidly growing small infants with low body stores of iron.

POSTMATURITY

Infants born 7 or more days after the normal gestational period are termed postmature. Placental dysfunction is frequently associated with postmaturity. Clinical features reflect an apparent recent weight loss. The infant is alert and generally the behavior is that of a 1-2-week-old infant. Long nails, dry skin, and absence of vernix caseosum are characteristic features.

Mortality is significant in instances of prolonged gestation when postmaturity exceeds 3 or more weeks. Early obstetrical intervention has markedly reduced the mortality rate.

Normal newborn care is all that is necessary in most postmature infants.

SMALL FOR GESTATIONAL AGE BABIES

Infants weighing less than their predicted weight for the gestational age are termed small for gestational age babies. A great deal of attention has been focused on these infants recently, particularly those weighing less than 2500 g (low birth weight), who were formerly simply classified as premature infants. It is now clear that these two groups of infants - the premature ones (born before 37 weeks) and the small for gestation age babies - differ in terms of their etiologies, their immediate neonatal problems, and their long-term prognosis. The smallness of the newborn with respect to gestational age has been attributed to intrauterine growth retardation. Various factors are thought to produce the growth retardation. In a small percentage of cases, the growth retardation is explained on the basis of some intrinsic disorder of the fetus itself, e.g., infection of fetus with rubella or cytomegalic viruses, *Toxoplasma gondii,* and chromosomal aberrations as in trisomies D or E. Associated congenital anomalies are common in this group of babies. The incidence of congenital anomalies seems to increase as the weight for the gestational age decreases. The cause, however, seems to be extrinsic in nature in the majority of these infants. This may be in the form of defective uteroplacental support to the growing fetus. Fetal malnutrition describes this situation. Long-term follow-up evaluation studies indicate that the incidence of impaired growth and development is more often seen in the group of children with associated congenital anomalies than the ones without them. Genetic, socioeconomic, and a host of other factors profoundly affect the ultimate growth and development of these infants. Maternal smoking and alcohol consumption result in intrauterine growth retardation. The fetal alcohol syndrome is very common and has distinguishing features. The affected infant has small palpebral fissures, long upper lips, low birth weight and length, and small head circumference.

Physical findings and neurological performance of these infants are compatible with their gestational age (Figure 2-1). Soft tissue wasting is apparent. Vigorous activity is common with unusually frequent demands for feedings. Hypoglycemia and hypocalcemia are noted in many of the infants. Generally, the weight gain in these infants is more rapid than with true premature babies. There is little or no postnatal weight loss.

Management consists of carefully monitoring blood glucose and treating hypoglycemia if it should develop. (See p. 22.) Prevention of hypoglycemia may be attempted by instituting early feedings. However, po feedings cannot be relied upon to forestall or treat hypoglycemia, and intravenous therapy must be utilized when hypoglycemia occurs. Other problems related to congenital anomalies should be promptly attended to.

LARGE FOR GESTATIONAL AGE BABIES

Infants born to diabetic mothers are characteristic of this group. The mortality and morbidity are closely related to whether they are born preterm or at term. The mortality is particularly high in those infants born at 24–28 weeks of gestation weighing more than 2500 g.

Postterm large for gestational age infants are not infrequently encountered (15/1000 births). Much work remains to be done with this group of infants to identify the etiological factors responsible for their large size, and to assess their long-term growth and developmental patterns.

INFANT OF THE DIABETIC MOTHER

The metabolic abnormality in a pregnant mother with diabetes profoundly affects the growing fetus. The mortality and morbidity associated with infants born to diabetic mothers are significantly higher than those born to nondiabetic mothers. Characteristically, most infants are large for their gestational ages by weight as well as by length. They can be plethoric with a Cushingoid appearance and the resemblance to one another is remarkable. The large body is liberally coated with vernix caseosa. The umbilical cord is plump and hypertrophic.

Hypoglycemia (blood glucose less than 30 mg/100 ml in term infants and less than 20 mg/100 ml in premature infants) occurs frequently in these infants within a few hours after birth. The majority of the infants are asymptomatic in spite of significant degrees of hypoglycemia. Those who develop symptoms may do so within a few hours after birth or may not exhibit any symptoms until 12-24 hours of age. The symptoms of hypoglycemia include tremors, cyanosis, convulsions, irregular respirations, limpness, refusal to feed, and apathy.

Hypocalcemia with tetany as measured by serum calcium (less than 7 mg/100 ml) and electrocardiographic (ECG) changes (prolonged QT intervals) may be noted in a significant number of infants.

The incidence of hyperbilirubinemia is higher in these infants as compared to infants of comparable weight and gestational age born to nondiabetic mothers. Some infants may develop the respiratory distress syndrome. (See p. 47.) Other problems of these infants include renal vein thrombosis, a variety of congenital anomalies, intracranial hemorrhage, and congestive cardiac failure.

The majority of the infants tend to have an uneventful neonatal course. The overall survival rate is excellent. Control of maternal diabetes and interruption of pregnancy between 35 and 37 weeks have contributed significantly to the improved mortality rate. The prenatal mortality seems to be related not so much to the duration of the disease in the mother, as to the severity and control of her disease.

MANAGEMENT

Management includes the following:

1. The internist, endocrinologist, obstetrician, and pediatrician should closely collaborate in the overall management of a pregnant mother with diabetes. Referral to a perinatal center should be considered.
2. Stable and satisfactory maternal environment for the fetus should be established by careful control of diet, activity, and use of insulin throughout pregnancy.
3. Interruption of pregnancy between 35 and 37 weeks of gestation is recommended for insulin-dependent diabetic mothers to accomplish the highest infant survival rate.
4. The pediatrician should be present at the delivery and be prepared to place an intravenous line immediately. A umbilical artery catheter or peripheral line promptly placed can avoid morbidity in the newborn. A peripheral line is preferred as being of lesser risk.
5. The initial management of the infant consists of expert care in an intensive care unit, careful regulation of temperature, humidity, and oxygen concentration. Aspiration of stomach contents shortly after birth (to detect intestinal obstruction, if any, and possibly to prevent respiratory distress syndrome), frequent estimation of blood glucose levels during the first 6–8 hours, and initiation of early (within 12 hours) oral feedings with glucose or fructose solutions are recommended.
6. Hypoglycemia can be managed as follows:
   a) Intravenous glucose initiated at 6 mg/kg/min which can be gradually increased to a maximum rate of 15 mg/kg/min to achieve euglycemia. Acute symptoms can be relieved by a bolus infusion of 25% glucose at a rate of up to 4 ml/kg followed by a continuous 10% glucose infusion.
   b) Pharmacologic therapy is indicated for patient needs exceeding the above therapy: hydrocortisone 5 mg/kg/day IV or po, or prednisone 2 mg/kg/day. ACTH offers no advantage over the above glucocorticoid therapy. Glucagon 30 mg/kg may result in a sustained hyperglycemia. The agent can be used as initial therapy at 300 mg/kg. Phenobarbital increases CNS glucose and, therefore, has greater therapeutic value than its use solely as a sedative. Most frequently, parenteral glucose infusion titrated to the infants needs is all that is required.

7. Concurrent hyperphosphatemia (serum phosphorus above 8 mg/dl) and/or hypomagnesemia (serum magnesium less than 1.5 mg/dl) should be sought and corrected.
8. Hypocalcemia (serum calcium 7 mg/100 ml or less or ionized calcium below 3-3.5 mg/dl) should be treated with a continuous intravenous infusion. Calcium gluconate 75 mg/kg/day given over 48 hours is effective. Calcium gluconate 10% can be given po q 4-6 h afterward avoiding the risk of necrotizing enterocolitis associated with hypertonic solutions.
9. Respiratory distress syndrome and hyperbilirubinemia may be managed as detailed elsewhere in this chapter.

JAUNDICE IN NEWBORN

Jaundice in the newborn results from increased accumulation of bilirubin in the blood. With the breakdown of hemoglobin, the heme portion is converted to the unconjugated form of bilirubin which is transported in the serum bound to albumin. In the liver, bilirubin is conjugated with glucoronic acid to form conjugated bilirubin. The enzyme glucuronyl transferase is responsible for the conjugation reaction. The increased accumulation of either form of bilirubin may be due to excessive production of bilirubin as a result of increased destruction of RBCs, reduced hepatic uptake and conjugation, and impaired excretion of conjugated bilirubin.

KERNICTERUS

Accumulation of varying levels of unconjugated bilirubin produces the neurological syndrome, kernicterus, in some infants. The syndrome is due to diffusion of unbound bilirubin into the CNS producing toxic encephalopathy. The syndrome is characterized by lethargy, refusal to feed, convulsions, rigidity, and opisthotonos. Surviving infants may show evidence of frank brain damage or subtly signs of impaired neurological development.

Levels of bilirubin at which kernicterus may develop vary depending on certain associated factors such as low birth weight, level of serum albumin, asphyxia, acidemia, hypoglycemia, and respiratory distress. Because the bilirubin bound to albumin does not diffuse into the CNS, the risk of kernicterus is greater in infants in whom the bilirubin-binding capacity of albumin is compromised either as a result of low levels of serum albumin (prematurity) or due to presence of factors in the blood that compete with albumin-binding sites (sulfonamides, salicylates, unesterified fatty acids, etc.) Hypoxia and acidosis also predispose the infant to kernicterus by decreasing the albumin-binding capacity. In addition, hypoxic states may render the CNS cells more susceptible to damage by bilirubin. The presence of hypoxia and/or acidemia places the infant at greatest risk of kernicterus regardless of the serum bilirubin level. Because of frequent association of most of the aforementioned factors with prematurity, premature infants are at a greater risk of developing kernicterus than full-term infants.

PHYSIOLOGICAL JAUNDICE

This is a phenomenon noted in a majority of newborn infants during the first week of life. Jaundice is due to accumulation of unconjugated bilirubin and does not usually appear before 24 hours of life. The serum level of bilirubin may go up as high as 10 mg/100 ml in full-term babies and 12-14 mg/100 ml in premature infants. Accumulations beyond these levels may indicate presence of other factors that might be aggravating the physiological jaundice. The jaundice may last for about 1-2 weeks.

The following factors have been postulated as causes of physiological jaundice: increased production of bilirubin due to excessive destruction of red blood cells, defective uptake of bilirubin by the liver cells, impaired conjugation due to deficiency of glucuronyl transferase activity and, primarily, increased enterohepatic circulation of bilirubin.

Most infants are asymptomatic and the diagnosis is made by exlusion of other common causes of jaundice during this period. (See Table 2-3).

DIAGNOSTIC WORKUP

1. Hemoglobin, serum bilirubin, both direct and indirect
2. Reticulocyte count
3. Examination of peripheral smear
4. Infant's and parents' Rh and blood grouping
5. Coombs' test, both direct and indirect

6. In the absence of blood group incompatibilities:
   a) Blood, urine, cerebrospinal fluid (CSF), and other
      culture to rule out sepsis
   b) Urinary sediment examination for cytomegalic in-
      clusion cells
   c) Viral studies as indicated
   d) Test for specific IgM antibodies
   e) Serum enzymes
7. Electrophoretic and enzyme studies of red cells as indicated

MANAGEMENT

The primary goal is the prevention of kernicterus. This can
be accomplished by promptly identifying the cause of the
jaundice and treating it whenever possible, correcting factors that may promote bilirubin movement into the tissues,
e.g., hypoxia, acidosis, lack of carbohydrate, dehydration,
low serum albumin, etc., and by keeping serum concentration of indirect bilirubin below a level that is most likely to
cause kernicterus. The critical levels of serum bilirubin
above which a significant number of newborns develop
kernicterus vary according to the predisposing factors referred to above. It is generally agreed that accumulation
of 20 mg% or more of unconjugated bilirubin in any newborn infant whose jaundice is due to hemolytic disease is
dangerous. Perhaps the critical level is even lower in premature infants.

Measures adopted to prevent bilirubin concentrations
from reaching critical levels include hydration and the use
of blue light which oxidizes bilirubin to less toxic metabolites. Therapy with phenobarbital apparently increases
the hepatic excretion of bilirubin by stimulating glucuronyl
transferase activity.

Phototherapy can be used in the management of infants
with hyperbilirubinemia. The effectiveness of this modality
of treatment in reducing the preexisting and expected
further increases in serum bilirbuin levels has been established. However, because there is a wide gap in the knowledge concerning the possible short- and long-term adverse
effects of phototherapy, a decision to subject an infant to
phototherapy should not be made lightly. Selection criteria
for phototherapy seem to vary from one medical center to

Table 2-3 Diagnostic Features of Some Causes of Jaundice in the First Week of Life

Diagnostic Consideration	Clinical Data	Laboratory Data	Remarks
Physiological jaundice	Onset: full term 2-3 days, premature 3-4 days.	Elevated indirect bilirubin. Peak bilirubin concentration: full term 10-12 mg%; premature 12-14 mg%.	Otherwise well newborn with no blood group incompatibility.
Hemolytic diseases 1. Rh incompatibility	Onset: usually within 24 hours. Hepatosplenomegaly. Petechiae.	Anemia. Reticulocytosis. Peripheral smear: increased nucleated red cells, polychromasia, anisocytosis. Positive direct Coombs' test. Elevated indirect serum bilirubin.	Rh-negative mother. Rh-positive infant. Occurrence in the first born infrequent. Severity increases with subsequent pregnancies.

2. ABO incompatibility	Onset usually within 24 hours. Mild anemia and hepatosplenomegaly.	Mild anemia. Mild reticulocytosis. Peripheral smear: mild elevation nucleated red cells, microspherocytosis. Direct Coombs' test: usually negative or weakly positive. Indirect Coombs' test: positive in most. Elevated indirect bilirubin.	Usually mother O blood group and infants have either A or B group.
3. Congenital spherocytosis	Early onset. Jaundice may be severe. Pallor, splenomegaly. Variable.	Mild anemia. Reticulocytosis. Peripheral smear: spherocytes. Coombs' test: negative. Elevated indirect bilirubin.	If there is also an ABO set up, hemolysis due to ABO incompatibility may be difficult to differentiate.

Table 2-3 (Cont'd.) Diagnostic Features of Some Causes of Jaundice in the First Week of Life

Diagnostic Consideration	Clinical Data	Laboratory Data	Remarks
4. Hemolytic disease due to enzyme deficiency, e.g., G-6PD deficiency, pyruvate kinase deficiency	Pallor, jaundice usually does not appear before 24 hours. Splenomegaly may be present.	Anemia. Reticulocytosis. Peripheral smear: normoblasts, spherocytes, poikilocytes, crenated and fragmented cells.	
5. Infantile pyknocytosis	Jaundice may not appear until after first week.	Reticulocytosis. Progressive anemia and indirect bilirubinemia. Pyknocytes in peripheral blood.	

Infections

1. Sepsis: bacterial	Other manifestations of sepsis, e.g., fever, hyper- or hypothermia, lethargy, vomiting, hepatospleno-megaly, etc.	Blood, urine, and other cultures may be positive. Both direct and indirect bilirubin elevated.
2. Viral infection a. Congenital rubella syndrome	Low birth weight infant. Multiple congenital anomalies.	Both direct and indirect bilirubin elevated. Diminished platelets.
b. Cytomegalic inclusion disease	Often premature infants. Jaundice may appear within a few hours of birth. Petechiae, hepatosplenomegaly.	Cytomegalic inclusion cells in urine. Diminished platelets. Bile in urine. Elevated normoblasts. Both direct and indirect bilirubin elevated.
3. Toxoplasmosis	Hepatosplenomegaly. Skin hemorrhage.	Bile in the urine may be present. Anemia. Diminished platelets. Specific IgM antibodies. Elevated direct and indirect bilirubin.

Table 2-3 (Cont'd.) Diagnostic Features of Some Causes of Jaundice in the First Week of Life

Diagnostic Consideration	Clinical Data	Laboratory Data	Remarks
Neonatal hepatitis	Jaundice may be present at birth. Liver enlargement. Males outnumber females.	Both direct and indirect bilirubin elevated. Elevated SGOT and SGPT.	Presumed viral etiology. Differentiation from biliary atresia difficult.
Biliary atresia	Jaundice usually appears late. Females outnumber males.	As above. Low excretion of ^{131}I-labeled rose bengal in the stool.	Early exploration, operative cholangiogram, and liver biopsy indicated to establish diagnosis.
Enclosed hemorrhage	Cephalohematoma most common cause.	Elevated indirect bilirubin with anemia.	

Crigler-Najjar syndrome	Jaundice appears in the first 2-3 days.	Elevated indirect bilirubin, glucuronyl transferase activity diminished or absent.	Glucuronyl transferase deficiency. Autosomal recessive inheritance.
Drug-related jaundice, e.g., vitamin K	Jaundice may appear early.	Elevated indirect bilirubin.	Increased hemolysis or/and interference of hepatic conjugation.
Breast milk jaundice	Well children. Significant degree of jaundice appears between 4 and 7 days of life.	Elevated indirect bilirubin.	Competitive inhibition of glucuronyl transferase by 5-beta pregnane-3 alpha, 20-beta-diol in breast milk.

Other causes of jaundice in the first week include transient familial neonatal hyperbilirubinemia, jaundice associated with hypothyroidism, galactosemia, pyloric stenosis, and maternal diabetes.

another. Figure 2-3 provides guidelines for its use and for exchange transfusion. It should be emphasized that where there are identifiable causes of jaundice they promptly should be attended to (antibiotics for sepsis, etc.). Also it must be remembered that phototherapy is not a substitute for exchange transfusion when there are indications for the latter.

Exchange transfusion is still the most important mode of therapy for both hemolytic and nonhemolytic hyperbilirubinemia. Several parameters such as cord bilirubin and hemoglobin levels, bilirubin, total protein ratio, and a rate of rise of bilirubin are considered useful in arriving at a decision to perform exchange transfusions. In practice, careful assessment of clinical circumstances and use of a table of guidelines as depicted in Figure 2-3 are valuable guides in determining the need for exchange transfusion.

NARCOTIC WITHDRAWAL SYNDROME IN THE NEWBORN

Many infants born to mothers addicted to narcotic drugs such as heroin and morphine develop characteristic withdrawal symptoms soon after birth. Infants born to mothers who are on methadone maintenance programs for heroin addiction also have been noted to exhibit withdrawal manifestations. The pathogenesis of the symptomatology is not clear. Mortality among treated infants is usually insignificant. The majority of infants tend to be small for their gestational ages. Associated congenital anomalies, although reported in the literature, are relatively rare. The symtoms make their onset usually within 24 hours after birth and may last for several weeks. Infants rarely are depressed at birth.

The principal clinical manifestations include irritability, restlessness, flushing of the skin, sweating, gastrointestinal distrubances such as diarrhea and vomiting, respiratory symtoms such as tachypnea and grunting respirations. Elevation of temperature and nasal congestion may be present in some infants. Diagnosis can be sometimes difficult since the mother's history is often unreliable.

Sepsis, cardiorespiratory problems, CNS disorders, hypoglycemia, and hypocalcemia are some of the conditions considered in the differential diagnosis.

Several drugs are in use to control the symptoms. Phenobarbital or paregoric in varying dosages is usually effective

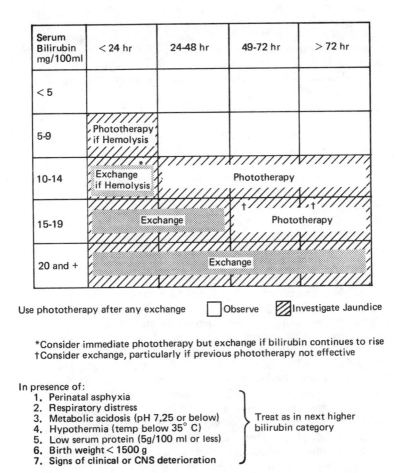

Serum Bilirubin mg/100ml	< 24 hr	24-48 hr	49-72 hr	> 72 hr
< 5				
5-9	Phototherapy if Hemolysis			
10-14	Exchange if Hemolysis*	Phototherapy		
15-19	Exchange		† Phototherapy †	
20 and +	Exchange			

Use phototherapy after any exchange   ☐ Observe   ▨ Investigate Jaundice

*Consider immediate phototherapy but exchange if bilirubin continues to rise
†Consider exchange, particularly if previous phototherapy not effective

In presence of:
1. Perinatal asphyxia
2. Respiratory distress
3. Metabolic acidosis (pH 7.25 or below)
4. Hypothermia (temp below 35° C)   } Treat as in next higher bilirubin category
5. Low serum protein (5g/100 ml or less)
6. Birth weight < 1500 g
7. Signs of clinical or CNS deterioration

Figure 2-3 Guidelines for the management of hyperbilirubinemia. (From Brown, A. K.: Neonatal hyperbilirubinemia. In Behrman, R. E., ed., Neonatology, C.V. Mosby Co., St. Louis, 1973. Reproduced with publisher's permission.)

in the majority of the infants. Duration of the therapy depends on the severity of the illness. Usually therapy may be needed for a period between 2 and 4 weeks. Care should be taken to discontinue the medications gradually to avoid

recurrence of symptoms. Plans should be made to permit
close developmental assessment from birth through infancy.

THE SICK NEWBORN: NEWBORN INFECTIONS

SEPSIS

The morbidity and mortality associated with untreated sepsis
in neonates are extremely high. The diagnosis is often difficult to establish early. Early diagnosis and treatment are
crucial in reducing the morbidity and mortality. Because of
these reasons, every sick child in a newborn nursery should
be presumed to have sepsis until proven otherwise.

Sepsis may be early (onset within 48 hours) or late (onset
later than 48 hours, nursery-incurred) and is caused by organisms which are usually nonpathogenic in older children.
In early sepsis, the infecting organism may involve the placenta and infect the fetus in utero, e.g., *Listeria monocytogenes.* More commonly, the fetus becomes infected by
swallowing and/or aspirating infected amniotic fluid. The organism then penetrates the mucosa of intestinal and respiratory tracts with resulting sepsis. Increased incidence of
amniotic infection is associated with premature rupture of
the membrane (for over 24 hours before the birth of the
baby), prolonged and difficult second stage of labor, and complicated deliveries requiring excessive manipulation. The
infection may also be acquired by aspiration of contaminated
vaginal secretion during delivery. *Escherichia coli, Klebsiella, Aerobacter,* enterococci, and streptococci are the
commonly encountered organisms in early neonatal sepsis.
Late sepsis is a result of infection acquired after the birth
of the baby. Contaminated equipment in the nurseries and
nursery personnel with infections are the primary sources of
infection. In addition to the spread of infection via the
gastrointestinal and respiratory tract, the spread may be
initiated via the umbilical vessels. Ruptured skin at the site
of venipuncture may constitute the portal of entry for the
infecting organisms. Organisms commonly associated with
late sepsis are *Pseudomonas, Klebsiella, Aerobacter,
Staphylococcus aureus,* and *Streptococcus B.*

Increased susceptibility of infants to infection in the
newborn period has been explained by the deficiency of im-

immunoglobulin and nonimmunoglobulin plasma factors and possible impairment or immaturity of a variety of immune responses.

Practical Points

1. Lack of specific signs and symptoms makes the diagnosis of sepsis difficult in early stages. A few newborns, particularly premature infants, may be totally asymptomatic. A high degree of suspicion, based on historical information (e.g., premature rupture of membrane, resuscitation, poor Apgar score, history of maternal infections just prior to the delivery of the baby, maternal fever, purulent amniotic fluid, fetal anoxia), along with appearance of any of the following manifestations must alert the physician to the possibility of sepsis:
   a) Lethary
   b) Poor feeding
   c) Fever or hypothermia
   d) Jaundice
   e) Respiratory distress
   f) Vasomotor instability
   g) Hepatosplenomegaly
   h) Tachypnea
   i) Cyanosis
   j) Vomiting
   k) Abdominal distention
   l) Irritability
   m) Diarrhea
   n) Hypotonia
   o) Petechiae or purpura
   Pallor, grunting, and irregular respiration and mottling of the skin may also be seen in those with far advanced septicemia. Careful search for any associated infection should be made, e.g., infected skin and umbilicus, which may be the focus of infection from which the generalized septicemia is ensuing.
2. Because the signs and symptoms are nonspecific in nature, the differential diagnosis may include a number of conditions where these manifestations are commonly encountered, e.g., intracranial hemorrhage (convulsions, irregular respirations, cyanosis), hypoglycemia, electrolyte imbalance (convulsions, cyanosis), cardiac

decompensation, hyperbilirubinemia (lethargy, poor feeding), hyaline membrane disease, pneumonia, pneumothorax (respiratory distress), narcotic withdrawal syndrome (irritability, vomiting, diarrhea).

3. Certain clinical manifestations may help in differentiating bacterial infection from viral infection, e.g., microcephaly, hydrocephalus, chorioretinitis, intracranial calcification, and other malformations suggest nonbacterial infection such as cytomegalovirus infection, toxoplasmosis, and rubella syndrome.

4. When other causes explaining the symptomatology cannot be found, a presumptive diagnosis of sepsis must be made and the newborn treated after taking appropriate cultures. Laboratory findings help substantiate the physician's suspicion of septicemia when positive. Absence of any of the positive laboratory findings will not rule out the possibility of sepsis. When sepsis is suspected, blood, urine, and spinal fluid cultures must be obtained. Blood cultures are often negative but, when positive, establish the diagnosis. Bladder aspiration is to be preferred to collecting urine for culture. Staining and microscopic examination of urine should be performed. Presence of bacteria and 10 or more white blood cells per high power field are significant findings. About one-third of infants with sepsis will show positive cerebrospinal fluid findings.

5. Presence of bacteria and polymorphonuclear leukocytes in the gastric aspirate indicates that the newborn has aspirated infected amniotic fluid and is, therefore, at high risk to develop sepsis. Presence of these findings in a child with clinical manifestations of sepsis must be considered significant.

6. Peripheral blood examination may show either leukopenia or leukocytosis. Thrombocytopenia may be seen in some cases. Peripheral blood smear may occasionally show evidence of hemolysis as a complication of septicemia.

7. Performance of a lumbar puncture may introduce bloodborne bacteria into the CSF. Appropriate use of antibiotics at an early stage of disease is crucial under these circumstances.

Management of Neonatal Sepsis

Generally, treatment must be started before having identified the infecting organisms. Therefore, the antibiotics
selected should cover most pathogens likely to cause septicemia.

Ampicillin (50 mg/kg/day in two doses for infants under
1 week of age and 100-150 mg/kg/day for older neonates in
three doses) and kanamycin (7.5 mg/kg/day) in two divided
12 hourly doses, form the combination of choice in sepsis of
unknown etiology. In institutions where *E. coli* has shown
resistance to kanamycin, gentamicin sulfate may be substituted for kanamycin in the dose of 2.5 mg/kg/day in two
doses for infants under 1 week of age and 7.5 mg/kg/day in
three doses for older neonates. Both kanamycin and gentamicin are given IM. Ampicillin can be given both IV and IM
depending on the condition of the infant.

Methicillin (50 mg/kg/day under 2 weeks and 50-75 mg/
kg/day over 2 weeks old) IM or IV divided into four 6 hourly
doses must be substituted in situations where staphylococcal
infection is suspected. Likewise, gentamicin (and/or car-
benicillin) should be substituted for kanamycin if *Pseudomonas* is a likely pathogen. Once the organism is identified, only one antibiotic to which the organism is sensitive
should be continued as follows:

1. Penicillin G (100,000 U/kg/day) for groups B and non-
   enterococcal D streptococci
2. Kanamycin for *E. coli, Klebsiella*
3. Gentamicin for kanamycin-resistant organisms and *Pseudomonas*
4. Ampicillin for *Proteus mirabilis, Lysteria monocytogenes,*
   and other gram-positive organisms except penicillin-
   resistant staphylococci
5. Methicillin for penicillin-resistant staphylococci
6. Vancomycin 30 mg/kg/day IV in q 12 h doses for patients
   allergic to penicillin or staph-resistant to methicillin
7. Treatment should continue for a period of 7-10 days
8. Infants with meningitis or visceral involvement should be
   treated longer, i.e., 2-3 weeks. In addition, intraven-
   tricular administration of gentamicin in a daily dose of
   2-3 mg may be considered if ventriculitis is diagnosed

Other supportive measures include adequate maintenance of skin temperature between 36 and 37°C (rectal temperature 37-38°C), administration of oxygen when necessary, maintenance of fluid, and electrolyte balance by IV infusion of electrolyte solutions.

STAPHYLOCOCCAL INFECTIONS

Hemolytic staph 80/81 phage type is the usual pathogenic strain although less virulent phage II staphylococci increasingly are being isolated in recent years. Immediately after birth, the skin and umbilical cord of the newborn become colonized by these organisms. Subsequently, colonization appears to spread to the nares from where infection may become generalized. Prevention of this phenomenon of colonization would, thus, be a deterrent to the spread of staph infection.

The incidence of staph infection was one of the major hazards in newborn nurseries across the nation until bathing all newborns immediately after delivery and daily thereafter with 3% hexachlorophene (HCP) soap became a nursery routine. This practice dramatically reduced the incidence of staph infections. Recently, however, reports have been published raising serious questions concerning the toxicity of hexachlorophene soap used for total body bathing of newborns. Animal studies, in which monkeys were washed daily for 90 days with 3% HCP, showed blood hexachlorophene levels high enough to cause central nervous system damage. At present, this and several other reports with similar implications have sufficiently alarmed neonatologists, and the practice of total body bathing with hexachlorophene is being discontinued. The fear that this will lead to increased incidence of nursery epidemics with staph has not been borne out in clinical practice. Clinical manifestation of staph infection may vary from blebs and pustules of the skin to exfoliative dermatitis (Ritter's disease and meningitis).

Prevention

In light of the recent controversy concerning the use of 3% hexachlorophene, the Committee on Fetus and Newborn of the American Academy of Pediatrics has recommended the

following procedure for practice in nurseries, as a method
to prevent staphylococcal infections.

> At the present the Committee recommends dry
> skin care; washing with plain, nonmedicated soap
> and tap water; or washing with tap water alone for
> skin care of the newborn infant. It should be em-
> phasized that the two most important factors in the
> transmission of infection from infant to infant are
> hand contact and breaks in technique. These fac-
> tors can be minimized by scrupulous hand washing
> before entering the nursery as well as just before
> and just after handling each infant. An iodophor
> preparation, 3% hexachlorophene emulsion, or any
> other cleansing agent may be used. Pediatrics 49:
> 625-626, 1972.

Triple dye daily applied to the umbilical cord area and
bacitracin to circumcision sites help control S. aureus colonization. Personnel handwashing and the avoidance of
cross-contamination of bassinets and infant supplies are the
mainstay of S. aureus control.

For minor infections of the skin, suspected and diagnosed
early, daily scrubbing with hexachlorophene and local application of ointment containing bacitracin may be all that is
necessary.

For more severely infected infants, pending the results
of sensitivity tests, IV methicillin 50-75 mg/day, in four
divided doses should be started promptly. Methicillin may
be replaced by penicillin G, if the strains are penicillin-
sensitive.

GROUP B STREPTOCOCCAL INFECTION

This has become a new challenge in neonatal infections. Two
types of clinical syndromes have been described: (1) the
early onset ($\leq$ 5 days) septicemic type, and (2) the late onset
meningitic type. In the early onset form, infants are either
born with severe signs of septicemia and respiratory distress
or develop them within 72 hours of birth. Unexpected apnea
and shock frequently are the earliest manifestations. Cardiomegaly and small pleural effusions often are found. Pneumonia is a frequent finding (40%). The course is rather

fulminant and mortality high (about 55%). Aspiration of infected amniotic fluid and/or vaginal discharge either in utero or during delivery probably causes the infection. In the late onset meningitic form, infants begin to manifest symptoms of sepsis and meningitis after the first week and as late as 12 weeks of life. The appearance of symptoms is gradual and the prognosis is better (mortality is about 25%). It is probably that the infants acquire infection vertically in the birth canal. Diagnosis is best made by culture of blood, CSF, and other sites of infection (pleural fluid). Some promising results have been obtained with latex particle agglutination and counter-current immunoelectrophoresis. Aqueous penicillin G is the drug of choice. The meningitic form should be treated with 300,000-400,000 U/kg/day; nonmeningitic forms with 200,000-250,000 U/kg/day. Ten to fourteen days is sufficient therapy for nonmeningitic forms; 2-3 weeks is needed for meingitis. Effective prophylactic measures still have not been developed.

INFECTIONS CAUSING DIARRHEA

A number of viral and bacterial agents are responsible for the nursery outbreaks of diarrhea, which fortunately are less frequent today than in the past. Isolated cases of diarrhea, however, are not infrequently seen, particularly in overcrowded nurseries.

Although shigella, salmonella, echoviruses, and adenoviruses can cause diarrhea, most of the epidemics are attributed to the pathogenic strain of *E. coli.*

Listlessness, refusal to feed, weight loss, and dehydration follow the onset of diarrhea. Vomiting is an uncommon feature. If the diarrhea continues, the infant becomes progressively weak and irritable. Marked lethargy and abdominal distension may precede the onset of shock with signs of pronounced dehydration. In most instances, normal temperature is maintained. Rarely, marked elevation of temperature may accompany the symptomatology. The degree of metabolic acidosis that most infants develop during the course of illness depends on the severity of the illness. The clinical symptoms are misleading insofar as predicting the degree of acidosis, as they are often absent. The limitations of renal function in newborns make them particularly susceptible to

develop hypernatremia under the stress of diarrhea. The
stools vary in consistency. Greenish–yellow, watery stool
may be mixed with mucus and blood.

Prevention and Treatment

Scrupulous hand washing by nursery personnel, careful isolation and observation of suspected newborns, and strict
barring of all personnel with possible intestinal infections
from coming in contact with newborns are some of the important measures that contribute to the prevention of
dangerous epidemics. Prompt reporting of diarrhea in a
recently discharged infant by a visiting health nurse, or any
other health personnel coming in contact with such an infant, is extremely important. Once an initial case has been
diagnosed in a nursery, the unit must be closed for any new
admissions and all infants given antibiotics, if appropriate.
After the nursery is cleared of all the treated infants,
thorough cleaning of the nursery and its equipment must be
made before reopening it again.

The treatment of affected infants consists of adequate
maintenance of fluid and electrolytes and administration of
antibiotics orally where indicated. Neomycin, 12.5–25 mg/
kg po q 6 h, given orally was the drug of choice for *E. coli*
diarrhea. However, most infants are treated supportively
without antibiotics. Ampicillin 100 mg/kg/day is effective
against shigella and salmonella infections. Parenteral administration of specific antibiotics must be administered for
systemic manifestations of the disease.

TUBERCULOSIS

1. Infants born to a mother with a history of active tuberculosis at the time of delivery:
   a) Isolate the infant until the mother is under effective
      treatment and acid–fast stains of her sputum are nega-
      tive. This is usually 2 weeks. A thorough investigation
      of family members and therapy, as indicated, should
      render the home environment noninfectious before the
      infant is discharged. If poor compliance places the in-
      fant at risk, then BCG vaccination is given in the first
      week of life and the baby discharged at age 6 weeks.

BCG protects against widespread disease but does not offer complete protection against tuberculosis. The physician must be watchful for tuberculosis infection.

b) Children without any evidence of infection, give isoniazid (INH) 10 mg/kg/day for 3 months. Check tuberculin test and x-ray after this period. If negative, give BCG.

c) Children with evidence of infection, give INH 10-15 mg/kg/day and rifampin 15 mg/kg/day; both are given po in two doses. In severe cases, streptomycin 20 mg/kg/day IM in bid doses can be added. INH and rifampin are given for 1-2 years with careful monitoring for hepatic, hematologic, and otologic side effects. More severe infections, such as meningitis, require increased drug doses and appropriate consultation and comanagement.

2. Infants born to a mother with a history of tuberculosis but no active disease at the time of delivery:

a) Evaluate the mother carefully for evidence of reactivation. If she is found to have a reactivated lesion, follow procedure above.

b) If the mother maintains an arrested state, evaluate the child periodically with tuberculin testing, the first one scheduled at 2 weeks of age and every 3 months thereafter until age 1 year. Consider BCG vaccination after ruling out a tuberculosis infection in the infant.

BCG Vaccination

Reliability in terms of its effectiveness is questioned in some cases. In the majority of infants, it does give protection against disseminated disease in the high risk group (refer to categories above). Opinions vary regarding its use as an alternative to prophylaxis with antituberculosis agents. One major objection to its use is that it becomes difficult to interpret a tuberculin reaction after its administration. BCG is given in 0.1 ml dose intradermally. The patient must be tuberculin tested after 6 weeks. Revaccinate if the test is negative. Contraindication: gammaglobulin deficiency states or history of such in the family.

CONGENITAL SYPHILIS

The fetus is infected transplacentally during the second and third trimester of pregnancy. Early infection causes death of the fetus in utero. Usually the infants are born apparently normal but show manifestations of the disease during the first week or two after birth.

Early symptoms include snuffles, and the characteristic copper-colored maculopapular rash. The rash is predominantly seen over the perioral-perinasal regions, diaper area, and on the soles and palms. As the rash becomes generalized, moist lesions at the mucocutaneous junction (mouth, anus, vulva) may be noted. The systemic manifestations include hepatosplenomegaly with anemia and jaundice, generalized lymphadenopathy, pseudoparalysis with osteochondritis and periostitis. X-ray examination of the bones reveals areas of radiolucency giving the bones a moth-eaten appearance, metaphyseal density, and periosteal elevation. Examination of the cerebrospinal fluid may reveal pleocytosis and an elevated protein content.

The diagnosis is established by demonstrating elevated IgM antibody levels, and more specifically, identifying the syphilis IgM antibodies. Caution must be exerted in interpreting a positive serologic test for syphilis (VDRL-Venereal Disease Research Laboratory, or RPR - rapid plasma reagin) in the newborn as it may be on the basis of passively transferred reagin from the mother who may or may not have been treated during pregnancy. Usually the passively transferred reagin will gradually disappear from the infant's blood by about 2 months. If, on the other hand, the titer shows a rise, it implies that the infant actually has the disease. If a positive serologic test is found, this should be confirmed by the more sensitive fluorescent treponemal antibody-absorbed assay (FTA-ABS).

Prevention is accomplished by early recognition of infection in the pregnant mother followed by vigorous therapy with penicillin. For the infected infant, treatment with procaine penicillin G in a dosage of 20,000–30,000 U/kg and administered once daily for 10 days should be initiated. Higher doses of penicillin for a longer period of time should be given to infants with evidence of neurosyphilis.

HERPES SIMPLEX

Herpes virus hominis type II is most often responsible for infection in the newborn. Rarely, type I is incriminated. The infection is transmitted transplacentally late in pregnancy and more often during birth from the vaginal lesions of the mother.

The illness generally becomes manifest during the first 1-3 weeks of postnatal life. The initial findings consist of vesicular lesions on the skin and mucous membranes of the throat and keratoconjunctivitis. These may be followed by symptoms referable to the central nervous system such as seizures. Systemic dissemination of the disease is marked by lethargy, fever, anorexia, jaundice, respiratory difficulty, and cyanosis. Hepatosplenomegaly and pulmonary findings are prominent at this stage. Bleeding tendency with anemia, petechiae, and thrombocytopenia is also noted.

Diagnosis is established by demonstrating the virus from the scrapings of the lesions. The level of IgM is increased and herpes-specific IgM can be detected using indirect fluorescent antibody technique. Prevention can be attemped by delivery of infants by cesarean section once herpetic lesions are recognized in the vaginal passage of the mother. For infants with proven infection, 5-iodo-2-deoxyuride (IDU) (50-100 mg/kg/day IV) or cytosine arabinoside is being used with varying degrees of success.

CONGENITAL RUBELLA

Teratogenic effects of this virus on the fetus are well established. The most pronounced effect is seen when the fetus is infected during the first 8 weeks of pregnancy. Table 2-4 presents the clinical manifestations of the rubella syndrome.

Diagnosis is established by the isolation of rubella virus from the nasopharyngeal secretions or from the spinal fluid. (The excretion of virus occurs for several months after birth). The IgM level in the infant is elevated indicating intrauterine infection, and specific rubella IgM antibodies can be demonstrated.

Eradication of rubella is a realistic result of current vaccination programs in the United States today. The incidence of rubella has decreased over 95% since 1969.

Table 2-4   Manifestation of Congenital Rubella

Common	Uncommon or Rare
History of maternal rubella	Jaundice
Low birth weight	Dermatoglyphic "abnormality"
Cataracts	Glaucoma
Microphthalmia	Cloudy cornea
Retinopathy	Myocardial damage
Deafness	Hepatitis
Congenital heart disease	Generalized adenopathy
Thrombocytopenic purpura	Hemolytic anemia
Hepatomegaly	Hypoplastic anemia
Splenomegaly	Cerebrospinal fluid pleocytosis
Bone lesions (metaphyseal rarefaction)	Spastic quadriparesis
Large anterior fontanelle	
Psychomotor retardation	

From Cooper, L.Z. and Krugman, S.: Diagnosis and management: Congenital rubella, Pediatrics 37:336, 1966. (Reproduced with permission of American Academy of Pediatrics, Evanston, IL.)

This disease is controlled in persons 14 years of age or younger. High school and college youth are now the age group of risk. Clinicians today cannot rely solely on their clinical judgment in the diagnosis of rubella; serial HI titers must be done to confirm the diagnosis. Many enteroviruses produce a morbilliform rash.

The present vaccine RA 27/3 induces a broad range of antibodies and has no demonstrated teratogenesis or arthralgias. A theoretical risk of congenital rubella syndrome with the vaccine is almost nonexistent, much less than the 20-30% risk of wild rubella in first trimester infection. These risks can be reduced to a negligible level in the near future with aggressive implementation of a vaccination program which includes young adults at risk for infection. If vaccination inadvertently occurs in the first trimester of pregnancy, the risk of congenital rubella syndrome (CRS) is negligible and is not an indication of interruption of pregnancy.

CYTOMEGALOVIRUS INFECTION

Cytomegalovirus infection has been documented as occurring in 3-5% of all pregnant women. The women are rarely symptomatic, thus escaping detection. Only a very small percentage of infants from these mothers acquire the disease. The infection is transmitted via the placenta but occasionally an infant may acquire it postnatally.

Clinical symptomatology varies. Most children do not show any evidence of infection during the first few months of postnatal life. In mild infections, symptoms are minimal and follow-up findings in these infants may be microcephaly and mental retardation. Only rarely do infants manifest a severe form of illness. In these instances, they are often born prematurely and shortly after birth develop symptoms of disseminated disease. Anemia, jaundice, hepatosplenomegaly, pulmonary involvement, convulsions, chorioretinitis, and bleeding tendencies with thrombocytopenia are some of the manifestations seen in these newborns.

Diagnosis is established by isolating the virus from nasopharyngeal secretions, urine, and CSF. Characteristic inclusion bodies (owl's eye cells) can be demonstrated in the cells of the urinary sediment. IgM levels are increased and specific cytomegalovirus antibodies can be demonstrated.

No specific treatment is currently available for general use. Studies are being conducted to assess the efficacy of some new drugs. Symptomatic treatment for the severely affected infants include blood transfusion for anemia and exchange transfusion for significant hyperbilirubinemia.

TOXOPLASMOSIS

The infection is transplacentally transmitted from infected pregnant women who are often asymptomatic. The clinical picture in newborns with the severe form of the disease includes severe jaundice, hepatosplenomegaly, purpura with thrombocytopenia, seizures, hypotonicity, chorioretinitis, microcephaly, or hydrocephalus. In the less severe form, the disease may escape detection for the first few months after birth. Diagnosis is often made in the infants when manifestations such as microencephaly, hydrocephalus, cerebral calcification, and psychomotor retardation are detected.

Diagnosis is established by demonstrating specific IgM for toxoplasmosis and by isolation of the organism in mice.

Prognosis for children who survive the acute form of the disease is normally poor with severe psychomotor retardation, neurological defects, and visual impairment.

Prevention of infection in the pregnant mother is difficult. Since uncooked meat has been shown to harbor the organism, avoidance of eating raw meat by pregnant women should be encouraged. Pregnant women should be careful when handling cats as organisms are also isolated from cats' excreta. Combined treatment with pyrimethamine and sulfadiazine may be effective in infected infants.

RESPIRATORY DISTRESS SYNDROME
(Hyaline Membrane Disease)

This is a developmental disease of the lungs seen in premature infants characterized by alveolar instability and, therefore, alveolar collapse at the end of expiration resulting in progressive distress, hypoxia, and acidemia. Intrauterine anoxia and postnatal hypothermia have been incriminated as the two major predisposing factors in the development of this syndrome. Infants dying of the disease show formation of hyaline membranes in the alveoli and hence the name hyaline membrane disease.

Alveolar stability is dependent on the production by the fetus of a surface-active lecithin. Although lecithin production can be detected in the fetus as early as the twenty-second week of gestation, the more stable type of lecithin is produced by the fetus only around the thirty-sixth week of gestation. Premature infants born before this period of gestation and who are exposed to any of the predisposing factors mentioned above are likely candidates to develop the respiratory distress syndrome.

Lack of the stabilizing surface-active factor results in collapse of the alveoli at the end of each expiration. This state of alveolar collapse demands a high opening pressure at each inspiration not unlike the pressure noted as the first breath of life begins. Due to abnormally high intrathoracic and intraalveolar pressures that are maintained during respiration, there is exudation of fluid into the alveoli from the pulmonary circulation. As the disease progresses, the exudate combines with the damaged alveolar cells to form the hyaline membrane. As the alveolar spaces get progressively compromised, worsening hypoxia and acidosis will eventually lead to death.

Respiratory symptoms become manifest immediately after birth as rapid shallow respirations. A downhill clinical course is marked by severe sternal, suprasternal, and intercostal retractions. This excessive respiratory effort is accompanied by an audible expiratory grunt. Later in the course of the disease, extreme fatigue, as a result of the intense respiratory efforts, is characterized by cessation of any spontaneous activity and the appearance of paradoxical respiration with xiphoid retractions. In severe cases, infants may die within a few hours after the onset of symptoms. Those who survive will show gradual signs of improvement by 3-4 days.

Examination of the infant may reveal rapid heart rate, diminished air exchange, and scattered rales over both lung fields. Blood gas studies show values consistent with hypoxemia and respiratory acidosis. Roentgenographic examination of the chest shows a fine reticulogranular pattern throughout the lung fields, reflecting the diffuse collapse of alveoli in both lungs.

The treatment is entirely supportive and primarily directed towards correction of inadequate pulmonary exchange of oxygen and carbon dioxide and the correction of acid-base imbalance, another major feature of the disease entity. The correction of inadequate pulmonary exchange of oxygen and carbon dioxide includes the maintenance of a clear airway by frequent suctioning of tracheal secretions, careful regulation of skin temperature at a level (36-37°C) to keep the oxygen consumption minimal, and administration of oxygen to maintain a satisfactory arterial oxygen tension (50-70 torr). The skin temperature at 36-37°C can be maintained by adjusting the incubator temperature between 32 and 34°C at a relative humidity of 80-90%. Oxygen therapy must be constantly evaluated by measuring arterial oxygen.

The toxic effects of a high concentration of oxygen on the retina of the premature infants and on the lungs, especially when it is administered by positive pressure respirators, have been clearly established. On the other hand, too little administration of O_2 will only perpetuate the state of hypoxia. Samples for analysis can be obtained from an indwelling plastic catheter inserted through one of the umbilical arteries sufficiently far enough so that the tip is just above the bifurcation of the aorta. (This distance is approximately equal to half the length between the lateral end of the clavicle and a point directly below it at the level of the umbilicus.) The position must be ascertained radiologically. Samples from temporal or radial arteries are even preferable inasmuch as they reflect more accurately the O_2 tension of blood perfusing the retina but repeated sampling is impractical.

Adequate humidity must be maintained during administration of high concentrations of O_2 in order to prevent inspissation of the accumulated secretions in the trachea.

Some type of assisted ventilation becomes mandatory in most infants. An arterial O_2 tension of less than 50 mmHg or arterial CO_2 tension of more than 70 mmHg when breathing 100% O_2 constitute the primary indications for use of assisted ventilation. The relative advantages and disadvantages of positive pressure respirations and mask and bag resuscitations have been extensively discussed in the literature.

Correction of Acid–Base Imbalance

Gradual correction of acid-base imbalance with either sodium bicarbonate ($NaHCO_3$) or THAM should be attempted on the basis of repeated blood gas measurements. The amounts of base to be used can be calculated on the following formulas:

$$NaHCO_3 \ (7.5\%) \ in \ ml = mEq/L \ of \ base \ deficit$$

$$x \ wt \ in \ kg \ x \ 0.3$$

$$THAM \ (0.3M) \ in \ ml = mEq/L \ of \ base \ deficit$$
$$x \ wt \ in \ kg$$

The umbilical vein may be used for infusion of this solution during the initial period of correction. Care must be taken to see that a good circulation is maintained (if necessary by external cardiac massage) in order to avoid toxicity to the liver. The umbilical vein infusion may be discontinued once the initial acid-base correction is accomplished. Further, $NaHCO_3$ may be added, if necessary, to the IV infusion to maintain the required acid base equilibrium.

Antibiotics are not recommended routinely. It must be remembered that these infants, subjected as they are to various procedures, are most susceptible to developing infections secondarily. Where such a diagnosis is apparent, appropriate antibiotics must be used.

Fluid and electrolyte needs can best be met in the initial stage by IV infusion of a balanced electrolyte solution (1/3-1/5 isotonic solution). Oral formula feedings in small amounts should be attempted as soon as possible in order to provide more calories.

The complexity of the management of this condition demands expertise and sophisticated equipment generally available only in regional neonatal centers.

NECROTIZING ENTEROCOLITIS

This neonatal clinical entity is emerging as a fairly common problem in some intensive care nurseries. The problem is mainly seen in low birth weight infants. The etiology of this disorder is not entirely clear. A combination of vascular insufficiency of the bowel leading to necrosis and septicemia is thought to produce the clinical manifestations. These include abdominal swelling with tenderness, bloody, loose stools, and other findings generally associated with sepsis. X-ray examination of the abdomen reveals the presence of pneumatosis intestinalis. The initial management is directed towards correcting the fluid and electrolyte imbalance and administration of appropriate antibiotics to treat septicemia. Parental alimentation is necessary to maintain the nutritional status. If no clinical improvement is observed by the medical regimen within 24-48 hours, surgical exploration and resection of the nonviable bowel with ileostomy or colostomy are performed. Even with proper management the mortality rate of this condition is still high.

INFANT BOTULISM

Since the original report of botulism occurring in infants,
some 100 cases have been identified, and the incidence has
been estimated at a minimum of 250 cases yearly in the
United States. Affected infants generally have been full
term ranging in age from 3 to 26 weeks with a common
problem of constipation occurring days to weeks prior to
the onset of neurological signs. Clinical symptomatology
is similar to that found in older age groups: generalized
weakness, specific motor nerve paresis or paralysis with a
uniform involvement of cranial nerves 7, 9, 10, and 11.
Diminished head control is a striking finding and respiratory
muscle failure the cause of death. In the Eastern United
States, type B prevails while type A is more common on the
West Coast. Electromyography (EMG) often reveals an
augmentation of amplitude of the evoked muscle action
potential at nerve stimulation frequencies greater than 10
Hz. Most cases also exhibit a positive response. The diagnosis is made more certain by isolating the organism or
demonstrating the toxin in the stool. The serum is generally
negative for toxin in infants.

Treatment includes support of the respiratory function
and general nutrition at centers equipped to handle these
problems well. The use of type-specific antitoxin is of uncertain efficacy and it is possible that tissue binding of the
toxin may defeat attempts to neutralize it with antioxin.
In addition, serum sickness and other allergic reactions occur frequently with horse antitoxin use. Human antitoxin
as yet has not become available. An antibiotic (penicillin)
to destroy clostridia organisms in the gastrointestinal (GI)
tract is theoretically useful, but no differences in clinical
course have been found in penicillin-treated patients. Also
it is possible that the rapid destruction of organisms may
serve only to release more toxin. Purgatives appear to
speed the excretion of organisms from the GI tract. Definitive treatment still awaits the results of more investigation. Prevention of infant botulism can be achieved by pro-
hibiting honey or corn syrup (Karo and similar syrups) under
one year of age.

COMMON SURGICAL PROBLEMS OF THE NEWBORN

INTESTINAL OBSTRUCTION

Common causes of obstruction are:

1. Atresias (e.g., esophageal, duodenal)
2. Stenosis (e.g., pyloric, annular pancreas)
3. Malrotation
4. Meconium ileus
5. Meconium plug syndrome
6. Others (e.g., intussusception aganglionosis, duplication of intestinal tract)

Practical Points

1. Suspect intestinal obstruction in the newborn if hydramnios is diagnosed in the mother. Obstruction, particularly of the proximal portion of the intestinal tract, prevents the normal intrauterine process of ingestion, absorption, and excretion of the amniotic fluid.
2. The ability to aspirate more than 10-15 ml of the gastric contents is strongly suggestive of proximal obstruction.
3. Vomiting is an important sign. Since most obstructions are distal to the ampulla of Vater, the vomiting is usually bile stained. Projectile vomiting seldom is seen. Blood may occasionally be noted in the vomiting.
4. Abdominal distension usually comes on gradually. Marked generalized distension usually suggests distal obstruction. A visible intestinal pattern is almost a sure sign of obstruction.
5. Nonpassage of meconium within 24 hours of birth should arouse concern. In high obstructions, one may note passage of meconium despite obstruction.
6. During x-ray examination, swallowed air gives a good enough contrast to judge the level of obstruction. Normally, air descends to the level of the colon within 18-24 hours after birth. Loops proximal to the obstruction are distended with air while the distal loops are airless. Barium studies rarely are necessary. Characteristic findings include:
   a) Large distended stomach which suggests pyloric obstruction.

b) Double bubble appearance (one, that of the stomach, and the other of the duodenum) which indicates duodenal obstruction.

c) Ground glass appearance (tiny air bubbles mixed with viscous meconium) is characteristic of meconium ileus.

d) Rectosigmoid narrowing with a dilated proximal segment of colon is indicative of Hirschsprung's disease.

Specific Conditions

1. Atresias: multiple 15%; ileum 50%; duodenum 25%. Found less frequently in the jejunum, rare in the colon. Esophageal atresias are associated with maternal hydramnios. Feeding results in regurgitation, choking spells, and cyanosis. When associated with the H type of tracheoesophageal fistula, diagnosis may be delayed. Recurrent pneumonia and respiratory difficulty after feeding are common features in such cases. Diagnosis is made by passing a radiopaque catheter through the nasopharynx, then taking an x-ray to ascertain the level of obstruction. In duodenal atresia the atretic segment is most commonly located near the ampulla of Vater. Vomiting is an early sign. Duodenal atresia is frequently associated with mongolism.

2. Stenosis: pyloric stenosis is rarely diagnosed before 2 weeks of age. It occurs most often in male infants. Progressive, projectile vomiting leads to hypochloremic, hypokalemic alkalosis. If careful examination is made, the characteristic pyloric "olive" can be palpated in the epigastric area to the right of the midline in the majority of affected infants. Severe duodenal stenosis can be caused by an annular pancreas.

3. Malrotation is a failure of normal rotation of the cecum during embryonic development. It usually is associated with omphalocele or congenital diaphragmatic hernia. Demonstrating the ectopic position of the cecum by barium studies establishes the diagnosis.

4. Meconium ileus occurs in 10% of children with cystic fibrosis. The meconium is maintained in a highly viscid and mucilaginous state due to lack of pancreatic enzyme. This inspissated meconium fills the intestinal lumen resulting in obstruction. The area near the ileocecal valve is most often the site of obstruction. Perforation results

in meconium peritonitis. Abdominal distension with a characteristic doughy consistency and vomiting are principal early findings. Surgical correction can be occasionally avoided by instilling acetylcystein into the intestinal tract in an attempt to dissolve the meconium.

5. The meconium plug syndrome is not associated with cystic fibrosis. Obstruction occurs most often in the distal colon or rectum. A tenacious meconium plug is the cause of the obstruction. This type of obstruction can be mistaken for anorectal atresia. Digital examination usually will distinguish between the two. An association of Hirschsprung's disease with this syndrome has been noted. Digital stimulation of the rectum often results in the expulsion of the meconium plug with relief of the obstruction.

6. Hirschsprung's disease is characterized by the absence of ganglion cells in the parasympathetic nerve plexus of the distal colon and rectum. Rarely the entire colon may be involved. Constipation or diarrhea is the presenting symptom in early infancy. Lack of peristaltic movements at the aganglionic level prevents propulsion of the meconium resulting in obstruction. Diagnosis is made by barium enema studies. The intestinal lumen proximal to the aganglionic segment is distended while the affected segment shows characteristic narrowing. Diagnosis is confirmed by demonstrating an absence of ganglion cells in a rectal biopsy specimen. A two-stage operation consisting of an initial colostomy followed by a pull-through procedure later at 1-2 years of age constitutes the surgical management.

7. Intussusception is very rare in the newborn period. Usually, the ileum is the site of the obstruction. While symptomatology varies, vomiting and blood-stained meconium are most often noted. Abdominal distension and tenderness very often are absent. Occasionally, a palpable mass may be detected. A flat film of the abdomen will show evidence of obstruction. Prognosis depends on the promptness in diagnosing the problem. Treatment is surgical if an attempt to undo the intussusception using hydrostatic pressure of a barium mixture under fluoroscopy does not succeed.

Chapter 3

INFANT AND CHILD HEALTH CARE

GROWTH AND DEVELOPMENT

An understanding of the principles of the growth and development of the child is the foundation upon which the practice of pediatrics must be based. While the two terms are closely interrelated and often interchanged, a practical approach to this subject is to define growth as an increase in the physical size of the child's body or any of its components. Growth, therefore, can be observed and measured in terms of inches or centimeters, pounds or kilograms. Normal development can be defined as a functional process increasing in complexity and dexterity until the full potential of an individual's abilities are reached.

The normal processes resulting in progressive growth and development are powerful forces, yet, a wide range of interfering factors frequently may block these forces. Genetic aberrations, malnutrition, a wide range of acute and chronic infections, endocrine abnormalities, psychological problems, and a noxious environment among other causes may interfere with normal growth and development.

A strong word of caution must be expressed concerning the interpretation of various charts, tables, and schedules depicting "normal" rates of growth and development. Individuality is the key word and, as such, each child must be so judged.

Finally, it must be emphasized that it is the duty and responsibility of the pediatrician to contribute this special knowledge and training and join with parents, teachers, and other professionals to see that each child has the opportunity to reach his full potential.

Growth and development charts and standards may be found in the Appendix.

FEEDING OF INFANTS AND CHILDREN

Understanding the fundamentals of nutrition is a prerequisite for professionals responsible for guiding parents in the proper feeding of their infants and children. Improved knowledge as to the nutritional needs of children and the techniques by which these needs are met in the individual child constitutes one of the most important advances in the field of child health.

Proper feeding habits not only result in normal physical growth but also strongly influence the psychological and emotional well-being of the infant and child. Feeding time should be a pleasurable and satisfying experience for both mother and child. The individual who counsels the mother must impart a practical interpretation of nutritional needs as well as emphasize the wide range of variation in the appetite and the feeding behavior of growing babies and children.

For the majority of parents of normal babies, a self-regulatory feeding schedule is most effective during the first month or so of life. For most babies an acceptable schedule will be adopted by 4-6 weeks of age. For parents who have a special need for order, a more formal schedule should be provided.

BREAST FEEDING

Despite the relative lack of popularity of breast feeding and despite the availability of excellent commercial formulas, breast feeding continues to be a practical and psychologically sound method of feeding young infants. Breast feeding

Table 3-1   Approximate Daily Requirements of Children for Calories, Protein, and Water

	Calories* per kg	per lb	Protein g/kg	ml/kg	oz/lb
Infancy	110	50	3.5-2.0	150	2-4
1-3	100	45	2.5-2.0	125	2
4-6	90	41	3.0	100	1 1/2
7-9	80	36	2.8	75	1.0+
10-12	70	32	2.0	75	1.0+
13-15	60	27	1.7	50	3/4
16-19	50	23	1.5+	50	3/4
Adult	40	18	1.0	50	3/4

*At least 10% variation

To convert g/kg to g/lb divide by 2 and subtract 10% of the quotient. Thus 4 g/kg is equivalent to 1.8 g/lb.

First weeks lower; first 6 months relatively higher than last 6 months

From Nelson, W.E., Vaughan, V.C., McKay, R.J.: Textbook of Pediatrics, 9th ed. W.B. Saunders Co., Philadelphia, 1969. (Reproduced with publisher's permission.)

should be offered as one method of feeding to all mothers in whom no contraindications exist either on her part or on the part of the infant.

Advantages of Breast Feeding

1. Breast milk is always available wherever mother is. No preparation is needed and bacterial contamination does not exist.
2. Feeding difficulties such as colic, "spitting up," and allergic reactions are fewer in breastfed babies.

Table 3-2   Recommended Daily Dietary Allowances,[1] Food and Nutrition Board, National Academy of Sciences—National Research Council, Revised 1974

	Age (years)	Weight (kg)	Weight (lb)	(cm)	(in.)	Energy ((kcal)[2])	Protein (g)	Vitamin A Activity (RE)[3]	Vitamin A Activity (IU)	Vitamin D (IU)	Vitamin E Activity[4] (IU)
Infants	0.0-0.5	6	14	60	24	kg x 117	kg x 2.2	420	1,400	400	4
	0.5-1.0	9	20	71	28	kg x 108	kg x 2.0	400	2,000	400	5
Children	1-3	13	28	86	34	1,300	23	400	2,000	400	7
	4-6	20	44	110	44	1,800	30	500	2,500	400	9
	7-10	30	66	135	54	2,400	36	700	3,300	400	10
Males	11-14	44	97	158	63	2,800	44	1,000	5,000	400	12
	15-18	61	134	172	69	3,000	54	1,000	5,000	400	15
	19-22	67	147	172	69	3,000	54	1,000	5,000	400	15
	23-50	70	154	172	69	2,700	56	1,000	5,000		15
	51+	70	154	172	69	2,400	56	1,000	5,000		15
Females	11-14	44	97	155	62	2,400	44	800	4,000	400	12
	15-18	54	119	162	65	2,100	48	800	4,000	400	12

19–22	58	128	162	65	2,100	46	800	4,000	400	12
23–50	58	128	162	65	2,000	46	800	4,000		12
51+	58	128	162	65	1,800	46	800	4,000		12
Pregnant					+300	+30	1,000	5,000		15
Lactating					+500	+20		6,000		15

[1] The allowances are intended to provide for individual variations among most normal perons as they live in the United States under usual environmental stresses. Diets should be based on a variety of common foods in order to provide other nutrients for which human requirements have been less well defined.

[2] Kilojoules (kJ) = 4.2 x kcal.

[3] Retinol equivalents.

[4] Assumed to be all as retinol in milk during the first 6 months of life. All subsequent intakes are assumed to be half as retinol and half as β-carotene when calculated from international units. As retinol equivalent, three-fourths are as retinol and one-fourth a β-carotene.

[5] Total vitamin E activity, estimated to be 80% as α-tocopherol and 20% other tocopherols.

Table 3-2 (Cont'd.) Designed for the Maintenance of Good Nutrition of Practically All Healthy People in the U.S.A.

	Water-Soluble Vitamins						Minerals					
Ascorbic Acid (mg)	Folacin[6] (µg)	Niacin[7] (mg)	Riboflavin (mg)	Thiamin (mg)	Vitamin B6 (mg)	Vitamin B12 (µg)	Calcium (mg)	Phosphorus (mg)	Iodine (µg)	Iron (mg)	Magnesium (mg)	Zinc (mg)
35	50	5	0.4	0.3	0.3	0.3	360	240	35	10	60	3
35	50	8	0.6	0.5	0.4	0.3	540	400	45	15	70	5
40	100	9	0.8	0.7	0.6	1.0	800	800	60	15	150	10
40	200	12	1.1	0.9	0.9	1.5	800	800	80	10	200	10
40	300	16	1.2	1.2	1.2	2.0	800	800	110	10	250	10
45	400	18	1.5	1.4	1.6	3.0	1,200	1,200	130	18	350	15
45	400	20	1.8	1.5	2.0	3.0	1,200	1,200	150	18	400	15
45	400	20	1.8	1.5	2.0	3.0	800	800	140	10	350	15
45	400	18	1.6	1.4	2.0	3.0	800	800	130	10	350	15
45	400	16	1.5	1.2	2.0	3.0	800	800	110	10	350	15
45	400	16	1.3	1.2	1.6	3.0	1,200	1,200	115	18	300	15
45	400	14	1.4	1.1	2.0	3.0	1,200	1,200	115	18	300	15
45	400	14	1.4	1.1	2.0	3.0	800	800	100	18	300	15

45	400	13	1.2	1.0	2.0	3.0	800	800	100	18	300	15
45	400	12	1.1	1.0	2.0	3.0	800	800	80	10 8	300	15
60	800	+2	+0.3	+0.3	2.5	4.0	1,200	1,200	125	18+	450	20
80	600	+4	+0.5	+0.3	2.5	4.0	1,200	1,200	150	18	450	25

6The folacin allowances refer to dietary sources as determined by *Lactobacillus casei* assay. Pure forms of folacin may be effective in doses less than one-fourth of the recommended dietary allowance.

7Although allowances are expressed as niacin, it is recognized that on the average 1 mg of niacin is derived from each 60 mg of dietary tryptophan.

8This increased requirement cannot be met by ordinary diets; therefore, the use of supplemental iron is recommended.

From Nelson, W.E.: Textbook of Pediatrics, 11th ed. W. B. Saunders Co., Philadelphia, 1979, p. 174.

3. Breast milk is the natural food for infants the first few months of life, supplying all nutritional requirements except vitamin D, fluoride, and iron.
4. Antibodies present in breast milk including high concentrations of IgA afford local gastrointestinal immunity against pathogenic organisms.

Contraindications to Breast Feeding

1. Fissures or cracking of nipples results in temporary cessation if breast shields are not satisfactory.
2. The resumption of menstruation is not a contraindication to the continuance of breast feeding.
3. Serious maternal illnesses such as septicemia, active tuberculosis, malaria, nephritis, and chronic or debilitating conditions such as poor nutrition, convulsive disorders, severe neurosis, and postpartum psychosis are contraindications for breast feeding.

Tips on Successful Breast Feeding

Practical Points

1. Complete emptying of the breast is the only effective methoid of stimulating the secretion of milk. Emptying should be accomplished by the vigorous sucking of the infant but artificial suction should be used if necessary.
2. Breast feeding should be begun as soon as practical after birth, preferably within 6-12 hours.
3. Infants should be fed on both breasts until the milk supply is adequate for a complete feeding.
4. The first 2 weeks are crucial for establishing successful breast feeding. When early supplemental bottle feedings are given, breast feeding is usually doomed. The baby finds it far easier to get milk from a bottle than from the breast.
5. If a normal infant is satisfied at the completion of a nursing period ahd sleeps 3-4 hours, it can be assumed that the milk supply is sufficient.

FORMULA FEEDING

There are many forms of cow's milk formulas and milk sub-
stitutes available. Fed in proper amounts with proper technique, infants will thrive on most of them providing deficient requirements such as vitamins and iron are included
in the formula or given as a supplement. Composition of
breast milk and some commonly used milk and milk sub-
stitutes is shown in Table 3-3. Whole milk or reconstructed
evaporated milk without added carbohydrate may be substituted for formula at 4-5 months of age.

Vitamins and Iron

The required daily intake of vitamins C, D, and possibly A
must be supplied via fortified formulas or by water-miscible
preparations of these essential nutrients. Vitamin D, 400 IU,
vitamin C (25-50 mg ascorbic acid), and vitamin A 3000-
5000 IU should be given from early in the neonatal period
through 12-18 months of life. The physician must be
familiar with the vitamin content of commercial formulas
and supplement the amount taken by the infant with an appropriate vitamin preparation.
    A supplemental source of iron other than from solid
foods should be given in the amount of 12 mg/day from 6
weeks through age 18 months. The iron in ferrous form
may be provided by iron-fortified formulas or by oral iron
preparations.
    A convenient method is to utilize an oral vitamin pre-
paration containing the necessary amounts of vitamins and
iron.
    If fluoride is not present in adequate amounts in the
drinking water, it should be supplied in oral drops (0.5-1.0
mg/day).

SOLID FOOD FEEDING

Human milk or fortified formula provides all the necessary
nutrients for satisfactory growth in a full-term infant until
several months after birth. It is not therefore usually
necessary to start solid foods before 3-4 months of age.
All solid foods should be first approved in small amounts

Table 3-3   Composition of Milks and Formulas

	Normal Dilution Ratio	Cal/oz (kcal/oz)	Approximate Percentage Composition In Normal Dilution (G/100 ml)				Approximate Electrolyte Composition In Normal Dilution (Milliequivalents/L)			mg/L		
			Pro-tein	Carbo-hydrate	Fat	Minerals	Na	K	Cl	Ca	P^2	Fe
Human milk, mature, average	Undiluted	20	1.2	7.0	3.8	0.21	7	14	12	340	150	1.5
Cow's milk, market, average	Undiluted	20	3.3	4.8	3.7	0.72	25	35	29	1170	920	1.0
Commercial pre-modified milks:												
Enfamil with Iron, Mead Johnson	1:1	20	1.5	7.0	3.7	0.3	11	19	12	500	400	12.0
Similac PM 60/40 Powder, Ross	1:8	20	1.5	7.5	3.4	0.2	7	14	12	400	250	3.0

S-M-A, Wyeth	1:1	20	1.5	7.2	3.6	0.25	7	14	10	312	50	12.0
Hypoallergenic milk substitutes:												
Isomil, Ross (soya)	1:1	20	2.0	6.8	3.6	0.4	13	16	15	700	500	12.0
Nutramigen Powder, Mead Johnson	1:6	20	2.2	8.5	2.6	0.6	27	16	13	600	450	12.0
ProSobee, Mead Johnson (soya)	1:1	20	2.5	6.8	3.4	0.5	17	17	11	750	500	12.0
Milk substitutes–special formulas:												
Flexical, Mead Johnson	1:45	30	2.2	15.5	3.4	--	15	38	34	25	43	--
Isocal, Mead Johnson	Undiluted	30	3.2	12.1	4.0	--	17	31	29	600	500	9.0
Lonalac, Mead Johnson	1:6	20	3.4	4.8	3.5	0.6	1.1	27	14	1100	1000	1.0
Polycose, Ross	Undiluted	32/tbsp		9.4								
Pregestimil, Mead Johnson	1:7	20	2.1	8.7	2.8		13	17	13	600	450	12.0
Vivonex Standard, Eaton	1:3	30	2.0	23.9	0.15		37	30	51	500	500	5.5

(1-2 teaspoonfuls). Infants often push food out of their mouth with their tongue rather than to the back until they learn to swallow efficiently. This must be explained to the mother since she often feels that the baby is "spitting up" and discontinues the food. One food should be given until it is accepted and tolerated before another is added. Every week or two is often enough to introduce a new food. The infant's appetite will determine how much solid food he will take. There is no point in forcing any particular food when an infant definitely dislikes it.

FEEDING DURING THE SECOND YEAR OF LIFE

By the end of the first year of life, the infant is usually on a three meal a day schedule and is eating vigorously. As he enters the second year he begins a deceleration in his rate of growth and, hence, a gradual reduction in his caloric need. He often has temporary periods when he is not interested in eating food in general or certain types of food. If the parents are unprepared for this, they are often alarmed and attempt to force feed the child. His reaction is rebellion, and feeding and psychological problems may ensue. Mothers, fathers, siblings, and relatives should all be educated to the normal reduction in caloric needs in the toddler prior to his first birthday.

COLIC

Colic is a symptom complex characterized by excessive crying and apparent abdominal pain in infants under 3 months of age. Often the baby's legs are pulled up to his abdomen, his hands are tightly clenched, his feet often cold. While the cause generally is not known, numerous explanations have been given. These include underfeeding, overfeeding, failure to "burp," allergy, excessive carbohydrate fermentation, emotional problems in the mother or family. Intestinal obstruction and infection may mimic colic and should be ruled out.

Management is varied and often unsatisfactory. Therapeutic trials may include:

1. Hold baby upright or permit him to lie prone on a hot water bottle or heating pad.

2. Passage of flatus or fecal material with the aid of a suppository may help.
3. Review feeding techniques and formula preparation.
4. In prolonged attacks, sedation for infant and/or mother may be indicated.
5. In the most severe cases a short period of hospitalization, often with nothing more than separation from the mother, may be indicated.
6. Attempts to provide a stable emotional environment are helpful in both prevention and management.

IMMUNIZATION

Practical Points

1. Routine immunizations should not be given during the course of febrile illnesses. Mild, convalescent, or healing infections should not be absolute contraindications.
2. Other general contraindications for vaccination include (a) immunosuppressive therapy, e.g., steroids, cytotoxic agents, (b) pregnancy, (c) immunodeficiency disorders, (d) malignancies, (e) history of previous allergic reactions to the vaccine, (f) history of allergy to eggs, chickens, or ducks (for vaccines grown on chick's or duck's embryos).
3. The preferred site of injection is intramuscularly into the lateral thigh for infants, and the deltoid or triceps muscle for older children. Each injection should be given at a different site.
4. Deep injection followed by massage reduces the incidence of so-called antigenic cysts.
5. Aspirin or acetaminophen in appropriate dosages for the age will often prevent febrile reactions.
6. When a convulsion or other possible neurological manifestations follow a DPT injection, e.g., persistent screaming, further pertussis immunization is contraindicated. It is also inadvisable to give pertussis vaccine to infants with a history of seizures.
7. Anergy to tuberculin may develop and persist for a month or longer after administration of live, attenuated measles vaccine. A tuberculin test should, therefore, be accomplished prior to giving the measles vaccine.

8. Use of live measles vaccine is not recommended for children with debilitating disease such as leukemia or those receiving immunosuppressive drugs.
9. A personal immunization record such as the one designed by the American Academy of Pediatrics should be provided for each child.
10. Pregnant women should not be given live rubella virus vaccine. Routine immunization of adolescent girls and adult women may be undertaken if they are susceptible to the infection and agree to avoid pregnancy for at least 2 months after immunization.
11. Hemophilus B polysaccharide vaccine is now available for all 24 month olds and high risk 18 month olds (asplenia, sickle cell disease, immunosuppressed).

Tables 3-4 and 3-5 give recommendations for routing immunizations.

Table 3-4 Recommended Schedule for Active Immunization of Normal Infants and Children

2 mo	DTP[1]	TOPV[2a]
4 mo	DTP	TOPV
6 mo	DTP	2b
1 yr		Tuberculin test[3]
15 mo	Measles,[4] rubella[4]	Mumps[4]
1 1/2 yr	DTO	TOPV
4-6 yr	DTP	TOPV
14-16 yr	Td[5]—repeat every 10 years	

[1]DTP—diphtheria and tetanus toxoids combined with pertussis vaccine.

[2a]TOPV—trivalent oral poliovirus vaccine. This recommendation is suitable for breastfed as well as bottlefed infants.

[2b]A third dose of TOPV is optional but may be given in areas of high endemicity of poliomyelitis.

[3]Frequency of repeated tuberculin tests depends on risk of exposure of the child and on the prevalence of tuberculosis in the population group. For the pediatrician's

Table 3-4 (Cont'd.)

office or outpatient clinic, an annual or biennial tuberculin
test, unless local circumstances clearly indicate otherwise,
is appropriate. The initial test should be done at the time
of, or preceding, the measles immunization.

[4]May be given at 15 months as measles-rubella or measles
mumps-rubella combined vaccines.

[5]Td—combined tetanus and diphtheria toxoids (adult type)
for those more than 6 years of age, in contrast to diphtheria
antigen. *Tetanus toxoid at time of injury:* For clean, minor
wounds, no booster dose is needed by a fully immunized child
unless more than 10 years have elapsed since the last dose.
For contaminated wounds, a booster dose should be given if
more than 5 years have elapsed since the last dose.

Concentration and Storage of Vaccines

Because the concentration of antigen varies in different
products, the manufacturer's package insert should be consulted regarding the volume of individual doses of immuniz-
ing agents.

Because biologics are of varying stability, the manufacturer's recommendations for optimal storage conditions
(e.g., temperature, light) should be carefully followed.
Failure to observe these precautions may significantly reduce the potency and effectiveness of the vaccines.

From Report of the Committee on Infectious Diseases, 18th
ed., Copyright American Academy of Pediatrics, 1977. (Reproduced with publisher's permission.)

Table 3-5   Primary Immunization for Children Not Immunized in Early Infancy*

Under 6 Years of Age

First visit	DTP, TOPV, tuberculin test
Interval after first visit	
1 mo	Measles, † mumps, rubella
2 mo	DTP, TOPV
4 mo	DTP, TOPV ‡
10-16 mo or preschool	DTP, TOPV
Age 14-16 yr	Td—repeat every 10 yr

6 Years of Age and Over

First visit	Td, TOPV, tuberculin test
Interval after first visit	
1 mo	Measles, mumps, rubella
2 mo	Td, TOPV
8-14 mo	Td, TOPV
Age 14-16 yr	Td—repeat every 10 yr

---

*Physicians may choose to alter the sequence of these schedules if specific infections are prevalent at the time. For example, measles vaccine might be given on the first visit if an epidemic is underway in the community.

†Measles vaccine is not routinely given before 15 months of age (see Table 3-4).

‡Optional

From Report of the Committee on Infectious Diseases, 18th ed., Copyright American Academy of Pediatrics, 1977. (Reproduced with publisher's permission.)

Chapter 4

COMMON GENETICALLY
DETERMINED SYNDROMES

There are now more than 2000 congenitally determined syndromes described. Some of the more common and characteristic ones are outlined in this chapter. The salient features of several syndromes and their specific diagnostic tests, where available, are listed below:

DOWN'S SYNDROME (MONGOLISM)

1. Findings
   a) Upward palpebral slant
   b) Brushfield spots
   c) Protruberant tongue
   d) Abnormal dermatoglyphics (Simian crease)
   e) Clinodactyly of fifth digit
   f) Generalized hypotonia
   g) Mental retardation
2. Helpful tests
   a) X-ray: Iliac index under 1 year of age
   b) Karyotyping: Extra 21 chromosome (most cases)

71

TRISOMY-13 SYNDROME

1. Findings
   a) Polydactyly, hyperconvex fingernails
   b) Facial and forebrain defects
   c) Scalp defects
   d) Abnormal dermatoglyphics (Simian crease)
   e) Mental retardation
   f) Cardiac defects
   g) Cleft lip and palate
   h) Microcephaly
2. Helpful tests
   a) Karyotyping: Extra chromosome 13

TRISOMY-18 SYNDROME

1. Findings
   a) Overlapping second and third digits
   b) Abnormal dermatoglyphic pattern (simple arches)
   c) Small mouth
   d) Narrow palpebral fissures
   e) Micrognathia
   f) Short sternum
   g) Hernias
   h) Cardiac defects
   i) Mental retardation
2. Helpful tests
   a) Karyotyping: Extra chromosome 18

TURNER'S SYNDROME (XO)

1. Findings
   a) Neck webbing and low-set hairline
   b) Shield-like chest with widely spaced nipples
   c) Cubitus valgus, short stature
   d) Lymphedema, amenorrhea
   e) Sometimes mental retardation, cardiac defects
2. Helpful tests
   a) Karyotyping: XO sex chromosome pattern
   b) Buccal smear: Absent Barr body

KLINEFELTER'S SYNDROME (XXY)

1. Findings
   a) Cryptorchidism or atrophic tests
   b) Infertility
   c) Gynecomastia
   d) Sometimes mental retardation
2. Helpful tests
   a) Karyotyping: XXY chromosome
   b) Buccal smear: Extra Barr body

MUCOPOLYSACCHARIDOSES
(General Findings Common To All)

1. Findings
   a) Mild to marked facial changes
   b) Joint stiffness (except generalized gangliosidosis)
   c) Kyphosis (Hunter rarely, Sanfilippo and Scheie's never)
   d) Mental retardation except Scheie's and Maroteaux— Lamy syndrome
   e) Short stature
2. Helpful tests
   a) Autosomal recessive (except X-linked Hunter's syndrome) metachromatic staining

HURLER'S SYNDROME TYPE I

1. Findings
   a) Cloudy cornea
   b) Marked facial changes
   c) Heart defects
   d) Clawhand
   e) Age at onset 6-18 months
2. Helpful tests
   a) Dermatan sulfate in urine

HUNTER'S SYNDROME TYPE II

1. Findings
   a) Clear cornea
   b) Marked facial changes
   c) Clawhand

    d) Deafness
    e) Hepatosplenomegaly
    f) Age at onset 2-4 years
2. Helpful Tests
    a) Heparin sulfate in urine

SANFILIPPO'S SYNDROME TYPE III

1. Findings
    a) Clear cornea
    b) Mild facial changes
    c) Mild skeletal changes
    d) Onset in early childhood
2. Helpful tests
    a) Heparin sulfate in urine

MORQUIO'S SYNDROME TYPE IV

1. Findings
    a) Cloudy cornea
    b) Mild facial changes
    c) Knock-knee
    d) Age at onset 1-3 years
2. Helpful tests
    a) Keratosulfate in urine

SCHEIE'S SYNDROME TYPE V

1. Findings
    a) Cloudy cornea
    b) Broad mouth
    c) Clawhand
    d) Retinal pigment
    e) Cardiac defect
    f) Onset in early-to midchildhood
2. Helpful tests
    a) Dermatan sulfate in urine

MAROTEAUX–LAMY SYNDROME TYPE VI

1. Findings
    a) Cloudy cornea
    b) Mild facial changes

c) Knock-knee
d) Hepatosplenomegaly
e) Onset in early- to midchildhood, 1-3 years
2. Helpful tests
a) Heparin and dermatan sulfate in urine

GENERALIZED GANGLIOSIDOSES

1. Findings
a) Marked facial changes
b) Renal abnormalities
c) Clawhand
d) Cherry red spot in macula
e) Only syndrome present at birth

ACHONDROPLASIA

1. Findings
a) Large head, saddle nose
b) Short extremities
c) Lumbar lordosis
d) Dwarfism
e) Occasional hydrocephalus
f) Normal intelligence
2. Helpful tests
a) Autosomal dominant inheritance

MARFAN'S SYNDROME

1. Findings
a) Cubitus valgus
b) Tall, thin body type
c) Arachnodactyly
d) Lental subluxation
e) Cardiovascular abnormality (aortic aneurysm)
2. Helpful tests
a) Autosomal dominant
b) Cytoplasmic metachromatic granules

CORNELIA DE LANGE SYNDROME

1. Findings
a) Short stature

    b) Mental retardation
    c) Microbrachycephalic
    d) Bushy, confluent eyebrows
    e) High-arched palate
    f) Micrognathia
    g) Hirsutism
    h) Micromelia

PROGERIA (HUTCHINSON-GILFORD SYNDROME)

1. Findings
    a) Alopecia
    b) Hypoplastic nails
    c) Loss of subcutaneous fat
    d) Stiff joints
    e) Skeletal hypoplasia
    f) Delayed dentition
    g) Atherosclerosis
2. Helpful tests
    a) Elevated serum cholesterol

LAURENCE-MOON-BIEDL SYNDROME

1. Findings
    a) Obesity
    b) Mental retardation
    c) Polydactyly, syndactyly
    d) Retinitis pigmentosa
    e) Genital hypoplasia

PRADER-WILLI SYNDROME

1. Findings
    a) Short stature
    b) Obesity
    c) Mental retardation
    d) Hypotonia
    e) Small feet and hands
    f) Hypogonadism
    g) Cryptorchidism

ATAXIA TELANGIECTASIA (LOUIS-BAR SYNDROME)

1. Findings
   a) Growth lag
   b) Ataxia
   c) Choreoathetosis
   d) Mental retardation (50%)
   e) Telangiectasia (especially the conjuctiva)
   f) Frequent infections
   g) Lymphoid hypoplasia
2. Helpful tests
   a) Lymphopenia
   b) Low or absent serum gamma 1-A globulin

TREACHER-COLLINS SYNDROME

1. Findings
   a) Antimongolian palebral slant
   b) Malar and mandibular hypoplasia
   c) Lower lid coloboma
   d) Absence of lower eyelashes
   e) Malformation of ears
   f) Conductive deafness
   g) Scalp hair on cheeks
2. Helpful tests
   a) Autosomal dominant inheritance pattern

WAARDENBURG'S SYNDROME

1. Findings
   a) Hypertelorism
   b) Broad nasal bridge
   c) Medial hyperplasia of eyebrows
   d) White forelock
   e) Deafness
   f) Heterochromia of eyes
2. Helpful tests
   a) Autosomal dominant inheritance pattern

STURGE–WEBER SYNDROME

1. Findings
   a) Facial hemangiomata
   b) Meningeal hemangiomata
   c) Seizures
   d) Mental deficiency
2. Helpful tests
   a) Cerebral calcification on x-ray

TUBEROUS SCLEROSIS (ADENOMA SEBACEUM)

1. Findings
   a) Seizures
   b) Mental retardation
   c) Fibrous-angiomatous facial lesions
   d) Bone "cysts" sclerosis
   e) Renal rhabdomyomas
   f) Shagreen patches
2. Helpful tests
   a) Autosomal dominant pattern
   b) Cranial calcification on x-ray
   c) Bone and kidney abnormalities on x-ray

NEUROFIBROMATOSIS
(Von Recklinghausen's Disease)

1. Findings
   a) Cafe au lait spots
   b) Multiple neurofibromas
   c) Scoliosis, osteosclerosis
   d) Sometimes acromegaly
   e) Sometimes sexual precocity
2. Helpful tests
   a) Autosomal dominant pattern
   b) X-ray bones

ELHERS–DANLOS SYNDROME

1. Findings
   a) Hyperextensible joints
   b) Easy bruisability
   c) Hyperelastic skin

d) Small stature
e) Hernias
f) Poor wound healing
2. Helpful tests
    a) Autosomal dominant pattern

Chapter 5

GENETIC COUNSELLING

With the decline in this country of infectious illness and the nutritional deficiency states, genetically determined disease has assumed a relatively more important position in the morbidity-mortality tabulations. Concomitantly, more sophisticated methods of diagnosing and predicting genetic illness have become available. In the wake of these developments has come an increase in the demand for genetic services, particularly counselling. Estimates of the number of newborns afflicted with inherited disease range from 2.5 to 5% of all live births

As an outcome of the rapid development in this area, the pediatrician's role is an important one. As a result, the physician must be knowledgeable regarding the general principles of genetics and their application to common diseases; should recognize the importance of an accurate family history, which, in most instances, need not be more than two or three generations of immediate relatives, and be able to obtain and interpret such; should recognize unusual clusters of disease, such as early-onset coronary artery disease or cancer, and question the possible implications; should be aware of the fact that specific genetic diseases may be more common in certain ethnic and racial groups; should be able to counsel patients, including families, for common disorders and refer complicated cases to appropriate experts; should recognize the possibility of a genetic disorder and obtain appropriate specimens for analysis or refer such patients to experts; should be knowledgeable regarding genetic screening and be aware of recommendations concerning newborn screening and carrier detection; should be familiar with indications for intrauterine diagnosis; and should be aware of the back-up resources for diagnosis, counselling, and treatment in the local community.

There are three essential ingredients:

An accurate diagnosis. There is no point in calculating risk factors for an illness the child does not have.

Familiarity, not only with the fundamentals of genetics but an awareness of the most recent developments in the field.

Good laboratory resources, to confirm diagnostic impressions and provide an accurate basis for subsequent counselling.

A most important component is thorough knowledge of the family. Construction of an accurate family geneology involving not only parents, siblings, and children, but also grandparents, uncles, aunts, and first cousins is a necessity. Information gathered by questioning one or two members of the family is often not accurate enough. Medical records of family members, death certificates, and data contributed by family physicians are useful sources of information for the counselor.

Once these prerequisites are met, the counselor relies on information derived from three sources. The first of these is provided by basic mendelian theory. For those genetic illnesses that closely follow mendelian principles, risk factors can be accurately obtained by merely applying Mendel's laws. Here the parents' genotypes must be known and the genetic disorder must be at a single site only. There are approximately 3000 conditions that may be encountered in this class of genetic disorder. Some of the most common are sickle cell disease, hemolytic disease of the newborn, and glucose-6-phosphate dehydrogenase deficiency. It is often possible for the physician without special expertise in genetics to provide accurate counselling without the aid of professional counselors in this class of genetic disease provided he can meet the prerequisites listed above. An excellent reference source to aid him in this is MuKusick, *Medelian Inheritance in Man, Catalogs of Autosomal Dominant, Autosomal Recessive, and X-linked Phenotypes,* 5th ed., Baltimore, Johns Hopkins Press, 1978.

The second source of information is derived from empirical studies of large population samples. Information related to gene frequencies, mutation rate, penetrance, and expressivity may then be applied in calculating risk factors. This method is most useful for those diseases that are genetically determined but do not clearly display discernible inheritance patterns, e.g., pyloric stenosis. Calculation of the risks involved may be complicated and involve considerable mathematical probabilities for interpretation. Professional counselling is advisable for the accurate evaluation of risk.

A third method of gathering information is based on careful analysis of the patient's pedigree. Risk factors may become more obvious by observing what has already occurred in the family. A situation arising from a spontaneously mutant gene may be distinguished from one arising from an inherited abnormal gene. Of course, any two or all three of the methods may be needed in solving a particular problem.

The final step in the process is educating and advising the family of the risks involved. This entails a clear exposition of the probability of both carrying an abnormal gene and transmitting either the carrier state or the disease to the progeny; but counselling does not end here. An awareness of the problems that are likely to be encountered should one bear an afflicated child must also be clearly understood. It is one thing to risk having a child with a hare lip; quite another to have one with a Duchenne-type muscular dystrophy.

In addition, all possible alternatives must be presented to the family so that decisions may be reached. The possibility of abortion for those diseases diagnosed by analyzing cells obtained from amniocentesis must not be forgotten. It is possible, for example, for a mother to terminate the pregnancy of classic sex-linked hemophilia if the sex of an infant is determined to be male while allowing a female fetus to be delivered at term. Future developments will increase the importance of these alternatives.

An adequate follow-up period is necessary. This may very well be carried out by the family physician who is made aware of the genetic counselor's analysis and opinion. The physician may then reinforce the education of the family, insure their full comprehension of the facts, and help answer any questions that may arise as time goes by.

There are three basic patterns of inheritance encountered in genetic disease: the autosomal dominant, autosomal recessive, and sex-linked recessive. A fourth, sex-linked dominant condition has also been described and is relatively rare, e.g., hypophosphatemia and vitamin D resistant rickets. The characteristics of each pattern can be briefly summarized.

AUTOSOMAL DOMINANT CHARACTERISTICS

This is the most frequent type; more than 1500 are described.

1. The abnormal gene may be located on any chromosome except the sex chromosomes (X and Y).
2. The abnormal gene is derived from one parent only and the affected individual is a heterozygote.
3. Unless a spontaneous gene mutation has occurred in the affected individual, other members of the family will be found to exhibit the illness. The trait appears in each generation.
4. Risk:
   a) to siblings of affected individual, 50% affected
   b) to children of affected individual, 50% affected
5. Males and females are affected equally. The carrier state is unimportant since the abnormal gene is dominant.
6. Pitfalls. Genes vary in the way they express themselves. People with the same genotypes may differ greatly in phenotype. This is referred to as the expressivity of a gene. When a gene has poor or minimal expressivity it is referred to as a gene of low penetrance or nonpenetrance. Nonpenetrance may make it difficult to identify affected individuals in a pedigree. In such instances, less than 50% of siblings and children may be found with the illness and an entire generation may be seemingly unaffected. It should be remembered that in certain illnesses affected individuals who appear to be normal may be found to have biochemical abnormalities consistent with the disease (porphyria).

7. Counselling. Counselling is not difficult when the pedigree clearly shows a pattern. When low penetrance is
encountered it becomes more difficult to ascertain risk
factors. When no other member of the family is affected
and low penetrance can be reasonably excluded, the individual affected is demonstrating a spontaneous gene
mutation. In this case, the risk to siblings is very low
although the risk to the affected individual's children
remains 50%. The more common autosomal dominant
conditions are achondroplasia, Alport's syndrome, an-
iridia, acute intermittent porphyria, hemophilia, hereditary hemorrhagic telangiectasia, multiple intestinal
polyposis, myotonic dystrophy, and neurofibromatosis.

AUTOSOMAL RECESSIVE CHARACTERISTICS

The 1100 autosomal recessive conditions described to date
make this the second most frequent type of genetic disease.

1. Abnormal genes occur on autosomal chromosomes only.
2. Inheritance of two abnormal genes, one from each parent,
   makes the patient homozygous.
3. The parents appear to be normal since they are heterozygous and the abnormal gene is recessive.
4. Consanguineous mating increases the risk of inheriting
   autosomal recessive conditions.
5. Risk:
   a) to siblings of an affected individual, 25% are affected,
      50% are carriers.
   b) to children of an affected individual, negligible risk
      exists since the trait is recessive and the same re-
      cessive gene is unlikely to be encountered in a future
      spouse. All the children will be carriers, however, and
      males and females are affected equally.

The more common autosomal recessive conditions are
adrenogenital syndrome, albinism, ataxia telangiectasia,
cystic fibrosis, cretinism, homocystinuria, Laurence-Moon-
Biedl syndrome, Niemann-Pick disease, phenylketonuria,
Riley-Day syndrome, sickle cell anemia, Tay-Sachs disease,
Werdnig-Hoffman disease, and Wilson's disease.

It should be realized that it may be possible to detect
heterozygotes with appropriate testing.

SEX-LINKED RECESSIVE CHARACTERISTICS

There are approximately 200 of these conditions.

1. An abnormal gene occurs on the sex chromosomes only (X or Y). No genetic disease has yet been described for the Y chromosome. In practice only the X chromosome abnormalities are considered.
2. The affected individual inherits an abnormal gene situated on an X chromosome. The abnormal gene generally behaves as a recessive, thus in the case of a female with a second (and normal) X chromosome, gross clinical manifestations will usually be, but are not always, lacking. In the case of a male who has only one (and an abnormal) X chromosome, the clinical symptomatology will be present.
3. Many more males than females are affected.
4. Females are carriers and are only rarely symptomatic, e.g., Fabry's disease.
5. Risk:
   a) to siblings of affected individual, 50% of male siblings are affected
   b) to children of an affected male, none of males affected, 100% of females are carriers
   c) to children of a female carrier, 50% of males affected, 50% of females are carriers.
6. Counselling. The probability of the mother being a carrier must be carefully assessed. If at least one male sibling of the mother, and one male offspring exhibit the illness, she may be considered a carrier. Common X-linked conditions are hemophilia (factor VIII and factor IX deficiencies), G-6-PD deficiency, ectodermal dysplasia, (anhidrotic variety) Duchenne muscular dystrophy, Lesch-Nyhan syndrome, nephrogenic diabetes insipidus, ocular albinism, and X-linked ichthyosis. It should be realized that the carrier state is often detectable because of the high rate of inactivation of the X chromosome carrying the mutant gene (50%). The ability to do so increases the precision of predicting risk in both autosomal recessive and X-linked recessive conditions. (See Table 5-1.)

Table 5-1   Predicting Risk of Carrier States

	Type	Means of Carrier Detection
Ocular albinism	X-linked	Retinal depigmentation observable
Sickle cell anemia	Autosomal recessive	Hb electrophoresis detects S Hb
Hemophilia A	X-linked recessive	80% have decreased levels of factor VIII
Duchenne muscular dystrophy	X-linked recessive	Serum creatine kinase levels elevated in 80% of carriers

SEX-LINKED DOMINANT CHARACTERISTICS

These conditions are rare.

1. The abnormal gene is situated on the X chromosome and behaves as a dominant. Gross clinical manifestations may occur in females.
2. Twice as many females are affected as males.
3. Homozygous females will transmit the disease to all their children; heterozygotes to half theirs.
4. Males will transmit the disease to their sons.

MULTIFACTORIAL INHERITANCE

It is recognized that many traits, malformations, and diseases appear to run in families with no evidence of mendelian inheritance. The nature of the familial component is unclear. In many instances there appears to be an interaction between hereditary and environmental influences.

The term used to explain this phenomenon is multifactorial inheritance. The term polygenic also is frequently used.

Technical advances have made possible the diagnosis of virtually all chromosomal aberrations, more than 100 inborn errors of metabolism, neural tube defects, and a number of other congenital malformations, and certain hemoglobinopathies. Prenatal diagnostic techniques include amniocentesis, placentocentesis, fetoscopy with fetal visualization, blood sampling and/or skin biopsy, amniography and fetography, analysis of maternal serum and urine, ultrasonography, and roentgenography.

The indications for prenatal detection of genetic disorders are as follows:

1. Maternal age greater than 35 years
2. Previous child with a chromosomal aberration
3. Chromosomal abnormality in either parent
4. Fetal sex determination for X-linked recessive disorders in which the precise diagnosis is not possible
5. Inborn errors of metabolism, more than 100 of which can now be detected in either cultivated amniotic fluid cells or cell-free amniotic fluid
6. Neural tube defects
7. Certain hemoglobinopathies

It should be realized that transabdominal amniocentesis, performed during the second trimester, carries a risk of abortion of approximately 1/200.

Chapter 6

COMMON COMMUNICABLE DISEASES

MEASLES (RUBEOLA)

ETIOLOGY AND EPIDEMIOLOGY

Agent: Measles virus, a paramyxo virus, one antigenic type. Source: Respiratory tract secretions, blood and urine of infected patients. Transmission: Generally direct contact with droplets from an infected person; may be airborne or by indirect contact with freshly contaminated articles. Incubation period: 10-12 days.

PERIOD OF COMMUNICABILITY

From 4 days prior to the rash through 4 days after eruption. Highest period of communicability is during the prodromal period just prior to onset of the rash.

CLINICAL MANIFESTATIONS

The clinical course of measles is illustrated in Figure 6-1.

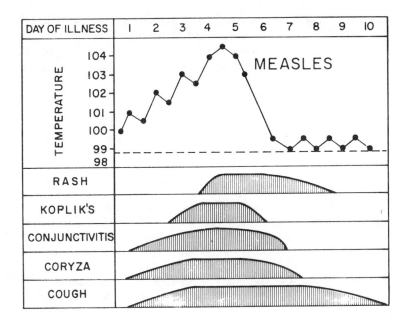

Figure 6-1 Schematic diagram illustrating clinical course of typical case of measles. The rash appears 3-4 days after the onset of fever, conjuctivitis, coryza, and cough. Koplik's spots usually develop 2 days before the rash. (From Krugman, S., and Ward, R.: Infectious Diseases of Children, 5th ed., C.V. Mosby Co., St. Louis, 1973. Reproduced with publisher's permission.)

DIAGNOSIS

The development of a maculopapular rash preceded by a 3-4-day period (occasionally as long as 7) of fever, conjuctivitis, coryza, and cough associated with pathognomonic Koplik's spots is diagnostic of measles. No confirmatory laboratory tests are needed.

In modified measles, either through the use of gamma-globulin or when maternally acquired antibodies are still present (in infants 5-10 months of age), diagnosis is much more difficult. Prodromal symptoms including Koplik's spots may be absent.

Diagnostic tests such as virus isolation or neutralization, complement fixation, or hemagglutination inhibition techniques demonstrate rising antibodies and may be utilized in the difficult diagnostic case.

DIFFERENTIAL DIAGNOSIS

The rash of measles must be differentiated from the rashes of rubella, roseola, enterovirus infections, toxoplasmosis, infectious mononucleosis, erythema infectiosum, scarlet fever, endemic typhus, and drug eruptions. Hemorrhagic measles may resemble meningococcemia and Rocky Mountain spotted fever.

Atypical measles in previously immunized patients who have received inactivated vaccine (which no longer should be used) may be manifested by a maculopapular, vesicular, urticarial, occasionally hemorrhagic rash which is often centrifugal in distribution. Since inactivated vaccine has not been used for more than a decade, the individual presenting with atypical measles is likely to be an adolescent or older.

COMPLICATIONS

Pulmonary complications are the primary cause of death in measles. Otitis media is one of the more common complications. Obstructive laryngitis may require tracheostomy. Acute encephalitis is a potentially crippling or fatal complication. Less common complications include purpura, thrombocytopenic and nonthrombocytopenic varieties, appendicitis (lymphoid hyperplasia in the appendix), and subacute sclerosing panencephalitis (Dawson's encephalitis occurs in 1/1000 cases).

IMMUNITY

One attack of measles is generally followed by permanent immunity.

TREATMENT

No specific therapy; antibacterial agents only for the treatment of secondary bacterial complication, otherwise supportive only.

PREVENTION

1. Active immunization, see immunizations (pp. 68-70.)
2. Passive immunization, immune serum globulin-ISG

Care of exposed susceptible children or adults: If previously unimmunized, give Edmonston B live measles vaccine with 0.04 ml/kg ISG at separate sites. An alternative method is to give a preventive dose of 0.25 ml/kg of ISG. ISG should be given as soon after exposure as possible and is to be followed in 8 weeks by live measles vaccine. If the exposed, susceptible child is known to have leukemia, disseminated malignancy, chronic immunosuppression, or "Swiss" type of agammaglobulinemia (lymphopenia with thymic agenesis) give 0.5 ml/kg not to exceed 15 ml. The Edmonston-B vaccine confers immunity in 95% (or more) of those inoculated. Subacute sclerosing panencephalitis occurs in approximately 1/million vaccine recipients.

ISOLATION OF PATIENT

Patients should be isolated from onset to prodromal period through the third day of rash. Quarantine of contacts not indicated except in hospital or institutional settings where children at usually high risk may be involved. If necessary, quarantine contacts from fifth day after known exposure until 12 days have passed (full incubation period).

RUBELLA (GERMAN MEASLES, 3-DAY MEASLES)

ETIOLOGY AND EPIDEMIOLOGY

Rubella is caused by a rubivirus virus, one of the togavirus family, which was isolated and cultivated in tissue culture in 1962. Rubella is worldwide in distribution. It is endemic in most urban areas. Epidemics occur in an irregular and unpredictable manner. Rubella is rare in infancy and uncommon in preschool children. There is a substantial incidence of the disease in older children, adolescents (outbreaks in colleges have been observed), and young adults. Since 1941, great attention has been given to this disease because of the association of congenital malformations when the disease occurs in pregnant women during early pregnancy (see p. 44). Incubation period: Usually 16-18 days with a range of 14-21 days.

SOURCE AND TRANSMISSION

By droplets or direct contact. Man is the sole source of the infection.

PERIOD OF COMMUNICABILITY

The maximal period of communicability extends from 7 days before to 5 days after onset of the rash. Infants with congenital rubella may be communicable up to 1 year of age. Repeat viral cultures, until negative, are useful to determine the end point of communicability.

CLINICAL MANIFESTATIONS

In the child, the usual first symptom is the rash. In adolescents and young adults, the rash is usually preceded by a 1-5-day prodromal period characterized by low-grade fever, headache, malaise, anorexia, mild conjunctivitis, sore throat, cough, and lymphadenopathy.

Practical Points

1. Lymph node enlargement may begin as early as 7 days before onset of rash.
2. Postauricular, cervical, and suboccipital lymphadenopathy to neck, arms, trunk, and lower extremities. The rash spreads much faster and clears more rapidly than the rash of measles.
4. The rash is generally a discrete pink to red, maculopapular eruption. On the trunk, it may become confluent the second day and resemble scarlet fever.
5. The rash may be evanescent, disappearing the first day, or it may persist for 5 days. Rubella without rash is not uncommon.

DIAGNOSIS

A diagnosis of rubella is considered where clinical features as described are present. Confirmation is by virus isolation or serologic testing. An acute and convalescent serum must be obtained for serological diagnosis. The acute serum should be obtained as soon as possible after the onset of the rash and the convalescent serum 2-4 weeks later. A four-fold rise in rubella antibody or seroconversion is indication of infection. The hemagglutination inhibition (HI) antibody test is the most useful and most rapid (results within 24 hours). The HI antibody test also is useful for demonstrating immunity.

COMPLICATIONS

Complications are unusual in rubella. Arthritis is common in adolescents and young adults, especially females. It has rarely been described in young children. The arthritis usually develops just as the rash is fading and may be associated with a return of fever, transient joint pain, or massive effusion in one or more joints. One or more larger or smaller joints may be involved.

Other complications are:

1. Encephalitis is very rare (1/6000 cases). Recovery is usually complete but fatalities have been described.
2. Purpura, thrombocytopenic or nonthrombocytopenic, has been described in a few cases.
3. In general, the prognosis of postnatally acquired rubella is excellent and is considered the most benign of childhood exanthematous illnesses.

IMMUNITY

One attack is generally followed by lifelong immunity.

TREATMENT

Symptomatic only. Arthritis is generally benefited by aspirin.

PREVENTION

Passive immunization should be considered only under specific circumstances in early pregnancy. The use of immune serum globulin (human), ISG, for the prevention of rubella may prevent or modify the acute illness if given in doses of 0.55 ml/kg. In pregnant women, there can be no guarantee that ISG will prevent congenital rubella; however, if abortion is out of the question, ISG does offer some hope. In any case, a determination of serum antibodies (HI) to rubella should be obtained prior to inoculation, if for no other reason than the reassurance that can be given to seropositive individuals.

ISOLATION AND QUARANTINE

Quarantine of contacts - none. Isolation of patient is ordinarily not indicated except in hospitals or to protect susceptible women in first trimester of pregnancy. In hospitals, rubella should be isolated from first sign of infection or on the seventh day after contact to 5 days after appearance of rash. All suspected cases of congenital rubella should be reported to the state department of health to assist surveillance efforts.

ROSEOLA INFANTUM (EXANTHEMA SUBITUM)

ETIOLOGY AND EPIDEMIOLOGY

Although final confirmation is not available, all evidence points to a virus as the infecting agent. More than 95% of cases occur between the ages of 6 months and 3 years. The disease occurs year-round with some concentration of cases in the spring and autumn months. It has been estimated that 30% of children under 3 years develop apparent disease. It is likely that the remaining 70% have either inapparent infection or fever without the rash. Incubation period: Difficult to determine because contact is rarely known. Information which is available indicates a range of 5-15 days.

CLINICAL MANIFESTATIONS

The typical course of roseola infantum is illustrated in the following diagram (see Figure 6-2).

Practical Points

1. Fever is high and continuous, often lasting 3 or 4 days.
2. Typically, the fever falls abruptly to normal levels after this period.
3. Generally, the rash develops at the time of disappearance of the fever. However, it may appear just prior to a drop in temperature or up to 24 hours after the temperature reaches normal.

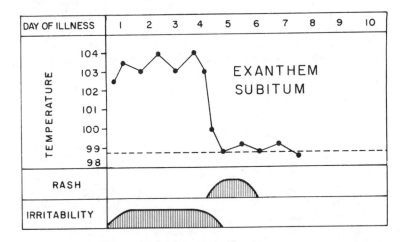

Figure 6-2 Schematic diagram illustrating typical clinical course of exanthema subitum. Between the third and fourth days the temperature drops to normal and a maculopapular eruption appears. (From Krugman, S., and Ward, R.: Infectious Diseases of Children, 5th ed, C.V. Mosby Co., St. Louis, 1973. Reproduced with publisher's permission.)

4. The rash is composed of rose-pink maculopapular lesions that tend to remain discrete. The rash characteristically appears on the trunk and may be limited to that area of the body. It may spread to the extremities, neck, and face.
5. The rash may be evanescent, disappearing in a few hours or it may pesist for 2 or 3 days.
6. Despite the marked elevation of fever, the child often does not appear ill and is quite playful. On the other hand, he may be quite irritable.
7. Puffiness of the upper eyelids is a clinical hint that one may be dealing with roseola.
8. Lymphadenopathy of the suboccipital, cervical, and post-auricular nodes is frequently present. A string of small nodes, the size of BB shot along the inferior aspect of the occipital bulge, in a child with markedly elevated temperature, and a paucity of physical findings, are very suggestive of roseola infantum.
9. It is not uncommon for the onset of roseola to be ushered in by a generalized convulsion.
10. A bulging fontanelle with normal cerebrospinal fluid findings may be present.

DIAGNOSIS

Chiefly based on clinical findings, a high index of suspicion, and a careful ruling out of more serious pathological processes. Toward the end of the febrile period, often a marked leukopenia develops with an increase in the percentage of lymphocytes and monocytes.

DIFFERENTIAL DIAGNOSIS

During the febrile stage when the rash is not present, all acute infectious processes must be considered, especially meningococcemia and sepsis. During the rash stage all conditions mentioned on p. 90 must be ruled out.

COMPLICATIONS

The most common complications are convulsive seizures which appear to parallel the incidence of other forms of

febrile convulsions. Spinal fluid findings are normal although occasionally the CSF pressure is elevated. Sequelae
are rare.

PROGNOSIS

The prognosis is uniformly excellent. However, the often
unexplained 3 or 4 day period of marked elevation of the
temperature in a small infant or child is of great concern to
both physicians and parents. The appearance of the rash,
therefore, is of great comfort.

TREATMENT

Treatment is purely symptomatic. Aspirin, or acetaminophen
are useful for their antipyretic effect. They may be repeated
at 4-hour intervals.

IMMUNITY

One attack probably confers permanent immunity. The fact
that the disease is rarely seen under 6 months of age suggests
that the infant is protected by passively acquired maternal
antibodies.

ISOLATION AND QUARANTINE

Neither is indicated.

CHICKEN POX (VARICELLA)

ETIOLOGY AND EPIDEMIOLOGY

The disease is caused by the varicella-zoster (VZ) virus. The
virus can be grown in tissue cultures using human embryonic
cells. Adequate evidence is available that the VZ virus is the
etiologic agent of both chicken pox and herpes zoster.
Chicken pox is predominantly a disease of childhood with the
highest incidence between 2 and 8 years of age.

Practical Points

1. Chicken pox may occur in early infancy despite maternal immunity.
2. Intrauterine infection may be followed by clinical chicken pox in the newborn infant. The majority of infants exposed to mothers who have chicken pox during labor develop the disease after an appropriate incubation period.
3. A patient with chicken pox may transmit the disease to susceptible individuals for 1 day before onset of rash and until all vesicles have become crusted. Direct contact with droplet transmission is the mode of spread. The period of infection varies between 5 and 10 days depending upon the severity of the individual case.
4. The encrusted scabs of chicken pox do not contain active virus as do the scabs of smallpox. Man is the only source of the disease.
5. Incubation period: 14-16 days; range 10-21 days.

CLINICAL MANIFESTATIONS

In children the disease usually begins with low-grade fever, malaise, and the appearance of the rash. A prodromal period of several days may precede the eruption in adults.

Practical Points

1. The lesions pass rapidly through the stages of macule, papule, vesicle, and crust, often in 6-8 hours.
2. The typical vesicle is superficial, dewdrop in appearance, with fragile, easily ruptured walls.
3. As the vesicle begins to dry, a umbilicated appearance (pseudoumbilication) may be apparent.
4. In a variable length of time, 5-20 days, the scabs fall off without scarring.
5. Scarring may be present if the lesion is excoriated or infected.
6. The distribution of the lesions is centripetal with the greatest concentration on the trunk.
7. All stages of the lesions can be seen at the same time as various crops erupt.
8. The number of lesions vary from 1 or 2 to thousands in individual cases.

Lesions appear on palms, soles, and mucous membrane surfaces.

10. Chicken pox is generally a mild disease in the newborn, but may be fulminating and fatal with widespread visceral lesions.

11. Chicken pox in adults is often a severe disease with a mortality between 10 and 30%. Varicella pneumonia is a relatively common complication in adults but is rarely seen in normal children.

12. Lesions of both herpes zoster and chicken pox may occur together in adults.

DIAGNOSIS

The typical case of chicken pox can be clinically identified without laboratory confirmation. In atypical cases, the virus may be readily isolated from the vesicular fluid within the first 3-4 days of the rash. Complement fixing antibody can be detected in serum obtained as early as 7 days after onset of rash. The white cell count is inconsistent and is not helpful in aiding in the diagnostic process.

DIFFERENTIAL DIAGNOSIS

Chicken pox must be differentiated from impetigo, insect bites, papular urticaria, herpetic dermatitis, scabies, rickettsial pox, eczema herpeticum and vaccinatum, and herpes zoster.

COMPLICATIONS

1. Secondary bacterial infection.

2. Encephalitis occurs in less than 1/1000 cases and generally is milder than postmeasles encephalitis. Chicken pox encephalitis may, however, be overwhelming, even fatal.

3. Varicella pneumonia occurs particularly in adults. It is also found in infants with varicella neonatorum. It may be identified by demonstrating intranuclear bodies in the sputum.

4. Fulminating, often fatal chicken pox occurs in children who received cortisone prior to contracting the disease or are immunocompromised. Reye's syndrome has followed a percentage of cases.

TREATMENT

Routine care includes:

1. Keep child cool by dressing lightly and controlling environmental temperature
2. Trim fingernails very short to prevent scratching and
   excoriation.
3. Daily, gentle bathing is recommended.
4. Pruritus may be relieved by the use of calamine lotion
   with or without added antihistamine.
5. Oral antihistamine preparations may reduce itching.
   Aspirin should be avoided for the possible association
   with Reye's syndrome.

Treatment of complications:

1. Bacterial - use appropriate antibiotic therapy.
2. Encephalitis - symptomatic therapy only. The effectiveness of steroids has not been demonstrated.
3. Varicella pneumonia - use supportive therapy. Assistive
   respiratory therapy may be lifesaving, especially when
   used with a respiratory depressant.

PREVENTION

Newborns, steroid-treated children, children receiving other
immunosuppressive medications, and susceptible adults
should be protected, if possible; ZIG (zoster immune globulin) may now be obtained from the American Red Cross.
It is effective in modifying varicella when administered
intramuscularly within 72 hours of exposure, at a dose of
1.25 ml/10 kg of body weight. Effectiveness of gamma
globulin (ISG) still is uncertain but is indicated in dosages
of 0.6-1.2 ml/kg of body weight in the above situations.
When ZIG is not available, ISG is not recommended for a
normal child. A live virus vaccine is available on a study
basis for immunocompromised children.

ISOLATION AND QUARANTINE

Isolation and quarantine procedures should be individualized.
The patient with chicken pox should be kept at home until

all lesions are crusted. Contacts generally should not be quarantined but only observed. On the other hand, rigid isolation procedures are necessary to protect the newborn and the child at high risk. Every attempt should be made to prevent contact with a definite or potential case of chicken pox.

SMALLPOX (VARIOLA MAJOR; VARIOLA MINOR) (ALASTRIM)

Although formerly worldwide in distribution, smallpox in recent years virtually has been eliminated. Despite the apparent control of this highly contagious disease, constant alertness must be practiced since the organism still exists in the laboratory and as a result at least one outbreak has occurred.

Practical Points:

1. Contraindications to smallpox vaccination include children and adults with eczema, other acute and chronic dermatologic conditions, lowered immune response (dysgammaglobulinemia, lymphoma, leukemia, therapy with steroids, antimetabolites, alkylating or ionizing irradiation). Pregnancy is also a contraindication. Routine vaccination is no longer practiced in the United States except in military personnel.
2. Vaccinia immune globulin (human - VIG) 0.12-0.24 ml/kg injected intramuscularly will prevent or modify smallpox if given within 24 hours after known exposure.
3. VIG (Hyland Laboratories, Los Angeles, California) is also used in the treatment of eczema vaccinatum, severe generalized vaccinia, and vaccinia necrosum. It is available through the Centers for Disease Control.

SCARLET FEVER

ETIOLOGY AND EPIDEMIOLOGY

Group A hemolytic streptococci are the etiological agents for a wide spectrum of clinical infections in children including scarlet fever, tonsillitis or pharyngitis, and erysipelas. Scarlet fever occurs in individuals who have not developed immunity against the erythrogenic exotoxin which is common to the 40 or more types of group A hemolytic streptococci. Antibacterial immunity, on the other hand, is type-specific so that an individual may have repeated streptococcal infections each caused only by a type to which the patient is not immune. The sequelae, rheumatic fever and acute glomerular nephritis, lend particular importance to this disease. Incubation period: 2-4 days.

CLINICAL MANIFESTATIONS

Many of the signs, symptoms, and laboratory findings of strep infections are described in Chapter 7, p. 128. Treatment is also covered in the same chapter. The clinical complications of acute rheumatic fever and glomerulonephritis are described in Chapter 16. In this section, only the characteristic signs and symptoms of scarlet fever itself will be described.

Practical Points

1. Scarlet fever is ushered in by fever, vomiting, sore throat, and headache.
2. Abdominal pain may be present early in the disease mimicking a surgical abdomen.
3. The typical rash generally develops within 12-48 hours after onset of the disease.
4. The degree of elevation and duration of the fever varies with the severity of the disease. With prompt diagnosis and penicillin therapy, the temperature drops precipitously to normal within 24 hours.
5. The exanthema, an erythematous, sometimes petechial involvement of the tonsils, pharynx, tongue, and palate, results in the classical but nonspecific tongue changes described in scarlet fever (white strawberry followed by the desquamated red strawberry tongue).
6. Distinctive features of the rash can best be seen by examining the skin with a source of light such as a penlight or otoscope directed horizontally to the skin. These features include:

a) Two apparent components: a diffuse erythema, blanching with pressure, which involves the papular lesions as well the intervening skin and the discrete, punctate, pinpoint papular lesions.
b) A rash that becomes generalized rapidly, usually over a period of 24 hours.
c) Contrary to many descriptions, the papular eruption may occur on the face although the lesions are very small. The erythema is prominent on the face with the characteristic circumoral pallor reflecting its absence about the mouth.
d) The papular eruption is best developed upon the inner aspects of the thigh.
e) Pastia's sign, transverse lines of small petechiae in the antecubital fossa, is a classic finding in scarlet fever.
f) The papular rash does not occur on the palms and soles which may be, however, erythematous and edematous.
g) Desquamation follows the disappearance of the rash and may be the only clinical sign of milder disease in which the rash was overlooked. Desquamation, especially of the hands and feet (often demonstrating a splitting of the skin at the free border of the nails of the fingers and toes), may occur 2 or 3 weeks after the onset of the disease. Such desquamation may be present during the course of acute rheumatic fever or glomerulonephritis, and indicates the prior streptococcal infection responsible for these conditions.

7. It should be kept in mind that the staphylococcus, particularly phage type 85, can also cause a similar clinical picture. Diagnosis and treatment are essentially the same as those of a streptococcal throat infection.

PERTUSSIS (WHOOPING COUGH)

ETIOLOGY AND EPIDEMIOLOGY

The causative agent of pertussis is *Bordetella pertussis (Haemophilus pertussis),* a small, gram-negative, nonmotile rod. *B. pertussis* is best isolated from the nasopharynx by means of the nasopharyngeal swab rather than the cough plate. The Bordet-Gengou medium (glycerin-potato blood agar) is still preferred for the greatest yield. The bacillus is isolated with greatest frequency during the catarrhal stage (first 1-2 weeks of illness).

The disease is worldwide in distribution and continues to be a serious health problem in all countries of the world. In many developing countries, the disease is a major problem with high morbidity and mortality. Females have a higher morbidity and mortality than males reversing the usual pattern of common childhood infectious diseases. A similar clinical picture is seen with *B. parapertussis* and *B. bronchiseptica* as well as some of the adenoviruses.

PERIOD OF CUMMUNICABILITY

This period can be considered to extend from 7 days after exposure to 3 weeks after the onset of the paroxysmal cough. The disease is spread via large droplets and frequently occurs before the whoops, i.e., before the disease is generally diagnosed. Incubation period: 7-10 days. Man is the only source of the organism.

CLINICAL MANIFESTATIONS

Practical Points

1. The catarrhal, or prodromal, stage manifests itself by nonspecific upper respiratory symptoms associated with a hacking cough which gradually becomes more severe. History of exposure to a case of pertussis is the only reliable finding indicative of possible whooping cough during this stage. There is little or no fever.
2. The paroxysmal stage lasts 4-6 weeks but may be prolonged to 10-12 weeks. It is characterized by the series of expiratory coughs climaxed in many children by an inspiratory whoop and often vomiting. Infants under 6 months of age and particularly immune individuals may be without the whoop.
3. During the convalescent stage, there is a gradual cessation of whooping and vomiting. However, with subsequent respiratory infections, the whoop and vomiting may recur over a period of 1-2 years.

DIAGNOSIS

During the paroxysmal stage the clinical picture and the frequent history of exposure point toward the diagnosis. When suspected in the catarrhal stage, the culture is most useful. The application of the fluorescent antibody technique offers a rapid method of identifying organisms although many false positives do occur.

The white blood count often aids in establishing a diagnosis. High counts (20,000-100,000) with a predominance of lymphocytes are characteristic. One must remember that young infants respond to a variety of viral and bacterial infections with lymphocytosis.

A culture on Bordet-Gengou media is confirmatory. This is best done during the catarrhal or early paroxysmal stages.

DIFFERENTIAL DIAGNOSIS

Differential diagnosis must include bronchiolitis, bronchopneumonia, fibrocystic disease, tuberculous tracheobronchial lymphadenopathy, foreign body in a bronchus, and parapertussis *(B. parapertussis)*.

COMPLICATIONS

The most common and generally the most serious complication is bronchopneumonia, especially in children under 3 years of age. The pneumonia is usually caused by secondary invaders but may be primary *(B. pertussis)*. Atelectasis and later bronchiectasis may follow.

Convulsions may occur secondary to gastric tetany, hypoxia, or hemorrhage. Often all these factors contribute to a diffuse encephalopathy with cerebral edema and subsequent cortical atrophy.

Hemorrhage may occur, e.g., conjunctival, epistaxis, skin petechiae, or ecchymosis. Other complications include prolapsed rectum, nutritional distrubances, and hernias.

IMMUNITY

As a general rule an attack of pertussis confers lasting, life-long immunity. Second attacks are rare, but do occur. The newborn infant is highly susceptible to this infection.

TREATMENT

Specific treatment in infancy includes the use of erythromycin 50 mg/kg/24 hr for 7-10 days.

Practical Points

1. Small infants are generally better off hospitalized. They require constant and expert nursing care.
2. Adequate nutrition should be maintained by using small frequent feedings, and refeeding after vomiting.
3. Moist oxygen is indicated for infants with respiratory distress with or without cyanosis.
4. Oxygen should also be given to children with convulsions.
5. Proper aspiration of secretions in the small infant may mean the difference between life and death.
6. Seizures are treated with sedation and oxygen.
7. Bronchopneumonia should be treated with appropriate antibiotics and supportive measures. Antistaphylococcal antibiotics may prove necessary.
8. Persistent atelectasis is an indication for bronchoscopic aspiration.
9. Isolation is indicated for 7 days after the start of antibiotic therapy. In the untreated, the disease may be communicated for 3 weeks after the onset of paroxysms. Cases should be reported to the state health department.

PROTECTION

Protection of exposed susceptibles may also be accomplished with a 10-day course of erythromycin (50 mg/kg/24 hr). Infants under 7 years of age who have been completely immunized should receive a booster dose of DPT as well as erythromycin. Incompletely immunized individuals will have to relay on erythromycin prophylaxis and should be suitably immunized if they escape active disease.

Active immunization can be accomplished with plain or alum-precipitated vaccine preferably given in infancy as combinations with diphtheria and tetanus toxoids. (See immunizations, pp. 68-70).

Recently revised recommendations include the following contraindications to pertussis vaccine:

1. History of a seizure within 48 hours of receiving pertussis vaccine
2. History of excessive somnolence, persistent screaming (> 3 hours), or temperature elevation > 105°F within 24 hours of receiving pertussis vaccine.

Other recommendations are not of the force of contraindications. It is advised to consider withholding pertussis vaccine for children with a history of seizures, whether following vaccination or not, and for children with certain neurological diseases that may predispose to seizures, like tuberous sclerosis. If pertussis vaccine is withheld, it is advisable to continue routine immunizations with DT (pediatric or adult formulation, dependent on age).

DIPHTHERIA

ETIOLOGY AND EPIDEMIOLOGY

The etiological agent is the *Corynebacterium diphtheriae,* a gram-positive bacillus which, when present in its virulent form, has the ability to produce a potent exotoxin which is responsible for most of the serious manifestations of the disease. Once the toxin is fixed in the cells of the body it cannot be neutralized by circulating antitoxin; hence it is mandatory to use antitoxin very early in the course of the disease. (See below.)

Diphtheria is a completely preventable disease since an effective vaccine is available. Unfortunately, while the incidence has been dramatically reduced since the general use of the vaccine began in 1923, epidemics are still occurring in this country today. For example, in 1970, in San Antonio, Texas, at least 201 cases were reported. Endemic and epidemic cases occur only when a nonimmunized or inadequately immunized population is available. Incubation period: 2-5 or more days.

Man is the sole source of the disease which is spread by intimate contact as well as by fomites. Communicability is generally less than 2 weeks but may extend for more than 4 weeks. In treated cases it is 2 days or less.

CLINICAL MANIFESTATIONS AND DIFFERENTIAL DIAGNOSIS

Practical Points

1. Nasal diphtheria is characterized by an excoriating sero-sanguinous discharge which may obscure the white membrane. A foreign body in the nose will produce a similar clinical picture.
2. Tonsillar and pharyngeal diphtheria is characterized by the presence of a "dirty gray" membrane which is present on the tonsils and/or pharyngeal wall and which may extend up to involve the uvula and soft palate. The membrane varies in color from white, to gray, to black, and if forcibly removed, will result in bleeding.

    Acute streptococcal tonsillitis with membrane formation is most often confused with diphtheria. A documented record of adequate diphtheria immunization is the most important historical fact in ruling out the possibility of diphtheria.

    Other conditions to be differentiated from pharyngotonsillar diphtheria are infectious mononucleosis, nonbacterial membranous tonsillitis, thrush, blood dyscrasias with oral and pharyngeal membranous lesions, and post-tonsillectomy faucial membranes.
3. Laryngeal diphtheria usually is the result of extension of the pharyngeal membrane but may occur as a single entity. The clinical picture is often indistinguishable from other forms of croup and laryngeal obstruction. The direct observation by laryngoscopy of the membrane generally differentiates this condition from other forms of infection, croup, spasmodic croup, angioneurotic edema of the larynx, and foreign body in the larynx.

DIAGNOSIS

A culture of the lesions confirms the diagnosis. Organisms are better retrieved by peeling off a portion of existing diphtheric membrane and culturing the denuded area. The membrane removed should also be cultured. Fluorescent antibody testing is also helpful for quick confirmations.

COMPLICATIONS

Myocarditis is the most frequent complication, especially in cases in which the administration of antitoxin has been delayed. Usually, myocarditis occurs during the second week of the disease but may occur as early as the first week and as late as the sixth week.

Neuritis, the most frequent being paralysis of the soft palate, may also result in ocular palsies, diaphragmatic paralysis and a widespread generalized paralysis indistinguishable from the Guillain–Barre syndrome. Onset of paralysis varies from soft palate during the third week to limb paralysis as late as the tenth to twelfth weeks.

PROGNOSIS

Practical Points

1. The gravis strain has a poor prognosis.
2. The more extensive the membrane, the poorer the outlook.
3. Laryngeal involvement may cause sudden death by producing complete respiratory obstruction.
4. The patient's status of immunity strongly affects the outcome.
5. The prognosis of any individual case of diphtheria is intimately related to promptness of recognition of the disease and early institution of optimal therapy, particularly the administration of antitoxin.

TREATMENT

Specific

Antitoxin is given even before culture results are available. The dose of antitoxin is estimated by the site of membrane, toxicity, and duration of illness. Diffuse cervical lymphadenitis suggests more than minimal toxin absorption. Suggested dose ranges are: in pharyngeal or laryngeal disease

of 48 hours' duration, 20,000-40,000 U; in nasopharyngeal
lesions, 40,000-60,000 U; in extensive disease of 3 or more
days' duration or in any patient with brawny swelling of the
neck, 80,000-120,000 U. IV administration of antitoxin
(after eye and skin tests for sensitivity) is given to neutralize toxin as much as possible before it fixes to tissues. If
the patient is sensitive to antitoxin, rapid desensitization is
undertaken. Antimicrobial therapy is a valuable adjunct to
antitoxin because it curtails multiplication of the organisms
and rapidly renders the patient noninfectious. It is not a
substitute for antitoxin. Erythromycin and penicillin are
the drugs of choice. Antibiotic therapy is given for 14 days.
Antitoxin is probably of no value for cutaneous lesions, but
topical antimicrobials, after cleansing the skin, constitute
the treatment of choice. Carriers should also be treated
with a 1-week course of antibiotics. Reculture should be
done to demonstrate eradication of the organism.

Nonspecific

For even the mildest case, strict bed rest for at least 3
weeks is indicated; electrocardiograms are repeated twice
weekly for 4 weeks; and regular check of the voice and gag
reflex is made (for evidence of paralysis). In severe cases
prednisone in a dose of 1-1½ mg/kg/day for approximately
2 weeks has been shown to lessen the incidence of myocarditis; a large dose of ascorbic acid (e.g., 500 mg) may
be useful, as is a diet very high in carbohydrate. Digitalization is recommended by some experienced clinicians for
myocarditis with cardiac enlargement. If respiratory obstruction occurs due to blockage of the airway by large
edematous tonsils or laryngeal membrane and edema,
tracheostomy should be carried out early before the patient
becomes exhausted.

Intimately exposed persons who have been immunized
should be cultured, given a booster dose of vaccine and
watched closely for 1 week. Unimmunized or incompletely
immunized individuals should be placed on erythromycin
(40 mg/kg) for 1 week, or benzathine penicillin 600,000-
1,200,000 U IM as well as close surveillance.

PREVENTION

The dramatic decline in the incidence of diphtheria is directly related to mass immunization with diphtheria toxoid. (See immunizations, pp. 68-70.) The failure to adequately immunize any segment of our population opens the door to local epidemics such as mentioned above.

MUMPS (EPIDEMIC PAROTITIS)

ETIOLOGY AND EPIDEMIOLOGY

Mumps is caused by a virus, *Myxovirus parotiditis,* which has predilection for glandular and central nervous system tissue. Mumps is generally an endemic disease especially in urban populations. Epidemics occur under conditions favorable to virus dissemination such as children's institutions or in military establishments. Epidemics do occur among adolescents and adults in the armed services. The disease may occur at any age from shortly after birth through extreme advanced age groups. Incubation period: 16-18 days.

Man is the only host. The illness is spread by direct contact. The period of communicability extends from 1 to 7 days prior to glandular swelling to 5 to 9 days after.

CLINICAL MANIFESTATIONS

In 30-40% of patients, mumps infection is clinically non-apparent. In clinically apparent cases there is a wide variety of clinical symptoms dependent upon the site or sites of the infection. In the majority of cases, mumps is characterized by involvement of one or both parotid glands. Submaxillary and sublingual gland involvement are next in frequency. Orchitis and meningoencephalitis are not uncommon. Pancreatitis, oophoritis, thyroiditis, and other glandular involvement are relatively rare.

Practical Points

1. Parotid mumps is frequently ushered in by fever, headache, and malaise. Often the child will complain of "earache" on the affected side prior to the onset of swelling.

2. While parotid mumps may be clinically unilateral, usually the opposite parotid gland becomes swollen several days after the first.
3. Maximal swelling generally occurs in 3 days and subsides over a 1-6 day period.
4. The orifices of the Stensen's ducts are frequently reddened and edematous. Wharton's ducts show similar findings when the submaxillary glands are involved.
5. Epididymoorchitis is a relatively common manifestation of mumps in postpubertal males occurring in 20-30% of the cases. While parotitis is generally present, orchitis may occur as the only manifestation of the disease. Fortunately, only 2% of orchitis cases have bilateral involvement. The adult male's frequent concern is that sexual impotence and sterility will follow testicular infection. There is no basis of fact for these fears even in the rare bilateral involvement since complete atrophy probably does not occur.
6. Meningoencephalitis is another common manifestation of mumps occurring in at least 10% of cases. It may precede. follow, or occur without the clinical picture of parotid mumps. The infection is characterized by a marked predominance of lymphocytes in the spinal fluid and by a generally favorable outcome.
7. Pancreatitis, thyroiditis, mastitis, dacryoadenitis, and bartholinitis are rare manifestations of mumps.

DIAGNOSIS

Clinical diagnosis is a very inaccurate process in mumps. A history of exposure, typical parotitis, or aseptic meningitis point to mumps as a likely diagnostic possibility but confirmatory tests are frequently indicated to establish a definitive diagnosis. The mumps complement fixation test utilizing acute and convalescent serum is the most practical test. The virus can also be grown in cell cultures and identified.

Serum amylase is elevated in 70% of cases of mumps parotitis and, thus, can be a helpful tool in ruling in or out the diagnosis of mumps.

DIFFERENTIAL DIAGNOSIS

Mumps may be confused with other conditions involving the parotid glands or regional lymph nodes. Conditions to be considered are anterior or preauricular adenitis, suppurative parotitis, and a calculus obstructing Stensen's duct. Recurrent parotitis, usually of unknown etiology, can best be differentiated by use of the complement fixation test. Meningoencephalitis without parotitis can be distinguished from other viral CNS infections only by viral or complement fixation tests.

IMMUNITY

One attack usually confers life-long immunity. Histories of recurrent mumps reflect improper diagnosis.

TREATMENT

Treatment is symptomatic and supportive. Antibiotics are not useful. Treatment of moderate and severe orchitis includes the use of corticosteroids which characteristically alleviate pain and may reduce swelling.

PREVENTION

The live, attenuated mumps virus vaccine is recommended (combined with measles and rubella vaccines) for all children and should be given at 15 months of age. (See immunization schedule, pp. 68-70.)

If the mumps vaccine is not given as part of a child's basic immunization it should be given to:

1. Boys who are approaching puberty
2. Adolescent and adult males
3. Children living in institutions, camps, etc.

Mumps vaccine is of no value in preventing the disease after exposure nor is mumps immune globulin.

ISOLATION AND QUARANTINE

Although many physicians believe that isolating the patient until parotid swelling has subsided has not been a very effective procedure, it should still be attempted. Isolation need not be prolonged beyond 9 days after onset of parotid swelling.

Chapter 7

COMMON INFECTIONS

UPPER RESPIRATORY INFECTIONS

The phrase, upper respiratory infections (URI), embraces a
number of older terms that specify the predominant site of
inflammation, i.e., rhinitis, pharyngitis, laryngitis. Since
the infectious process is rarely limited to one segment of
the upper respiratory tract, these terms are not strictly
accurate although they may remain useful to the clinician.

URI accounts for an estimated minimum number of 30
infections occurring in the average individual from birth
through adolescence. After maternal antibodies decline in
the infant (3-6 months) URIs occur with distressing regularity. This is particularly true in children who have contact with many other children, i.e., first year in school,
nursery school, or day care center. The physician is often
called upon to allay parental anxiety induced by frequent
URIs. Literally, hundreds of viruses have been demonstrated to cause URI while the most frequently encountered
bacterium is the beta hemolytic streptococcus. Less frequently, *Haemophilus influenzae,* pneumococcus, staphylococcus, and meningococcus can be cultured from upper airway passages. (See Table 7-1.)

Table 7-1 Acute Respiratory Tract Disease—Clinical Syndromes and Etiologic Agents

Clinical Syndrome	Etiologic Agents		
	Viral	Bacterial	Other
Common cold; coldlike illness; upper respiratory tract infection; coryza; rhinitis; rhinopharyngitis; acute catarrhal tonsillopharyngitis	Respiratory syncytial virus Parainfluenza viruses Rhinovirus (100+ types) Echo viruses Group A Coxsackie viruses Adenoviruses	*Haemophilus influenzae* *Bordetella pertussis*	*Mycoplasma pneumoniae*
Febrile nasopharyngitis (in infants)		Streptococcus, Group A	
Acute otitis media		Pneumococcus *H.influenzae* Streptococcus, Group A Others	*M.pneumoniae*

Acute tonsillopharyngitis with exudate or membrane	Adenovirus EB virus	Streptococcus, Group A *Corynebacterium diphtheriae*	
Acute tonsillopharyngitis with vesicles or ulcers	Herpes virus hominis (herpes simplex virus) Group A Coxsackie viruses		
Acute laryngitis; laryngotracheobronchitis (croup)	Parainfluenza viruses Influenza viruses Adenoviruses Rhinoviruses Respiratory syncytial virus	*C.diphtheriae* *H.influenzae*	
Acute epiglottitis (croup)		*H.influenzae* type B	
Bronchiolitis	Respiratory syncytial virus Parainfluenza viruses Adenoviruses Influenza viruses	*?H.influenzae*	*M.pneumoniae*

Table 7-1 (Cont'd.) Acute Respiratory Tract Disease–Clinical Syndromes and Etiologic Agents

Clinical Syndrome	Etiologic Agents		
	Viral	Bacterial	Other
Pneumonia	Respiratory syncytial virus Parainfluenza viruses Measles virus Adenoviruses Influenza viruses Herpes virus varicellae Cytomegalovirus Lymphocytic chorio- meningitis virus	Staphylococcus Pneumococcus Hemolytic strep- tococcus Other	*M. pneumoniae* *Pneumocystis carinii* *Psittacosis agent* *Coxiello burnetti* (Q fever) *Toxoplasma gondii* *Histoplasma capsulatum* *Coccidioides immitis*

Influenza-like illness	Influenza viruses
	Parainfluenza viruses
	Adenoviruses
	Group A Coxsackie viruses
	Lymphocytic choriomen-
	ingitis virus

From Krugman, S., Ward, R., and Katz, S. L.: Infectious Diseases of Children, 6th ed. C.V. Mosby Co., St. Louis, 1977. (Reproduced with publisher's permission.)

Symptoms include coryza, sneezing, tearing, and sore throat. Extension of infection to the paranasal sinuses will produce sinus headache, fever, and purulent discharge. Extension through the eustachian tubes can cause otitis media. Involvement of the respiratory tract produces cough, hoarseness, and sometimes respiratory stridor and is termed laryngitis in older children, croup in younger ones. Further spread into the trachea and main stem bronchi causes the persistent cough of tracheobronchitis.

Fever, when present, is seldom high in uncomplicated URI and while the children appear uncomfortable, they do not look sick. Mucous membranes of the nose and throat are injected. In the case of tracheobronchitis, coarse ronchi may be heard over the upper thorax.

The chief complication of URI is otitis media. Sinusitis is infrequent in young children. Bacterial organisms may invade these structures resulting in abrupt rise in temperature and local signs. (See p. 127.)

The course of illness is usually of short duration with complete recovery after 3-7 days. The cough in tracheobronchitis may continue for a longer period of time, several weeks not being uncommon.

The condition most frequently confused with URI is allergic rhinitis. Symptoms may be identical. Table 7-2 lists the differentiating features of both.

TREATMENT

Treatment is symptomatic, unless a bacterial pathogen is suspected or sinusitis and otitis media are encountered. (See Table 7-3.) Antihistamines, decongestants, and antitussives have been commonly used and their efficacy called into question almost as commonly. There is little evidence that antihistamines and decongestants provide significant relief from cold symptoms and even less that they prevent otitis media. A regular diet and fluids prescribed in accordance with the normal thirst mechanism of the child are all that need be done. Communicability is high but elaborate quarantine is not necessary for children who are well. Children with chronic, severe illnesses such as diabetes mellitus and cystic fibrosis must be restricted from contact with any infection including URI.

Table 7-2 Features Differentiating URI from Allergic Rhinitis

URI	Allergic Rhinitis
Short duration	Variable duration
Typical course	Variable course (one day better, one day worse)
Other siblings often sick too, or "catch cold"	Other siblings well and do not "catch cold"
Nasal mucosa injected, mucopurulent nasal secretions by third day of illness	Nasal mucosa pale, bluish, and edematous; clear watery nasal secretions
Neutrophils or lymphocytes on nasal smear	Eosinophils on nasal smear
No other signs of allergy	Possibly other sign of allergy (asthma)

Antibiotic therapy is not indicated except when a bacterial pathogen such as the streptococcus is isolated. Ampicillin or penicillin in combination with a sulfonamide are antibiotics of choice for acute otitis media.

Practical Points

1. In neonates and young infants who are obligate nose breathers, it is important to keep the nasal passage clear during URIs to prevent hypoxia. Saline nose drops and suctioning with a bulb syringe as needed may be employed at home. Respiratory syncytial virus, a cause of URI in older children, determines a more severe infection in infants, particularly in premature neonates.

Table 7-3 Choosing an Antibiotic According to Diagnosis

Condition	Preferred Antibiotic	Alternate
Strep. pharyngotonsillitis	Penicillin	Erythromycin
Pneumonia		
Aspiration	Penicillin	Erythromycin
Newborn	Methicillin and gentamycin	Erythromycin
Pneumococcal	Penicillin	Erythromycin
Mycoplasma	Erythromycin	Tetracycline
Staphylococcal		
Penicillin resistant	Methicillin	Vancomycin
Penicillin sensitive	Penicillin	Cephalosporin (Keflin)
Meningitis		
H.influenzae	Ampicillin (if sensitive)	Chloramphenicol
	Chloramphenicol (if resistant)	
Pneumococcus	Penicillin	Chloramphenicol
Meningococcus	Penicillin	Chloramphenicol
Neonatal meningitis		
Unknown etiology	Ampicillin and gentamicin	Penicillin and kanamycin

Neonatal sepsis		
Unknown etiology	Ampicillin and gentamicin	Penicillin and kanamycin
Gastroenteritis		
E. coli (pathogenic)	Neomycin	Polymyxin B colistin
Shigella	Ampicillin	TMP-SMX
		Chloramphenicol
Salmonella		
Simple gastroenteritis	No antibiotic	
Septicemia (salmonellosis) and typhoid	Ampicillin	Amoxicillin
		TMP-SMX
Otitis Media	Amoxicillin, ampicillin, or penicillin and sulfisoxazole	Erythromycin and sulfisoxazole
Urinary Tract Infection		
First episode	Amoxicillin, sulfisoxazole, or ampicillin	Cephalexin
Recurrent	Gentamicin, kanamycin, or TMP-SMX	
	Carbenicillin	

Table 7-3 (Cont'd.) Choosing an Antibiotic According to Diagnosis

Condition	Prefered Antibiotic	Alternate
Endocarditis		
Unknown etiology	Penicillin and streptomycin	
Streptococcus viridans	Penicillin and streptomycin	
Enterococcus	Ampicillin and gentamicin	Penicillin and streptomycin
Staphylococcus aureus		
Penicillin sensitive	Penicillin	
Penicillin resistant	Nafcillin	Vancomycin
Pericarditis		
Unknown etiology	Nafcillin	
H.influenzae	Ampicillin and chlorampheni-col	Chloramphenicol or cefamandole
Pneumococcus	Penicillin	
Skin Infection		
Impetigo		
Streptococcal	Penicillin	Erythromycin
Staphylococcal	cloxacillin	Cephalexin
or mixed		
Cellulitis	Penicillin or ampicillin (*H. influenzae*)	Erythromycin or cephalexin

Septic Arthritis		
Unknown	Methicillin	Nafcillin
Staphylococcus		
Penicillin resistant	Methicillin	Nafcillin
Penicillin sensitive	Penicillin	
H. influenza	Ampicillin and chloramphenicol	
Streptococcus	Penicillin	
Gonococcus	Penicillin	
Meningococcus	Penicillin	
Pneumococcus	Penicillin	
Osteomyelitis		
Unknown	Methicillin	Nafcillin
Staphylococcus		
Penicillin resistant	Methicillin	Nafcillin, vanomycin
Penicillin sensitive	Penicillin	
Salmonella	Ampicillin	
Syphilis		
Congenital		
Without CNS involvement	Benzathine penicillin	
With CNS involvement	Penicillin (procaine)	
Primary, secondary	Benzathine penicillin	Tetracycline

Table 7–3 (Cont'd.) Choosing an Antibiotic According to Diagnosis

Condition	Preferred Antibiotic	Alternate
Gonorrhea	Penicillin and probenecid	Tetracycline and spectin-omycin

Bronchiolitis and pneumonia are not uncommon manifestations. Nursery personnel with URI symptoms should be restricted from direct contact with neonates during respiratory syncytial virus (RSV) outbreaks.

2. Sinusitis in children under the age of 10 years is unusual since the sinuses are incompletely formed until the age of 7-10 years.

3. The most common cause of otitis media is bacterial. About 60% of these are due to the pneumococcus. *H. influenzae* accounts for a greater percentage of cases over the age of 4 years than was heretofore realized and cannot be ignored in therapy.

CONJUNCTIVITIS

The causes of conjunctivitis include a wide variety of agents varying from chemical and allergic to viral and bacterial. Common infecting organisms are *Staphylococcus aureus,* the Koch-Weeks bacillus, beta hemolytic streptococcus, pneumococcus, *H. influenzae,* and *Neisseria catarrhalis.* Gonococcal conjunctivitis is a particularly severe infection progressing, at times, to panophthalmitis. Herpes simplex also poses a serious threat to the preservation of sight when the conjunctiva is affected. (See p. 190.) In the newborn, sepsis is a possible complication of conjunctivitis.

With acute conjunctivitis, older children will complain of ocular burning or itching in one or both eyes, mild photophobia, tearing, or discharge. Visual acuity is not usually affected.

The conjunctiva are injected. The distribution of injected conjunctival vessels has great importance in differentiating this disease from iritis or iridocyclitis. In the latter the injected vessels are found predominantly around the iris whereas in conjunctivitis the entire conjunctiva are injected. Deformities of the pupil occur in otitis and not in conjunctivitis. A thin watery or frankly purulent eye discharge may be found. Ocular tension is normal and the cornea is clear thus helping to distinguish this entity from glaucoma. At times, particularly with viral conjunctivitis, tender and enlarged preauricular lymph nodes may be palpated. In the more severe forms of conjunctivitis (gonococcal), chemosis, pain, and eyelid edema may be prominent.

Helpful Laboratory Tests

1. Culture and sensitivity tests of the eye discharge
2. Conjunctival scraping and a Gram-stain smear to identify bacterial organisms, particularly gonococcus.

Treatment

1. Irrigation 3-4 times daily is indicated when thick purulent discharge is present.
2. Warm applications for the more severe forms of conjunctivitis, including patching of the eye, are helpful.
3. Zinc sulfate ophthalmic solutions may give relief in chronic catarrhal conjunctivitis due to the Morax-Axenfeld bacillus. IDU and vidarabine are specific therapies for herpes simplex.
4. Antibiotics are instilled in the eye when bacterial infection is confirmed or suspected. Sodium sulamyd, neomycin, bacitracin, polymixin B, chloramphenicol, and ampicillin have all been used with excellent results. Small infants may have an antibiotic ointment. Ambulatory children should receive the antibiotic drops so that visual acuity is not impaired. Ointments with their greater duration of action (up to 3-4 hours compared to 1-2 hours for drops) are indicated for use before bedtime.
5. Steroids may provide some relief in viral conjunctivitis; however, they are contraindicated in herpes simplex infection and in bacterial infections.

TONSILLITIS

Acute tonsillitis is one of the most common infections of childhood. Many viruses and a few bacteria cause the infection. The major bacterial organism encountered is the group A beta hemolytic streptococcus. Most of the 60 distinct M protein types can cause the disease, as well as rheumatic fever; about 12 can cause poststreptococcal glomerular nephritis. Meningococcus, pneumococcus, and H. *influenzae* are much less frequently cultured from tonsillar swabs and do not constitute common causes of tonsillitis. The major problem of management therefore is to determine whether the tonsillitis is streptococcal or viral in origin. Tonsillar involvement may be present in other less commonly encountered disease states, e.g., leukemia, diphtheria; and is one of the characteristic findings of infectious mononucleosis.

The only practical way of making a diagnosis of streptococcal tonsillitis (or of ruling it out) is by swabbing the tonsils and culturing the swabs. Clinical findings of exudate and tonsillar infection without cough, coryza, or other findings of viral diseases favor the diagnosis of streptococcal tonsillitis but etiological diagnoses based on these clinical findings are not entirely accurate. It should be realized that a significant false-negative rate occurs with throat culture techniques, even when flawless procedures are used. As many as one-third of single throat cultures may be falsely negative.

Once a bacterial etiology is established then antibiotic therapy must be employed. Penicillin, either orally or intramuscularly for 10 days, is the drug of choice for streptococcal infection. It is effective in meningococcal infection as well. Ampicillin is indicated for *H. influenzae.* For viral tonsillitis symptomatic treatment is all that is indicated. (See Table 7-3.)

Practical Points

1. Quantitating the number of colonies of streptococcus grown in a standard way is advocated by some investigators to help distinguish carriers from those with active streptococcal infection. Fewer than 10 colonies are considered likely to represent a carrier state unless the throat swab was not performed correctly or the infection is very early. A rise in ASO titers of the streptozyme test helps distinguish true infection from carrier states, but the information is available only after 2 or more weeks.
2. The chief problem in treating streptococcal tonsillitis is parent compliance with the 10-day course of treatment. As few as one-third of the patients may actually receive a full 10 days of treatment. Educating parents to the danger of rheumatic fever may increase parent compliance, but one can be certain that some patients will not receive the full course of therapy. A single long-acting IM injection of combined procaine and benzathine

penicillin insures an adequate duration of treatment. Care should be taken that sufficient benzathine penicillin is administered when using mixtures of short-acting and long-acting penicillin. The dose is 600,000 U of benzathine penicillin for children weighing 60 lb or less, 1.2 million U for those over 60 lb. The chief disadvantage to IM penicillin is that it is more sensitizing than oral penicillin. The use of IM penicillin is best suited to situations where patient compliance is likely to be poor. Oral penicillin G is effective when compliance is achieved. A daily dose of 800,000-1,000,000 U is sufficient. This may be given either 3 or 4 times a day for 10 days. Erythromycin is an excellent alternative for patients sensitive to penicillin.
3. Other complications of acute tonsillitis are uncommon. One rarely sees peritonsillar abscesses now. Cervical adenitis is seen infrequently. (See p. 131.) Rheumatic fever and acute glomerular nephritis remain the most serious poststreptococcal sequelae. (See pp. 351, 361.) Otitis media and sinusitis in older children are more common complications. Rarely pulmonary infection or septicemia occurs.
4. It is good practice to culture all family members and intimate contacts of patients with acute streptococcal throat infection. Those with positive cultures should receive a full 10-day course of antibiotic therapy as outlined above.

Differentiating Streptococcal from Nonstreptococcal Pharyngotonsillitis

1. Infectious mononucleosis
   a) Grayer, larger membrane
   b) Generalized lymphadenopathy
   c) Splenomegaly (50%)
   d) Atypical lymphocytes
   e) + Heterophile agglutination
   f) Negative throat swab
2. Herpangina (Coxsackie A virus)
   a) Petechiae developing to small shallow ulcer(s) on soft palate or anterior tonsillar pillars
   b) Less systemic illness
   c) Negative throat swab

3. Acute lymphonodular pharyngitis (Coxsackie A 10 virus)
    a) Nodular soft palate lesions
    b) Negative throat swab
4. Herpetic stomatitis
    a) Gingival, lingual, buccal, mucosal involvement
    b) Distribution primarily confined to anterior portion of oral cavity
    c) More severe pain on swallowing - drooling
    d) Negative throat swab
5. Pharyngoconjunctival fever (adenovirus)
    a) Conjunctivitis
    b) Anterior and preauricular lymph node enlargement
    c) Negative throat swab

CERVICAL ADENITIS

This inflammatory disease of the cervical lymph nodes is caused most commonly by beta hemolytic streptococci and staphylococci. Other less common bacterial causes are pneumococcus, mycobacteria tuberculosis, and the atypical or Battey strains of mycobacteria. (See tuberculosis, p. 172.)

Infection may be the result of a local inflammation of the scalp, face, and neck; however, it may also follow a preceding upper respiratory infection. Swelling, tenderness and, at times, redness over one or more cervical lymph nodes are characteristic. The nodes are discrete, indurated, mobile, and tender to palpation. In a later phase, they may soften, point, and drain. Systemic symptoms of fever, malaise, and anorexia are frequently present. Cervical adenitis must be distinguished from lymph node enlargement found in several disease states but primarily from systemic viral illness (rubella, infectious mononucleosis, mumps parotitis, etc.) and from neoplastic diseases (lymphoma, Hodgkin's, leukemia). In general, the lack of other findings characteristic of each of the viral illnesses serves to rule them out. A unilateral mumps parotitis, expecially when the accessory lobe of the parotid is involved, may cause some difficulty, but mumps swelling has no clear, palpable border and a "cystic feel" unlike the encapsulated indurated mass of cervical adenitis. The enlarged nodes in neoplastic disease are usually not tender, may not be localized to the cervical region alone, and have an entirely different clinical course.

A positive tuberculin test with or without a positive chest x-ray will help establish tuberculous adenitis.

The white blood cell count and differential typically show an increase of polymorphonuclear leukocytes. Organisms may be recovered from the lymph node by needle aspiration and culture or, less accurately, by throat culture.

Treatment is similar to that for pyogenic infections elsewhere in the body. Systemic antibiotics like penicillin or, in the event of a resistant staphylococcus, prostaphlin, cloxacillin, dicloxacillin, or methicillin are the drugs of choice. Erythromycin may be used for penicillin-sensitive patients, but staphylococcal resistance develops rapidly. A cephalosporin may be effective, but some patients allergic to penicillin are also sensitive to the cephalosporins. Antipyretics and analgesics may be useful as well. Incision and drainage are necessary if the node suppurates.

Practical Points

Dramatic responses to antibiotic therapy may not occur with cervical adenitis. Swelling, tenderness, and induration usually decrease very slowly over the course of 1-2 weeks or more, even with appropriate therapy.

MIDRESPIRATORY TRACT INFECTION

Two common forms of croup exist: an acute laryngotracheobronchitis causing progressive hoarseness, cough, and inspiratory stridor, and a spasmodic variety occurring in conjunction with a URI or respiratory allergy. The latter entity is termed spasmodic croup. Symptoms are similar between the two except that the hoarseness and stridor of spasmodic croup is abrupt in onset and tends to disappear rapidly, constitutional symptoms are absent, and a history of recurrent episodes is frequent. Spasmodic croup is a benign entity rarely requiring tracheostomy. Progressive croup is usually not serious but may be so in some instances. Particularly severe is the croup caused by the measles virus and *H. influenzae*. The latter may be suspected when constitutional symptoms are severe and peripheral white blood cell counts are elevated and consist predominantly of polymorphonuclear leukocytes. The classical picture of croup should be familiar to almost every parent as well as every physician responsible for the health care of children. A brassy cough, hoarseness, inspiratory stridor, suprasternal retractions, and flaring of the alae nasi, all more severe at night, are characteristic.

The more severely ill child may be cyanotic, tachypneic, and restless (air hunger). After a prolonged bout of croup the patient may become exhausted. These signs are danger signals and tracheostomy must be seriously considered when they occur.

Milder croup can usually be successfully managed by inhaling air saturated with water vapor. Fluid replacement and maintenance must be provided. In the case of a severely ill child, this is best accomplished by the intravenous route. Antihistamines and other drying agents are not indicated because they tend to inspissate laryngeal and tracheal secretions thus adding to the airway obstruction. Antibiotics are useful only when a bacterial pathogen such as *H. influenzae* is the causative agent.

Other entities must be considered in the differential diagnosis: diphtheria, epiglottitis, foreign body, tumors, laryngeal malformations (web, laryngeal malacia), and tracheal rings. Diphtheric membranes may be seen in the pharynx of a child with incomplete immunizations. (See p. 108.) The engorged, cherry red epiglottis is easily visualized in most children. This is a major emergency situation. (See p. 134.) A history of foreign body and the characteristically abrupt onset serve to distinguish this entity from croup. Malformations and tumors of the larynx and trachea cause recurrent problems in the absence of any sign of acute infection. Direct visualization by laryngoscopy confirms the diagnosis.

Practical Points

1. Cold steam vaporizers are better suited than warm steam vaporizers for the management of croup. Environmental temperature is not elevated by cold steam. The sauna effect of warm steam may actually have a partial drying effect and may serve to raise body temperature in a febrile child.
2. Spasmodic croup tends to recur until the age of 5 or 6 years. Parents should be prepared for this and educated to manage the problem when it occurs.

3. Pneumothorax and a collapsed lung must be searched for in children undergoing a tracheostomy; a chest x-ray following the procedure is a useful precaution.
4. Steroids have no place in the management of croup and no reliance can be placed on them. Similarly, sedation should be avoided because respiratory depression may ensue. The best sedative is a reassuring parent and physician.
5. Epiglottitis
   a) Epiglottitis is a severe, life threatening inflammation of the epiglottis and supraglottic structures of the larynx usually caused by *H. influenzae* type B. Symptoms are abrupt in onset and include inspiratory stridor, dysphonia or aphonia, fever, and a "toxic" appearance. Swallowing is difficult and the neck may be painful. A bright, cherry red epiglottis (often readily seen in young children) confirms the diagnosis but should be visualized only when the clinician is completely prepared for tracheostomy or intubation.
   b) With epiglottitis, there is a great danger of complete laryngeal obstruction, occurring abruptly. Immediate hospitalization and the availability of a physician skilled in performing tracheostomies or intubation are indicated. A lateral, soft tissue x-ray of the neck is a safer way of making the diagnosis.
   c) Ampicillin (IM or IV) together with chloramphenical and cold steam vaporization should be used.
   d) The pharynx should not be examined repeatedly and throat swabs must be taken only when a tracheostomy is functioning or intubation has been accomplished.
   e) Since the majority of children with epiglottitis will require tracheostomy or intubation, an artificial airway should be established as soon as the diagnosis is made.

LOWER RESPIRATORY TRACT INFECTION

BRONCHIOLITIS

Bronchiolitis is an inflammation of the small and terminal bronchioles and is a relatively common entity in children between 3 months and 3 years of age. It is most often

initiated by a viral agent but secondary bacterial invasion
may occur. Several viruses have been identified as causative organisms. Among the more frequent are the respiratory syncytial, influenzae B, adenoviruses, and parainfluenza
viruses. Symptoms develop gradually over a 1-3-day period
and are characterized by cough and increasing respiratory
distress with concomitant respiratory stridor in the more
severely afflicted. Fever is absent or low grade. Wheezing
may be heard. Physical findings are variable and largely
confined to the thorax. Respiratory distress, i.e., flaring of
alae nasi, dyspnea, suprasternal and substernal retractions,
and cyanosis, may be observed. Auscultatory findings range
over the whole gamut of possibilities. Classically, one hears
an expiratory wheeze and crepitant rales bilaterally. In
many instances coarse and sibilant ronchi are also heard.
Because of this variability, it is sometimes difficult to distinguish children with bronchiolitis from those with asthma
or pneumonia. Several points of differentiation should be
considered. (See Table 7-4.)

Practical Points

1. Laboratory tests are of little practical help. There may
   be a lymphocyte response present. Viral cultures and
   serological tests may eventually permit a specific, although retrospective, etiological diagnosis. The chest
   x-ray is the single most important tool. Findings are
   those of overinflated lungs. The lung fields are dark, the
   cardiovascular shadow small, and the diaphragms flattened. Small patches of atelectasis scattered throughout both lung fields are not infrequent.
2. Bronchiolitis follows the course of a viral disease usually
   lasting from 3 days to 1 week. In most instances the
   disease is mild, but severe and even fatal cases occur.
   Complications include pneumothorax, atelectasis, respiratory acidosis, electrolyte imbalances, dehydration,
   and cardiac failure.
3. Treatment is largely supportive. Many children are in
   severe enough respiratory distress to run a serious risk
   of aspiration during feedings. Often children will refuse
   an adequate intake of liquids. In these cases, IV fluids
   are necessary to prevent dehydration and electrolyte
   imbalance. Care must be taken not to overhydrate

Table 7-4 Features Differentiating Bronchiolitis from Asthma and Pneumonia

	Bronchiolitis	Asthma	Pneumonia
History			
	Child 3-36 months old	Few months to adulthood	Any age
	More common in cold weather	Any weather	More common in cold weather
	No previous history of attacks	Previous history of attacks	No previous history of attacks
	Low or no fever	Usually no fever	Moderate to high fever
Physical			
	Inspiratory and expiratory obstruction	Expiratory obstruction	Obstructive respiratory pattern usually lacking
	Prolonged expiratory phase with or without wheezing	Prolonged expiratory phase and audible wheezing	Dyspnea or tachypnea without prolonged expiratory phase

Respiratory distress usually marked	Respiratory distress varies from mild to marked	Respiratory distress varies from mild to marked
Diagnosis Wheezing, rales, or ronchi on auscultation	Wheezing on auscultation	Rales on auscultation
Hyperesonant on percussion (hyporesonant if atelectasis occurs)	Hyperesonant on percussion (hyporesonant if atelectasis occurs)	Hyporesonant over areas of consolidation
Bilateral chest findings	Bilateral chest findings	Chest findings unilateral or biateral
Course 3-7 days	Highly variable, usually short	7-10 days
Lab "Viral" white count and differential	Eosinophilia may be present	"Viral" or "bacterial" white count and differential

Table 7-4 (Cont'd.) Features Differentiating Bronchiolitis from Asthma and Pneumonia

	Bronchiolitis	Asthma	Pneumonia
X-Ray	Hyperaeration; no pneumonic infiltrates, occasionally patchy areas of atelectasis	Hyperaeration; no pneumonic infiltrates in uncomplicated asthma; occasionally atelectasis	Pneumonic infiltrate or consolidation; pleural effusion occasionally

because of the danger of cardiac failure. Increased base
(sodium bicarbonate or lactate) may be necessary if
blood gas studies indicate a state of respiratory acidosis.
4. Antibiotics are not helpful except in the seldomly encountered case of mycoplasma pneumonia. In these instances, erythromycin is the drug of choice.

Bronchodilators are disappointing; usually only temporary
relief is achieved and more often no relief at all. Mist and
oxygen for cyanotic children or those with a PaO_2 under 60
mmHg are useful therapeutic adjuncts. Digitalis may be
indicated for those children with right-sided heart failure.

PNEUMONIA

Pulmonary infections take a wide variety of pathological
forms from lobar consolidation to interstitial infiltrates.
The etiology embraces virtually all known pathogenic organisms from viruses to molds, and noninfectious pneumonias
may be associated with chemical agents, immune mechanisms,
and neoplastic disease. Clinical characteristics will differ
markedly depending on etiology and the child's age. The following are the more common types of pneumonia seen in
children.

Viral Pneumonia

Numerous viral agents may be implicated in pulmonary infection. The clinical picture is that of a preceding URI followed in 1-3 days by a worsening cough, increasing fever,
and occasionally symptoms of respiratory distress. Children
so afflicted are most often in the first decade of life.

Tachypnea, or dyspnea and flaring of the alae nasi, may
be observed. If large areas of bronchopneumonia exist, an
increase in vocal fremitus or a flat percussory note may be
detected. On auscultation often both ronchi and fine rales
are head. These findings may be confined to one side or a
portion of one hemithorax or be bilateral.

The single most important diagnostic tool is the chest
x-ray. Both a posterior-anterior (PA) and a lateral view
should be ordered to detect that portion of the left lung ob-
scured by the cardiac shadow in the PA view. X-ray findings
may consist of patchy infiltrates of bronchopneumonia, or

streaky, linear interstitial infiltrates. Viral cultures and serological studies are expensive and helpful only in retrospect since it takes 2 or more weeks for an answer to be forthcoming. There is a tendency for lymphocytic predominance and slight to moderate elevation of the white cell count in viral pneumonia, but other patterns may be discerned.

The most likely complication is atelectasis. Pleural effusion occurs but probably less often than in bacterial pneumonias. Pneumothorax is rare.

Treatment is symptomatic and supportive. Expectorants and antipyretics are employed. A mist tent is helpful for the dyspneic child, and oxygen is indicated for the severely dyspneic and cyanotic child with low PaO_2 values.

Bacterial Pneumonias

The symptoms and signs of the common baterial pneumonias, i.e., pneumonococcal, *H. influenzae,* streptococcal, and staphylococcal may be identical to those of viral pneumonia. However, these children are more likely to look seriously ill. Dyspnea and cyanosis occur with greater frequency as do the complications of pleural effusion and pneumothorax. Septicemia, lung abscess, emphysema, pneumatoceles, and bronchiectasis also may occur.

Peripheral white blood cell (WBC) and differential counts may reveal an absolute increase in polymorphonuclear leukocytes sometimes to a marked degree. This is especially true of staphylococcal pneumonia where WBC counts in excess of 20,000 are to be expected. Sputum cultures and Gram stains of tracheal secretions are difficult to obtain in children, yet valuable clues may be obtained from these tests. A Gram stain of sputum displaying many organisms with the morphological characteristics of staphylococcal pneumonia cannot be ignored. Antistreptolysin-O (ASLO) titers may be helpful in streptococcal pneumonia.

Culturing material obtained from lung punctures or from pleural fluid in cases of effusion is the best way to obtain the etiological agent. The fear of complications from the procedure restrains most clinicians from using the lung puncture method. However, recent information indicates that the complication rate may not be excessive. Blood cultures in seriously ill children may reveal the causative organism.

Again, the most immediate helpful diagnostic procedure available is the chest x-ray. The characteristic lobar consolidation of pneumonococcal pneumonia may be observed. Pneumatoceles appear commonly but not exclusively in staphylococcal pneumonia. These appear in the early stages as honeycomb areas of decreased opacification in the midst of a zone of consolidation. On serial x-rays, these areas will persist and enlarge, occasionally expanding enormously and virtually filling an entire hemithorax.

The course of illness will vary for many reasons. The bacterial agent, the extent of infection, the type of therapy, and the general condition of the child are the principal factors involved. Pneumococcal and streptococcal pneumonia will usually respond promptly to adequate therapy; *H. influenzae* and *K. pneumoniae* more slowly. Staphylococcal pneumonia may take 6 weeks or more to run its course even with optimal treatment. In additon, this type of pneumonia progresses more rapidly. A young child under 2 years of age with rapidly worsening pneumonia should always suggest the possibility of staphylococcal pneumonia.

Prognosis is generally good with early and adequate therapy and an otherwise healthy child. Complications occur most frequently with staphylococcal pneumonia, especially pleural effusions and lung abscess. Nonetheless, complete recovery can be achieved in the majority of these children.

Therapy of Bacterial Pneumonia

The most important therapeutic decision is the choice of a proper antibiotic. (See Table 7-3.) When the etiology is known this is not difficult. Penicillin 25,000-50,000 U/kg/day is the drug of choice for mild to moderate pneumococcal and streptococcal pneumonias. It is usually administered intramuscularly in 2 daily doses as the sodium or potassium salt of procaine penicillin. Therapeutic levels are achieved quickly (2 hours) and are maintained for a long period (18 hours). Critically ill children should have intravenous, aqueous penicillin by slow IV push every 4-6 hours. The dose is 20,000-100,000 U/kg/24 hr. A careful accounting of potassium intake will be necessary if the potassium salt of penicillin is used. This is especially true in infants and children with poor renal function. A total potassium intake from all sources should not exceed 40 mEq/L of fluid intake. Oral penicillin 50,000 U/kg/day (penicillin V or penicillin G) may be used after a clinical response has occurred and the child is out of danger. A 7-10-day course of therapy is adequate unless complications have occurred (emphysema). By this time serial chest x-rays have usually demonstrated complete resolution of the pneumonic process and the chest findings have virtually disappeared.

Erythromycin and cephalexin are also effective antibiotics and with the exception of the latter, may be safely used in penicillin-sensitive patients.

H. influenzae pneumonia should be treated with ampicillin unless resistance is encountered. This may be administered IM or IV initially depending on the severity of illness, and, following a favorable response, by the oral route. Treatment is usually necessary for a minimum of 2 weeks and may be required for longer periods. A dosage of 100-300 mg/kg/24 hr is adequate, depending on severity. Chloramphenicol 100 mg/kg/day is an excellent alternative with proper monitoring of possible hematological side effects, and is the drug of choice for resistant *H. influenzae* organisms.

The therapy of staphylococcal pneumonia is dependent on whether or not a penicillin-sensitive (nonpenicillinase-producing) organism is the cause of the pneumonia. Penicillin G (100,000 U/kg/day to 400,000 U/kg/day) is the drug of choice for the nonresistant staphylococcus. For initial therapy and when resistance is encountered or suspected (penicillinase-producing organisms), methicillin 200-300 mg/kg/24 hr given at 4-hour intervals is the drug of choice. Cloxacillin or dicloxacillin, nafcillin, and oxacillin may be used. In patients with penicillin allergy, cephalothin may be substituted keeping in mind the possibility of cross-sensitivity. Clindamycin and vancomycin are other alternatives but both can give serious side effects. Therapy should be for a minimum of 4 weeks and should continue until complete clinical and radiological clearing occurs. Surgical therapy in the form of closed waterseal drainage via a chest tube for large effusions or pneumothorax may be required.

The drug of choice for *K. pneumoniae* is largely dependent on sensitivity testing. Gentamycin or tobramycin are the most effective antibiotics before results of the sensitivity testing are known.

Mycoplasma Pneumonia

Pneumonia due to a nonencapsulated protoplastic bacterial form called M. *pneumoniae* (Eaton agent) is perhaps the most frequently encountered pneumonia in the 5-15-year-old age group. The disease occurs either sporadically or in epidemics usually sparing infants and younger children. The incubation period is 2-3 weeks and an asymptomatic carrier state can result lasting for several months. Symptoms tend to be milder than other types of pneumonia giving rise to the often used synonym "walking pneumonia." Chest findings are non-specific and may vary from a few scattered rales to bilateral severe involvement. Helpful laboratory tests include an elevated ESR but only an occasional absolute lymphocytosis. Sputum or tracheal culture may show the mycoplasma organism when grown on special cell-free agar, and the cold hemagglutinin titer may be in excess of 1:32 after the first week of illness. The complement fixation test becomes positive in the second to third week of illness and is the best single clinical test available because it is specific, unlike the cold hemagglutinin titer. Fluorescent antibodies also are demonstrable at this time.

The chest x-ray usually shows more striking findings than one would expect from the physical signs. An interstitial pattern denser at the hilum or patchy densities is most often found. Less commonly, lobar consolidation is observed. Pleural effusion is seen only rarely. The course of the illness is usually benign and many patients recover without having had recourse to a medical facility. However, an occasional child has required hospitalization and has had extensive pneumonitis, pleural effusion, and marked respiratory difficulty. The treatment of choice is erythromycin 40-50 mg/kg/24 hr in four divided doses orally until symptoms, signs, and x-ray findings disappear (usually 5-7 days). Tetracycline 25-40 mg/kg/24 hr is an equally effective alternative drug for children older than 8 years. (See Table 7-3.) It is recommended as a second drug because side effects, e.g., dental staining, to tetracycline exceed those of erythromycin, particularly in children under 8 years of age. Other family members and close contacts should be observed for the illness and treated early if symptomatic.

Pneumocystis Carinii Pneumonia

The cause of this variety of pneumonia is believed to be a
sporozoan although it still awaits definitive classification.
It is not normally an aggressive pathogen for humans but
may infect the malnourished and immunosuppressed.

It gives rise to an insidious illness characterized by fever
and increasing cough, leading to tachypnea, dyspnea, and
hypoxia. The disease is potentially life-threatening. Diffuse
bilateral interstitial infiltrates are seen on chest x-ray which
are often more striking than the clinical findings would suggest. The diagnosis is confirmed by identifying the organism
from bronchoscopic or lung biopsy.

Trimethoprim-sulfamethoxazole is effective. It may be
given also as a prophylactic agent to immunosuppressed patients. Another effective chemotherapeutic agent is penta-
midine isethionate. Patients with the disease should be isolated from others with immune disorders.

INFECTIOUS MONONUCLEOSIS

Infectious mononucleosis is a relatively benign but disabling
illness characterized by fever, weakness, anorexia, and
sore throat. Infectious mononucleosis is caused by the
Barr-Epstein virus, one of the herpes viruses. Man is the
only source of the infection. The incubation period is thought
to be a long one, extending from 10 to 50 days. Generalized
lymphadenopathy, splenomegaly (50% of the cases), upper
eyelid edema, and exudative tonsillitis dominate the findings.
Occasionally, a variable rash also is found, particularly in
those patients treated unnecessarily with antibiotics like
ampicillin. The diagnosis is relatively simple when more
than 5-10% of the lymphocytes are atypical lymphocytes, or
Downey cells are seen on a peripheral blood smear. The
heterophile agglutination test and a number of quicker
screening tests (mono test) are helpful in confirming the
diagnosis when they are performed at the end of the first
week of illness. Tests to detect various Barr-Epstein virus
antigens may also be available. The most common is the
viral capsid antigen test (VCA) which gives high titers early
in the course of the disease. The IGM anti-VCA test is useful to identify recent illness. These tests are useful in detecting the occasional heterophile/mono spot test negative

individual. Treatment is entirely symptomatic and consists of analgesics, antipyretics, maintenance of hydration, and bed rest.

Practical Points

1. The rash in mononucleosis takes many different forms. It can be scarlatiniform, maculopapular, or purpuric. Most commonly it is a maculopapular, morbilliform eruption.
2. Splenic rupture due to an overstretching of the splenic capsule is a rare but serious complication. Excessive or energetic palpation of the spleen is to be avoided as well as other activites that may damage the spleen, e.g., sports.
3. Communicability is of a relatively low order. Rather intimate exposure (popular synonym: "kissing disease") is needed to transfer the infection. Quarantine procedures are not necessary.
4. The duration of illness is approximately 1-2 weeks. Relapse is possible in the first year of convalescence. Second attacks are not considered to occur. Laboratory relapse without clinical symptoms of mononucleosis may occur during other acute illnesses.
5. Full recovery is the rule. Sequelae are unusual and death rarely occurs.
6. Jaundice and hepatomegaly may occur simulating hepatitis A or B.
7. Heterophile agglutinins occurring in infectious mononucleosis remain unabsorbed onto guinea pig kidney cells distinguishing them from other agglutinins. Unabsorbed titers usually reach 1:56 or more.
8. Deaths have been reported from airway obstruction induced by hyperplasia of pharyngeal lymphatic tissue. This may be prevented by emergency tonsillectomy or adenoidectomy, which is preferred over tracheostomy.

CAT SCRATCH FEVER

Cat scratch fever is known to be spread by cats who are believed to inoculate the as yet unidentified causative agent (possibly a gram-positive organism that loses its cell wall in vivo) by their scratch. The illness does not appear to be spread by humans. It has a wide range of incubation, 3-30 days with an average between 1 and 2 weeks.

The disease is characterized by lymph node tenderness and swelling in the areas draining the scratch site. Fever and malaise accompany the swelling in 30% of patients, and a small papule where the inoculation has occurred may precede other signs.

The course is generally benign but unusual complications have been reported, e.g., encephalitis, erythema nodosum and multiforme. The diagnosis is made clinically. Aspirated material from lymph nodes may be used to exclude other etiologies. An antigen skin test has been developed that is safe and reliable and awaits commercial distribution. Therapy consists of aspirating large, fluctuant lymph nodes or excising small ones if symptoms are severe. There are no specific therapies otherwise.

FIFTH DISEASE (ERYTHEMA INFECTIOSUM)

Fifth disease is an illness of unknown etiology characterized by mild systemic symptoms, e.g., fever and the appearance of malar flushing reminiscent of a slapped cheek. A confluent, reticular, erythematous rash may appear on the extensor surfaces of the upper extremities or trunk and arthralgia or arthritis may accompany it.

The disease is probably spread by droplet infection. It has an incubation period of 7-14 days and may occur in epidemics usually in the spring. The course is mild with virtually no complications and specific therapy does not exist.

GASTROENTERITIS

Diarrhea is more often found in the infant and younger child. Before the advent of effective hygienic methods of formula preparation and the development of fluid and electrolyte therapy, diarrheal disease with dehydration represented the major cause of infant mortality.

The etiology is protean. The more important pathogens, however, are viral agents (rotavirus, Echo, adenovirus, Coxsackie) and enteric bacteria, particularly *E. coli, Shigella* and *Salmonella,* less often *Campylobacter, Proteus, Paracolon, Pseudomonas, Klebsiella, Yersinia, Clostridium,* and *Staphylococcus* species. Important parasites are *Giardia lamblia* and *E. histolytica.*

The clinical picture is characterized by anorexia and diarrhea. Vomiting may occur and, at times, be severe. In mild cases constitutional symptoms are lacking; however, some children are quite sick with high fever and prostration. This latter picture is encountered more often with shigella, salmonella, and staphylococcal enteritis.

Varying degrees of dehydration also may be found depending on the amount of fluid the child has lost (in stools and vomitus and through insensible water loss), and his ability to replenish this loss by fluid intake.

Infants with dehydration present several common physical signs. Skin turgor is decreased so that a pinched fold of skin about the abdomen tends to remain tented longer than it normally would. The infant's mouth is dry, the eyes appear sunken in the orbital cavity, a large anterior fontanelle may be scaphoid. Lassitude, weakness, and poor cry are also part of the picture. The respiratory rate usually is increased since metabolic acidosis is generally present, and an acetone breath odor may be noted.

The prognosis is excellent with adequate therapy. The major danger is dehydration. Proper management will restore 99 of 100 infants to normalcy within a week or so. Less common but more difficult to manage is chronic gastroenteritis. The mortality here is significant despite all therapeutic measures.

Helpful values in assessing the clinical condition are:

1. Gastroenteritis with no dehydration, nontoxic child:
   a) Body weight at least daily
   b) One or more stool cultures
   c) Urinalysis
   d) Gross estimation of intake and output
2. Gastroenteritis with clinical dehydration and severely restricted oral intake (frequent vomiting, marked anorexia) or a toxic child:
   a) Body weight twice daily
   b) Complete blood count including hematocrit
   c) Three or more stool cultures
   d) Cultures to isolate pathogen from nose, throat, blood, urine
   e) Urinalysis including urine specific gravity
   f) Accurate intake and output
   g) Serum electrolytes - Na, K, Cl, Mg, Ca, P

h) Blood pH, pCO_2, bicarbonate and base excess
i) Body temperature 4 times daily
j) Stool pH
k) Rotozyme test for suspected rotovirus infection

THERAPY

A threefold approach is necessary: to eliminate specific pathogens; to maintain hydration while the infection is active; and to correct deficiencies in fluid, electrolytes, and acid-base balance that may have occurred.

Goal 1: Eliminate specific pathogen, if possible. Nothing is available to eliminate viral agents. In the event that a bacterial pathogen exists, specific antibiotics are often helpful. (See Table 7-3.) *E. coli* infection will respond to neomycin, and polymyxin B or E. Antibiotic-sensitivity testing should be employed in making a choice. *S. aureus* will respond to penicillin or a semisynthetic penicillin in the event of penicillinase-producing organisms. *Shigella* may be oblivious to all antibiotics but ampicillin or TMP-SMX appears to be effective.

Salmonella organisms are left untreated unless the child is toxic or has sickle cell disease, because therapy appears to prolong the carrier state. However, a child with salmonellosis and typhoid fever is preferentially treated with chloramphenicol. Treatment should be continued for at least 1-2 weeks until the pathogen is no longer recovered in stool cultures.

Some children are found to have concomitant bacterial infections in addition to their diarrhea (so-called parenteral diarrhea). Pneumonia, otitis media, and pharyngotonsillitis are frequently associated infections. Here treatment of the associated infections is indicated.

Goal 2: Maintain hydration during the acute infection. In children who have a reasonably unimpaired appetite for fluids (the majority of cases) the oral route is relied upon. It is merely necessary to offer enough fluids to the child to avoid dehydration. Balanced electrolyte solutions often are used but are not necessary. Ordinary beverages will do, such as diluted milk (1 part milk to 1 part water) or fruit juice, clear soup, soda beverages, and liquid Jello.

Goal 3: Correcting fluid, electrolyte, and acid-base imbalances. Most commonly, in dehydrated children, electrolyte loss is either equal to or in excess of fluid loss. The net result of this is isotonic or hypotonic dehydration. Less commonly, fluid loss exceeds electrolyte loss and hypernatremia results. This is a much more dangerous type of dehydration leading to CNS damage. Acid-base imbalances almost invariably occur in dehydrated children. The overwhelming majority of times, metabolic acidosis is present. (See p. 192 for fluid and electrolyte therapy.)

Practical Points

1. The virulence of *E. coli* organisms can no longer be inferred by serotyping.
2. Despite the many *Salmonella* serotypes, only a few cause clinical disease. As many as 25% are caused by *S. typhimurium*.
3. The presence of polymorphonuclear leukocytes in the stool suggests a bacterial etiology.
4. To maximize the yield of positives, multiple stool cultures should be obtained. Three rectal swabs quickly placed on culture media are considered adequate.

URINARY TRACT INFECTION

Urinary tract infections (UTI) are commonly caused by bacterial organisms although viral agents also have been implicated as pathogens. The infectious process does not usually confine itself to one anatomic subdivision of the urinary tract. Older terms like cystitis and pyelonephritis are, therefore, not accurate. They do, however, continue to be used to indicate the predominant site of infection. Thus, a child with urinary frequency, dysuria, and the absence of systemic manifestations like fever is considered to have cystitis; a child with fever and CVA tenderness, to have pyelonephritis.

The organisms most frequently encountered are the enteric bacteria. *E. coli* is the most common one, but *K.pneumoniae, Enterobacter, Pseudomonas, Proteus morgani* and *mirabilis* are also frequently isolated. Occasionally, *S. aureus* and *S. faecalis* also are seen.

The pathogenesis of urinary tract infection has never been well understood. Hematogenous and lymphatic spread

is possible but direct extension from outside through the
urethra in the form of an ascending infection would seem to
be a more likely way. Oddly enough, this mode of infection
has never been satisfactorily demonstrated.

Symptoms will depend on age. Infants tend to present
with the signs of sepsis and occasionally are jaundiced; older
children present with the symptomatology peculiar to "cystitis" or "pyelonephritis."

1. Cystitis: Common symptoms are urinary frquency,
   urgency, and burning on urination. Lower abdominal
   pain is present often, and tenderness over the bladder
   area may be elicited. Enuresis and tenesmus are somewhat less common in our experience. These children do
   not appear to be ill nor do they have fever as a rule.
2. Pyelonephritis: The symptoms of pyelonephritis tend to
   be less specific. That is, they mimic other acute febrile
   illnesses like gastroenteritis, salmonellosis, early meningitis, or acute appendicitis.

The diagnosis of UTI is confirmed by examining the urine.
Pyuria (WBCs in excess of 10/hpf), WBC clumps or casts of
white cells and bacteria seen on a Gram stain of a clean
catch specimen are all highly suggestive of UTI. A properly
collected clean catch urine placed on culture media within
15 minutes of voiding will provide identification of the infecting organism(s), and a colony count in excess of 100,000
colonies/ml is significant in untreated patients. The presence of WBC casts, leukocytosis, and elevated ESR points to
the kidney as the primary site of infection. Other laboratory tests are generally not very helpful and unless diagnostic confusion exists as to whether or not one is dealing with
another condition (glomerulonephritis, renal tuberculosis,
etc.) they need not be done.

An IVP and voiding cystourethrogram should be done in
all male patients and certainly in all female patients with
persistent or recurrent urinary tract infection. More authorities are recommending that these studies be done on females during their first UTI. Cystoscopy generally requires
the services of a urologist and a brief hospital stay. It should
be done where the infection has been difficult to control, is
recurrent, or where urinary tract anomalies are suspected.
The caliber of the urethral meatus should be measured

whenever treatment fails. Urethral meatal stenosis occurs frequently, and dilatation may provide a cure in some children.

TREATMENT

The approach to therapy will vary. Children with recurrent or persistent UTI, reflux, or meatal stenosis require more intensive therapy than those with an initial UTI. Table 7-5 outlines the basic therapeutic modalities employed.

The recurrence rate after the first episode of acute urinary tract infection is high. Approximately 40% will have a second episode within the first year of convalescence.

Prognosis is excellent if medical care is sought and adequate follow-up is provided. Fully 90% or more of the children will be cured permanently with little or no residual damage to the urinary tract. Follow-up should, as a minimum, include urine cultures monthly for 6 months and then every 2 months for an additional 6 months.

Practical Points

1. If clinical symptoms and/or bacteriuria do not improve after 48-72 hours of antimicrobial therapy, a change in medication should be considered. The most common mistake made in treating UTI is to persist in administering an ineffective antibiotic. The sensitivity test is usually available after 24-48 hours to guide the physician in selecting an appropriate antibiotic to switch to.
2. Bacteriuria may be intermittent and urine cultures taken by the clean catch midstream method are easily contaminated. Where possible, multiple cultures (three or more) should be obtained prior to starting antimicrobial therapy.
3. Sensitivity testing to sulfisoxazole is notoriously unreliable unless special culture media are employed. Many times a good clinical response is obtained when sulfisoxazole is used in spite of in vitro resistance. It is still an excellent drug for treating the first episode of UTI.
4. The most reliable method for culturing urine is by suprapubic puncture. The chance of urethral contamination is eliminated. This is especially true in small infants who cannot void on request. The clean catch method is adequate for children able to void on request.

Table 7-5 Therapeutic Approach to Recurrent UTI

Initial Acute UTI		
Pyelonephritis	—Antibiotics x 2 weeks	Sulfisoxazole 150 mg/kg/24 hr po
		Ampicillin 100 mg/kg/24 hr po
		Amoxicillin 20 mg/kg/24 hr po
		Cephalexin 25 mg/kg/24 hr po
		Tetracycline 25 mg/kg/24 hr po*
Cystitis	—Antibiotics (same as above) x 2 weeks	
	Analgesic—Pyridium x 2 weeks	
Persistent, Recurrent UTI		
Pyelonephritis	Antibiotics—chosen by sensitivity and given for 3 months or more followed by one of the long-term medications listed below for 1 year	

Cystitis

Furadantin 5–7 mg/kg/24 hr po
TMP–SMX, TMP 8 mg/kg/24; SMX 40 mg/kg/24 hr po
Mandelamine 7 mg/kg/24 hr po

Dilation of urethral meatus
Surgical correction of anomalies
Surgical correction of reflux

*Not suggested for children under 8 years of age.

MENINGITIS

Meningitis is an inflammatory process of the meninges of diverse etiology, distinctly related to age. The many causes include enteroviruses (Echo, Coxsackie), measles, mumps, varicella viruses, and four principal bacterial organisms (*H. influenzae B,* pneumococcus, meningococcus, tuberculosis). Age plays a definite role in the etiology, neonates being more liable to have enteric organisms (see newborn, p. 34), while children 3 months to 4 years of age are more likely to have *H. influenzae B* infections, and older children and adults pneumococcal infections. The meningococcus tends to have no particular age predilection.

Onset in children may follow or accompany symptoms of upper respiratory infection. *H. influenzae B* and pneumococcal meningitis should be suspected when otitis media, mastoiditis, or sinusitis is present. The classical signs of meningitis are fever, headache, vomiting, nuchal rigidity, and positive Brudzinski and Kernig signs. These signs may be absent in children under the age of 2 years, making the diagnosis difficult to establish without resorting to a lumbar puncture. In the under 2 years age group, the most consistent findings are fever, vomiting, and behavioral changes such as irritability or lethargy. In infants, a bulging fontanelle may help establish the diagnosis. Even when meningeal signs are present, the likelihood of a positive tap is slightly less than 50%. However, it is imperative to perform a lumbar puncture whenever suspicious signs and symptoms are present and no adequate cause for them can be elicited. Performed on this basis, lumbar puncture will be positive in about 10% of the cases. Conditions most likely to mimic early meningitis are pyelonephritis, exanthema subitum, salmonellosis, shigellosis, and meningismus occurring during a variety of other illnesses. While lumbar punctures have been routinely performed in children presenting with their first febrile seizure, meningitis seldom presents as a febrile episode with a convulsion of short duration and no other signs or symptoms.

A positive lumbar puncture confirms the clinical impression. To determine specific etiology and appropriate therapy, the following tests should be performed on the spinal fluid:

1. Total WBC count
2. Differential
3. CSF glucose + simultaneous blood glucose
4. CSF protein
5. Gram stain and/or Quellung reaction, fluorescent antibody test, countercurrent immunoelectrophoresis
6. Culture and sensitivity tests

A low spinal fluid glucose (less than 50% of glucose in a specimen of blood taken simultaneously with the lumbar puncture) indicates a bacterial etiology. A differential count of the white cells found in the spinal fluid may also offer an indication of etiology. Bacterial meningitis is more probable when the cells are predominantly polymorpho- nuclear, while viral meningitis is probable when the cells are predominantly mononuclear. There are numerous ex- ceptions, however. Early in the course of viral meningitis there may be a polymorphonuclear response before mono- nuclear cells predominate. Prior antibiotic therapy may possibly alter the cellular response.

A Gram stain of the spinal fluid may allow identification of bacterial organisms and the capsular swelling or Quellung test using specific serum antibodies to *H. influenzae* organ- isms will identify these organisms rapidly. Fluorescent anti- body techniques and countercurrent immunoelectrophoresis will also allow precise identification of organisms. The spinal fluid protein is generally elevated in all types of acute meningitis.

MANAGEMENT OF MENINGITIS

Meningitis is a medical emergency. Therapeutic measures must be applied with the least possible delay. The patient will require hospitalization and preferably intensive care facilities. The necessary monitoring is outlined in Table 7-6.

Antibiotic therapy is indicated when the etiology is suspected to be bacterial. (See Table 7-3.) In the newborn period, the drugs of choice are ampicillin or penicillin to- gether with kanamycin or gentamycin because of the prev- alance of enteric bacteria (see newborn, p. 37). In older children, when a specific organism has not been identified, ampicillin is the drug of choice. While the recommended dosage is 150/mg/kg/24 hr, it must be remembered that

Table 7-6   Therapeutic Approach to Meningitis

Cardiovascular
  Blood pressure
  Heart rate
  Central venous pressure

Respiratory
  Respiratory rate
  Airway patency

Neurological
  Level of consciousness
  Reflexes
  Sensory and proprioceptive sense
  Neurological signs
  Cranial nerve dysfunction
  Head size
  Funduscopic examination
  Fontanelle

Skin and mucous membranes
  Color
  Presence of petechiae or purpura

General body temperature
  Rectal temperature

State of hydration
  Weight
  Urine specific gravity and hematocrit
  Electrolyte balance—fluid intake and output

Hematological
  Hemoglobin, WBC
  Differential, coagulation factors (platelets
  prothrombin fibrinogin, factor V)

---

spinal fluid concentrations fall as meningeal inflammation recedes and therefore higher doses (200–300 mg/kg/24 hr) may be needed by the third day of therapy. It is important that the intravenous route be used to insure complete, rapid absorption. It is preferable that ampicillin be given by IV push every 4 hours rather than placed in an IV bottle where degradation may occur. The use of chloramphenicol in conjunction with ampicillin now has been recommended for therapy of suspected bacterial meningitis of unknown etiology wherever ampicillin-resistant *H. influenzae* organisms have been encountered. Table 7–7 lists the drugs of choice and alternates for the common bacterial meningitides.

Treatment is continued for at least 5 days after the temperature returns to normal with close observation of the patient for 2 more days thereafter. If there are doubts about the response to therapy, a second lumbar puncture should be performed. CSF cultures become negative and improvement in CSF glucose occurs early (first 24–48 hours) when therapy is effective. If the clinical response is good, a second lumbar puncture may be omitted in children older than 1 year.

Clinical problems that may arise early in the course of treatment include:

1. Continued infection with resistant organisms
2. Development of localized infection (brain abscess)
3. Disseminated intravascular coagulopathy
4. Septic shock or Waterhouse-Friderichsen syndrome
5. Status epilepticus and cerebral edema
6. Electrolyte imbalance, especially hyponatremia and dehydration (inappropriate ADH secretion)

Problems developing later on are:

1. Subdural effusions
2. Hydrocephalus
3. Neurological and behavioral sequelae

Practical Points

1. Petechiae and ecchymoses while commonly associated with meningococcal meningitis also may be found in sepsis with any organism. Identification may be made

Table 7-7   Bacterial Meningitis Antibiotic Therapy

H. *influenzae B*
  Ampicillin 200–300 mg/kg/day IV in q^6 h doses
  Chloramphenicol 100 mg/kg/day IV in q6 h doses

Pneumococcus
  Penicillin G 250,000 U/kg/day IV in q4 h doses
  Chloramphenicol 100 mg/kg/day IV in q6 h doses

Meningococcus
  Penicillin G 250,000 U/kg/day IV in q4 h doses
  Chloramphenicol 100 mg/kg/day IV in q6 h doses

Unknown bacteria
  Ampicillin 200–300 mg/kg/day IV in q6 h doses
  Chloramphenicol 100 mg/kg/day IV in q6 h doses

---

by scraping the petechial lesion and doing a Gram-stain smear and cultures of any blood obtained.

2. Children with neurological conditions such as hydro-cephalus, meningomyelocele, and previous skull fractures may be unusually susceptible to meningitis.
3. Children with sickle cell disease are also more suscept-ible to meningitis, especially the pneumococcal variety.
4. A full fontanelle may not appear in children who are de-hydrated.
5. Unusual organisms causing meningitis after the age of 2 months should alert the clinician to the presence of an unusual predisposition to develop meningitis. Immuno-logical defects, neurological defects, localized infections (sinusitis, mastoiditis, endocarditis), and trauma are other possible predisposing conditions.
6. Continued fever after the first 48-72 hours of antibiotic therapy is most likely due to bacterial resistance. Other causes are brain abscess, abscess or phlebitis in injection sites or areas of operative procedures (cut down site, tracheostomy site), subdural effusion, or drug fever.

7. Neurological defects may not be apparent in the convalescent period until 2 or more months after the acute infection.
8. Prophylactic therapy for household and nursery school contacts is necessary as soon as possible when the infecting organism is the meningococcus. Sulfisoxazole or sulfadiazine were recommended widely until reports of increasing resistance have made their use questionable. An increasing percentage of sulfonamide-resistant organisms are being encountered. Rifampin is still the drug of choice unless the organism is known to be sensitive to the sulfonamides.

   Dosage for Prophylaxis:
   For Sulfa-Sensitive Organisms

Sulfisoxazole	100 mg/kg/day, maximum of
Sulfadiazine	4 g/day given in four divided
	doses daily for 2 days

   For Nonsulfa-Sensitive Organisms and Where Sensitivity is Unknown

Rifampin	10 mg/kg/dose for four doses
	q12 h in children 1 month to 12
	years of age, not to exceed 1200
	mg/day. Half this dose for neo-
	nates to the age of 1 month.
	Older children and adults:
	1200 mg/day in two divided
	doses.

   Prophylaxis is recommended for relatives and close contacts of the patient. Unless the medical and nursing staff has rather intimate contact (mouth-to-mouth resuscitation), prophylaxis is not necessary. Meningococcal vaccines are also useful in preventing disease from group A and C organisms. Group A vaccine is effective in children older than 3 months; group C vaccine in children over 2 years of age.
   There is evidence now that household contacts of patients with *H. influenzae* meningitis have a higher incidence of contracting the illness if they are under 49

months of age. Some authorities are now recommending rifampin prophylactically for all household contacts* regardless of age, where there are children younger than 49 months. The dose of rifampin for this purpose is 20 mg/kg/day given once daily for 4 days. The maximum dose is 600 mg/day. Nursery schools and day care centers are considered as households for prophylactic therapy purposes. Pregnant women should not receive prophylactic rifampin (see hemophilus B polysaccharide vaccine, p. 68).

9. Isolation is necessary for at least 48 hours in the case of meningococcal meningitis. Isolation may be discontinued after 48 hours unless signs of acute infection (fever) have not dissipated by this time. Isolation for suspected bacterial meningitis of unknown etiology is indicated until a specific diagnosis is made, or in the event this proves impossible, until signs of acute infection abate.

10. Meningitis treated with antibiotics prior to lumbar puncture frequently occurs. In these instances, all usual efforts to isolate the bacterial pathogen fail. If the differential cell count and/or the spinal fluid glucose suggest a bacterial etiology, the patient must be treated with ampicillin as previously outlined. Procedures such as countercurrent immunoelectrophoresis, which do not require live organisms to be present, may permit accurate identification even after partial antibiotic treatment.

BOTULISM

A disorder caused by botulinum toxin usually present in food contaminated by *Clostridium botulinum* organisms. It results in a neurological disorder causing a rapidly progressive symmetric paralysis of motor nerves that may lead to respiratory paralysis and death.

In children (older than infancy) and adults, the toxin is usually ingested from canned goods, particularly home preserves, that have been contaminated with the heat-resistant anaerobe. In infants, the source is not always clear although spores found in honey and other improperly prepared infant

---

*Household contact = individual living with patient or who has been with the patient for 4 h/day for 5 of the 7 days preceding the patient's hospitalization.

foods apparently lead to colonization of the gastrointestinal tract with subsequent toxin formation.

There are several known neurotoxins elaborated by *C. botulinum* types. Types A, B, and E are of clinical importance. Types A and B are found in meat and vegetable products while type E is more likely to derive from fish.

Symptoms of motor paresis or paralysis involving the cranial nerves (especially the oculomotor) usually have their onset from 12 to 48 hours but may be delayed for as long as a week after ingestion. Gastrointestinal symptoms such as nausea, vomiting, or diarrhea are not necessarily associated with the neurotoxin. When present, they indicate the presence of other contaminating organisms in the spoiled food ingested. Swallowing and speech difficulties, hypothermia, constipation, blurry vision, headache, and dizziness are common symptoms.

The diagnosis is generally suspected on clinical findings and/or a history of eating tainted food and may be confirmed by isolating the organism or its toxin from the food source in the patient's blood and stool. In infants, a saline enema may help in obtaining stool since muscle weakness and hypotonia generally cause constipation.

A so-called staircase phenomenon has been described as highly characteristic of this disease on electromyography. This alludes to the increasing amplitude of muscle action as the frequency of nerve stimulation is raised abot 10 Hz.

The treatment for patients beyond the age of infancy consists of administering the antitoxin after skin testing for hypersensitivity. A trivalent preparation containing anti A, B, and E is available through the Center for Disease Control in Atlanta. The early induction of emesis or use of gastric lavage before neurological symptoms have developed is recommended. Enemas may also be helpful if no paralytic ileus is present.

In infants, antitoxin has not been helpful and antibiotics have produced mixed results. Ampicillin has been reported to eradicate the organism from the gastrointestinal tract in some infants. Supportive therapy in an intensive care environment is necessary in both infants and older patients particularly when paralysis of the respiratory and gastrointestinal systems are present. While mortality is high, early therapy is frequently successful and will lead to complete recovery.

VIRAL HEPATITIS

Hepatitis is an inflammatory disease of the liver with four acute forms and a variety of chronic forms. Infectious hepatitis is now commonly known as type A hepatitis. It is caused by a picorna virus and is characterized by a shorter incubation period, a usually shorter, more acute course, and greater comcunicability than serum hepatitis (type B hepatitis). The type B variety has been shown to be associated with the Australian antigen, and is caused by a DNA-containing virus. Table 7-8 contrasts the two major types. A third acute form, termed hepatitis non-A non-B, resembles type B more than type A. It frequently runs a chronic course and may be caused by more than one viral agent. A newly described fourth type, hepatitis D, is believed to be caused by a virus which can only replicate in the presence of hepatitis B virus. The illness it causes can be acute or chornic

Clinical characteristics of type A hepatitis include a sudden onset with fever, fatigue, anorexia, gastrointestinal disturbances, right upper quadrant tenderness, and varying degrees of icterus. Clinical characteristics of type B include an onset that is usually insidious. Fever is low grade or absent but other signs and symptoms are entirely similar to those found in type A. Anicteric forms exist in both types of hepatitis. In the epidemic form of type A as many as one-third of all cases are anicteric. Abortive forms also occur in both types. In these instances, symptomatology resembles a protracted gastrointestinal disturbance without icterus and with normal liver function tests. Occasionally (more often in adults) myalgia, arthralgia, or arthritis and urticaria are observed.

COURSE OF ILLNESS (BOTH A AND B TYPES)

1. The prodromal period is present in the majority of cases in both types A and B. It lasts a variable amount of time. Symptoms are usually only GI. The stool becomes acholic.
2. The preicteric period usually lasts 5-8 days. Symptoms include myalgia, fever, and right upper quadrant tenderness. The ESR, liver enzymes (SGOT, SGPT, etc.), and serum alanine aminotransferase usually peak at this stage.
3. Icteric period - with the advent of icterus, constitutional symptoms usually begin to abate gradually. Concomitantly, the urine begins to look dark and hepatosplenomegaly increases. Hyperbilirubinemia and bilirubinuria reach their peak during this period as does the cephalin

Table 7-8 Hepatitis Types A and B: Clinical, Epidemiologic, and Immunologic Features Compared

Features	Type A	Type B
Incubation period	15–40 days	50–180 days
Type of onset	Usually acute	Usually insidious
Fever	Common; precedes jaundice	Less common
Prodrome: arthritis and rash	Not present	May be present
Age group affected	Usually children and young adults	All age groups
Jaundice	Rare in children; more common in adults	Rare in children; more common in adults
Abnormal SGOT	Transient – 1–3 weeks	More prolonged; 1–8 + months
Thymol turbidity	Usually increased	Usually normal
IgM levels	Usually increased	Usually normal

Table 7-8 (Cont'd.) Hepatitis Types A and B: Clinical, Epidemiologic, and Immunologic Features Compared

Features	Type A	Type B
HBs/Ag (Australia antigen) in blood	Not present	Present in incubation period and acute phase; occasionally may persist
Virus in feces	Present during late incubation period and acute phase	May be present but no direct proof
Virus in blood	Present during late incubation period and early acute phase	Present during late incubation period and acute phase; occasionally persists for months and years
Immunity Homologous Heterologous	Present None	Present None

From Krugman, S. and Ward, R.: Infectious Diseases of Children, 6th ed., C.V. Mosby Co., St. Louis, 1977. (Reproduced with publisher's permission.)

flocculation test. The icteric phase usually lasts 4-6
weeks and results in complete cessation of symptoms in
the majority of cases. Children usually are not icteric.
4. Posticteric period - in this stage symptoms may return.
Anorexia and fatigue with GI disturbances predominate.
Liver and spleen size increase. The cephalin flocculation
remains elevated as does the thymol turbidity. After a
highly variable period of 2 weeks to several months all
symptoms abate and liver function tests return to normal.
The return of fever after a period of normalcy is indicative of possible relapse. The persistence of serum alanine
aminotransferase and HB surface antigen suggest chronicity in hepatitis B infection.

LABORATORY DIAGNOSIS
(See Figure 7-1)

1. Total, direct, and indirect bilirubin levels
2. Urobilirubin in the urine
3. Elevation of various enzymes, especially SGOT, SGPT, and
alkaline phosphatase
4. Alanine aminotransferase—positive at onset. Persists in
chronic case
5. Serum antigens in type B:
   HBsAg—positive early. Persists in chronic case
   HBeAg—positive early. Persists in chronic case
6. Serum antibodies in type A:
   Anti-HAV IgM—positive early in acute phase. Persists
   3-6 months
   Anti-HAV (NOPV IgM)—positive late in acute phase and
   convalescence
   Serum antibodies in type B:
   Anti-HBs—positive in recovery phase. Indicates full
   recovery
   Anti-HBe—positive in recovery phase and carrier state
   Anti-HBc (IgM)—positive early. Disappears in recovery
   phase
   Anti-HBc (IgG)-positive during and after recovery phase

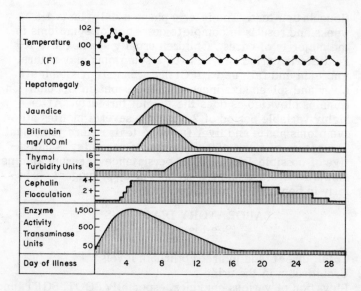

Figure 7-1 Comparison of the clinical findings with selected tests of liver functions. (From Krugman, S., Ward, R. and Katz, S.L.: Infectious Diseases of Children, 6th ed., C.V. Mosby Co., St. Louis, 1977. Reproduced with publisher's permission.)

DIFFERENTIAL DIAGNOSIS

1. Extra - and intrahepatic biliary obstruction
2. Hemolytic icterus
3. Icterus associated with various infections (infectious mononucleosis, Weil's disease, gonococcal hepatitis)
4. Icterus associated with drugs and medications (isoniazid, phenothiazines, oral contraceptives, indomethacin, erythromycin estolate)
5. Cholelithiasis
6. Congenital liver diseases (Gilbert's disease, Crigler-Najjar's syndrome, Budin-Johnson syndrome)
7. Wilson's disease
8. Poisoning (acetaminophen, mushroom)

COMPLICATIONS

1. Chronic hepatitis
2. Pneumonia
3. Myocarditis and pericarditis
4. Central nervous system disease, i.e., meningoencephalitis and polyneuritis; hematological conditions - hemiparesis, thrombocytopenia, and aplastic anemia
5. Pancreatic necrosis
6. Thyroiditis and arthritis

THERAPY

No specific therapy exists for hepatitis. The following measures have been found to be helpful:

1. Acute Course
   a) Bed rest during the symptomatic phase is no longer considered a necessity
   b) Diet - Limit on fat intake during acholic phase; vitamins, especially B complex
      Cholestyramine and/or an antihistamine if pruritus (bile salts) is a problem
   c) Antiemetics, if needed
   d) Analgesics such as Darvon, acetaminophen, but not aspirin
   e) Gradual resumption of physical activities in convalescence
2. Chronic Course
   a) Steroids: prednisone 10-40 mg/day slowly decreased over several weeks
   b) Azathioprine or Imuran has also been used
   c) In hepatitis treated with corticosteroids, the recurrence rate is high (20%)
3. Acute Hepatic Failure
   a) IV fluids
   b) Limit protein intake
   c) Sterilize bowel
   d) Hyperperfusion
   e) Monitor central venous pressure to make sure blood volume is maintained
   f) Mannitol if urine volume decreases

g) Steroids are of questionable value
h) Clotting factors for coagulopathies

PREVENTION (MODIFICATION)

Type A Hepatitis

Gamma globulin containing antibodies against hepatitis virus (immune serum globulin ISG) has been useful in at least modifying the course of type A hepatitis. ISG given prior to exposure or within 2 weeks of exposure to type A will prevent clinical symptoms. See Table 7-9 for indications governing the use of ISG. True prevention demands the avoidance of infection. The most important mode of transmission is the fecal-oral route. This should be interrupted. Isolating the patient during the acute phase of illness (up to 2 weeks after onset of illness) is an effective way of preventing further spread. Rigorous personal hygiene is also necessary; for those able to exercise it, stool control without isolation is all that is necessary. The disease is believed to be most communicable 2 weeks prior to the onset of jaundice.

Subclinical infection may occur even with the use of ISG. For example, active immunity is not prevented by giving ISG. However, a single dose has been found to be reasonably effective in preventing clinical symptoms of hepatitis for about 4 or 5 months. The present recommended dose is 0.02 ml/kg. Travelers to endemic areas staying longer than 2 months should receive 0.06 ml/kg.

Type B Hepatitis

Infection with type B hepatitis may occur from exposure to whole blood, red blood cells, plasma, platelet concentrates, fibrinogen, cryoconcentrates, and other materials containing the virus, e.g., semen. Airborne transmission is an unlikely mode of spread. Detecting HBsAg carriers among blood donors should be of preventive significance. A hepatitis vaccine is now available and is useful for high-risk patients. High titer ISG specific for hepatitis B (hepatitis B immune globulin, HBIG) is also available. It has proven to be 70% effective in the prevention of type B hepatitis and is being

Table 7-9 Indications for Prophylaxis with Immune Serum (Gamma Globulin)

Type of Exposure	Cases Given Gamma Globulin	Dose, ml/kg Body Weight	Comments
Household contact	All	0.02	
School contacts	Usually none		Immune serum globulin is given if the infection tends to spread
Work contacts	Usually none		Immune serum globulin is given if the infection tends to spread
Institutions, orphanages, day care centers, playing schools	All exposed	0.02	Immune serum globulin given if type of contact is similar to that of household contacts or poor hygiene is prevalent
Common source outbreaks	All exposed	0.02	As restricted as possible to individuals known to have been exposed

Table 7-9 (Cont'd.) Indications for Prophylaxis with Immune Serum (Gamma Globulin)

Type of Exposure	Cases Given Gamma Globulin	Dose, ml/kg Body Weight	Comments
Medical personnel	Usually none		Immune serum globulin given if cases occur among personnel
Travelers to countries with a high incidence of hepatitis			
Short-term travel (1-3 months)		0.02	
Extended travel (> 3 months)		0.06	Repeated every 4-6 months

Modified from Ringertz, O.: Prevention of infections with type A hepatitis virus, Am J Dis Child 123:427, 1972. (Reproduced with permission of American Medical Association.)

recommended in instances of accidental inoculation with contaminated material, contact with infectious patients, and transfusion with infected material. Evidence demonstrating its superiority over standard ISG is not yet clear.

Infants born of mothers with acute hepatitis B in the third trimester of pregnancy who are also HBsAg and HBeAg-positive should receive 0.5 ml/kg of HBIG (hepatitis B immune globulin) within 1 hour of birth. The simultaneous administration of hepatitis B vaccine is also recommended and will achieve protective levels even after ISG or HBIG has been given. The second and third inoculations of the vaccine are then given at age 1 and 6 months.

Management is symptomatic except in the chronic form. Stool precautions and/or isolation are not necessary; blood precautions are. The recommended dose of HBIG is 0.06 ml/kg as soon as possible after exposure with a second dose 1 month later.

Non-A/Non-B Hepatitis

Recently, a third type of acute viral hepatitis, the non-A non-B, serologically unrelated to hepatitis A or B, has been discovered. While not much is known about the illness, it appears to behave as a milder form of hepatitis B with an incubation period ranging between 2 and 22 weeks. Cyclic transaminase elevations seem characteristic of the disease which has been erroneously diagnosed as a new infection of type A or B. It is endemic especially in lower socioeconomic populations, is known to be spread by parenteral exposure, and most likely leads to an infectious carrier state.

Practical Points

1. Liver biopsy would be theoretically helpful but is contraindicated where a clear case of viral hepatitis exists. In cases of doubt and in the chronic forms of hepatitis, liver biopsy must be resorted to for definitive diagnosis.
2. Abdominal pain is quite common in children with hepatitis (approximately 60% of cases). It is occasionally so severe as to lead to exploratory laparotomy.
3. The return of fever after a period of normalcy is indicative of possible relapse.

4. Occasionally, an exanthematous maculopapular or erythematous eruption is observed in the acute phase of illness. Pruritus may be an associated finding.
5. The term chronic hepatitis should be reserved for those illnesses lasting 12 or more months.
6. Hepatitis B is more likely than type A to lead to chronic active hepatitis and cirrhosis. The incidence in the former approximates 10%.
7. Hepatitis B virus carrier states are associated with the persistence of HBsAg and anti-HBe and occur in about 10% of infected individuals. They may last from several years to a life-time.
8. In chronic active hepatitis, corticosteroids have been shown to reduce morbidity/mortality.

TUBERCULOSIS

Large urban areas in the United States provide a persistent reservoir of tuberculosis despite its near absence elsewhere. Population movements from countries of endemic infection into the cities make total eradication still an elusive goal. The inadequate health care delivered to the urban poor insure our failure in this direction. *Mycobacterium tuberculosis* is an acid-fast bacillus most often transmitted by droplet infection. Other body secretions, unpasteurized milk, percutaneous inoculation, or transplacental spread may also transmit the disease.

There are four common ways that tuberculous infection presents in childhood: as an adenitis (usually cervical), as a pneumonic process, as a meningitis, and as a fever of unknown origin. Other forms such as renal tuberculosis and gastrointestinal tuberculosis are not as frequently seen in this country. Still other uncommon forms are tuberculous infection of the eye, skin, bone, or peritoneum.

TUBERCULOUS ADENITIS

This condition presents as swelling and induration of one or more lymph nodes, usually cervical, that gradually enlarge and are not very painful. Unlike other types of bacterial adenitis, redness, tenderness, and fever are inconspicuous. In early stages the glands are palpated as separate masses.

In a later stage, coalescence and adherence to nearby structures are common. A chronically draining fistula may be the result of an inadequately treated infection. The Battey strain of tuberculosis is a very likely pathogen in this variety. Battey or atypical stains of mycobacteria usually do not give a positive tuberculin reaction when standard 5-10 tuberculin U are used. Some induration, usually less than 5-10 mm is often seen due to cross-reactivity. Specific testing material is available and greatly increases the likelihood of obtaining a positive reaction. Needle biopsy of the infected node will permit adequate culture material to confirm the diagnosis.

TUBERCULOUS PNEUMONIA

Unlike other bacterial pneumonias, it is often insidious in onset and respiratory symptoms may not predominate. Fever, anorexia, weight loss, or a failure to gain at a normal rate are the usual findings. A history of contact with an infected adult, usually a close relative, a positive tuberculin reaction, a suggestive chest x-ray, and failure to respond to antibiotics point clearly to the diagnosis of tuberculous infection. Another striking characteristic is the relative paucity of chest findings in comparison to the x-ray picture. Cough, night sweats, hemoptysis, and cavitary disease are not found frequently in childhood tuberculosis. Unilateral wheezing in a child should make one think of endobronchial tuberculosis as a major possibility; a positive tuberculin should help establish the diagnosis. Miliary pneumonia is seen occasionally and is suggested by the x-ray findings, toxic appearance of the child, and splenomegaly.

TUBERCULOUS MENINGITIS

The onset of tuberculous meningitis is usually slow and insidious. The characteristic history is of days, if not weeks, of illness with gradually increasing symptomatology. Behavioral changes, lethargy, headache, fever, and anorexia are the major presenting symptoms. On physical examination, cranial nerve signs such as upper eyelid ptosis suggest an involvement of the base of the brain. The spinal fluid reveals a pleocytosis with a predominance of mononuclear cells and a depressed spinal fluid glucose (less than 50% of the blood sugar). A Ziehl–Neelsen stain may show acid-fast organisms. Culture for ordinary bacterial organisms will be negative and cultural confirmation of a mycobacterial etiology should be forthcoming after 4–8 weeks. A considerable number of these children will have negative tuberculin reactions (as many as 50% in our experience). Frequently, the chest x-ray helps confirm the diagnosis as does a history of contact with the disease in an adult. Delay in starting therapy will significantly alter mortality; therefore, in children with a clinical picture suggestive of tuberculous meningitis but with a negative tuberculin reaction and a negative Ziehl–Neelsen stain, specific antituberculous therapy should be instituted.

THE INAPPARENT TUBERCULOUS INFECTION

The presenting complaint is usually an intermittent fever in a child who does not appear to be very ill. Anorexia is a frequent accompanying symptom. The physical exam is negative as is the chest x-ray. The diagnosis is generally made because the tuberculin reaction is positive.

THERAPY

1. Prevention – BCG vaccine for infants with continuous and intimate contact with an infected individual
2. Treatment for infected children:
   a) Positive tuberculin reaction, no other findings:
      (1) INH for 1 year for any child from infancy through adult age (35 years)
   b) Tuberculous adenitis:
      (1) Excise nodes where possible (discrete and few in number); needle aspiration for liquified nodes if surgery cannot be done
      (2) INH for 1 year or more
   c) Tuberculous pneumonia:
      (1) INH and rifampin for at least 1 year or INH and ethambutol or INH and PAS
      (2) In older children where retrobulbar neuritis is more easily detected, ethambutol 25 mg/kg/24 hr may be used more safely

(3) If no response to the above, add streptomycin and continue for 1 month

(4) If endobronchial involvement is present, particularly with atelectasis, steroids are added (prednisone 1 mg/kg/24 hr for 6-12 weeks)

(5) Miliary tuberculosis: INH for 18-24 months and rifampin plus streptomycin

(d) Tuberculous meningitis:

(1) INH for 18 months at 20 mg/kg for 4-6 weeks then 10 mg/kg and rifampin for 6 months then PAS for 12 months 500 mg/kg for < 6 year olds or ethambutol for 12 months for > 6 year olds

(2) Streptomycin for 1 month

(3) Prednisone 1 mg/kg/24 hr for 6-12 weeks

3. Dosage of antituberculous agents:

a) INH 10-20 mg/kg/24 hr not to exceed 500 mg daily

b) PAS 200 mg/kg/24 hr not to exceed 12 g daily

c) Streptomycin 20-40 mg/kg/24 hr not to exceed 1 g daily

d) Ethambutol 15-25 mg/kg/day not to exceed 1500 mg daily

e) Rifampin 10-20 mg/kg/day

4. Some of the newer antituberculous drugs being utilized more frequently and when resistance to INH and streptomycin is found:

a) Cycloserine 5-10 mg/kg/day

b) Ethionamide 10-20 mg/kg/day

c) Pyrazinamide 15-30 mg/kg/day

Practical Points

1. Patients who are positive tuberculin reactors and who are to receive steroids or other immunosuppressive therapy for any reason should be placed on prophylactic therapy (INH) during the course of treatment.

2. Children who have completed therapy should have a prophylactic course of treatment reinstituted when they reach puberty.

3. Since mycobacteria are acid-fast, they are one of the very few organisms able to survive in the highly acid secretions of the stomach. For this reason, culturing gastric washings from children unable to cough up sputum is helpful in isolating organisms.

4. Hematogenous spread during the course of tuberculous infection is a common occurrence. Bone marrow cultures, therefore, are frequently positive.
5. Miliary tuberculosis as well as the other complications of primary tuberculous infection usually occurs within 6 months to 1 year after initial infection. This is the critical time and constitutes the basis for treating recent converters for a 1-year period.
6. Communicability of childhood tuberculosis is of a very low order. Exceptions are the draining tuberculous lymph node and the uncommon occurrence of cavitary disease in untreated patients. Isolation in other instances need not be rigorously practiced.
7. It takes from 2 to 10 weeks after invasion for the tuberculin reaction to become positive. Usually symptoms coincide with the onset of tuberculous allergy. It is possible that findings may occur in the anergic stage and this possibility should be borne in mind when evaluating the results of the tuberculin test.
8. Various viral illnesses can suppress the tuberculin reaction. This is especially true of measles. It is during this time that a latent infection may be reactivated. This phenomenon occurs during vaccination with live measles virus vaccines as well. Positive reactors should receive INH before being vaccinated against measles.

SEPTIC ARTHRITIS

Primary arthritis caused by a bacterial organism is not an unusual occurrence. The common causative organisms are the streptococcus, S. aureus, and pneumonoccus. Meningococcus, H. influenzae B, and gonococcus infections occur less frequently. A close association between salmonella infection of bone and joints and sickle cell disease has been observed.

Symptoms of septic arthritis are pain, swelling, heat, redness, and limitation of joint motion. Systemic symptoms are usually present. Fever, generally high and spiking, a toxic appearance, and anorexia complete the clinical picture. Large joints are most frequently involved, i.e., hip, knee, ankle.

HELPFUL LABORATORY TESTS

1. A complete blood count to demonstrate polymorphonuclear leukocytosis and to help rule out sickle cell
anemia. A sickle cell preparation should be done if
anemia is present in a child of appropriate ethnic origin.
2. Cultures, Gram stain, and cell count of joint aspirate.
3. Cultures of blood.
4. X-ray of the joint will show widening of the joint space,
indicating an effusion. In later stages, destruction of
the joint cartilage may be seen.
5. Aspiration of involved joint: synovial fluid will commonly show an increase in white cells. Total counts
range from 25,000 to 225,000 with a predominance of
polymorphonuclear leukocytes. There is a substantial
decrease in glucose concentration compared to a simultaneous blood glucose. A Gram stain is helpful in rapid
identification of the causative organism.

TREATMENT

The most common error in management is to delay antibiotic therapy. A delay of hours can make a significant
difference in the outcome. Joint cartilage may be destroyed
quite rapidly leading to a permanently impaired joint. Splinting of the joint while local signs are most acute is mandatory.
However, increasing mobility of the joint is indicated when
local signs abate.

Incision and drainage are indicated for any large collection of pus in the joint, particularly in the hip. Needle aspiration, incision, and drainage are helpful when fever and
local signs show no improvement after 48–72 hours of therapy.

CHOICE OF ANTIBIOTICS

**Initial Antibiotic Therapy (Before Culture and
Sensitivity are Known)**

Antibiotics are best chosen on the basis of in vitro sensitivity. (See Table 7-3.) In the first 48 hours before the culture
and sensitivity are known, the choice is dictated by the Gram-
stain result of the joint aspirate and the organisms most likely
to be implicated.

Staphylococcus, Streptococcus, and pneumococcus must be covered. In children from 3 months to 3 years, *H. influenzae* type B is included. In infants under 3 months, the gram-negative organisms are a possible cause.

The use of one of the penicillinase-resistant penicillins like oxacillin 200 mg/kg/day, methicillin 200 mg/kg/day, cloxacillin or dicloxacillin 100 mg/kg/day will be effective for the three most common organisms. Ampicillin 200-300 mg/kg/day or chloramphenicol 100 mg/kg/day is added for the possibility of *H. influenzae*. Gentamicin 5-7.5 mg/kg/day is added in newborns and infants under 3 months of age for the gram-negative organisms. The child with sickle cell disease should be treated with ampicillin or chloramphenicol in combination with penicillin.

Definitive Antibiotic Therapy (After Culture and Sensitivity are Known)

After the results of the culture and sensitivity are known, antibiotic therapy should be readjusted. Thus, resistant staphylococcal organisms are treated with methicillin 100,000 U/kg/day. Streptococcus is treated with penicillin G, and *H. influenzae* with ampicillin or chloramphenicol. Antibiotic therapy should be continued for at least 4-6 weeks. Intravenous therapy should be used for the initial 2-3 weeks. Surgical drainage should be accomplished if there is no clinical response to therapy after 48 hours.

OSTEOMYELITIS

Osteomyelitis may be found in almost any bony structure; however, the most frequent sites afflicted are the long bones, particularly of the lower extremities. The usual causes are the pyogenic, gram-positive organisms, especially streptococcus, both group A and B, staphylococcus, and pneumococcus. Occasionally, one encounteres *H. influenzae* and salmonella organisms. The latter are associated with sickle cell disease.

Symptoms include both local and systemic manifestations. The local signs are point tenderness over the site of infection, swelling, redness, and heat which may vary from conspicuous to virtually absent.

Systemic signs are fever, anorexia, and a toxic appearance. These are late symptoms and may be entirely absent at the outset.

HELPFUL TESTS

1. CBC
2. Blood cultures
3. Culture of aspirate from the site of infection
4. X-ray and radionuclide scan (99^m technetium)

Early x-rays may not be diagnostic of osteomyelitis. It takes a week or longer for the characteristic periosteal elevation and new bone formation to occur. Some useful information may be obtained from early x-ray. Early changes of osteomyelitis are an indistinct subcutaneous-muscular border over the infected area and increased size of the muscle mass when compared with the opposite extremity. A deep seated myositis cannot be ruled out on the basis of these findings. The radionuclide bone scan is more effective to detect early changes than are standard x-ray techniques.

MANAGEMENT

Antibiotics, antipyretics, and analgesics are all useful. (See Table 7-3.) The principles discussed under antibiotic therapy for septic arthritis are applicable to osteomyelitis as well. The duration of therapy should be a minimum of 4-6 weeks and, depending on the type of response, may be considerably longer. The intravenous route is preferred in the early days (1-4 weeks) of treatment. Intramuscular or oral therapy is used subsequently depending on how rapid a response is obtained. Dicloxacillin is preferred for oral therapy of resistant staphylococcus because higher tissue levels can be achieved (400 mg/kg/24 hr, six doses). If a large collection of pus and dead bone forms, surgical intervention is indicated.

RICKETTSIAL DISEASES

MURINE OR ENDEMIC TYPHUS

The *Rickettsia mooseri* is the causative agent of endemic typhus. Like all the rickettsiae, this organism is pleomorphic and is usually transmitted by an arthropod vector, the *Xenopsylla cheopis* or rat flea. Direct transmission from animal (rat) to host is also possible. In the United States, the disease is found primarily along the Eastern sea coast and the South mostly in the summer months.

The symptoms of endemic typhus are milder than the epidemic form. There is a rash, but it is often localized and nonhemorrhagic. Vascular and visceral involvement is infrequent.

As a rule, recovery takes place within 10–14 days. Therapy: for children < 9 years old, chloramphenicol; > 9 years old, tetracycline.

LOUSEBORNE OR EPIDEMIC TYPHUS

Epidemic typhus is caused by *Rickettsia prowazekii* transmitted from body lice *(Pediculosus humanus)*. One animal host in the United States is the squirrel. The disease is found wherever poor social conditions with overcrowding favor the spread of body lice. Unlike endemic typhus, epidemic typhus is more common in winter months when opportunities for the transmission of the lice vectors are greater. The disease may be confirmed by detecting agglutinins against Proteus OX-19. A fourfold rise in complement fixing antibodies, which peak at 2 weeks, is diagnostic.

Management includes delousing procedures for both endemic and epidemic typhus. Pyrethrin, piperonyl butoxide, and lindane are effective.

Chloramphenicol for children less than 9 years of age and tetracycline for older children or adolescents are the antibiotics of choice. They are continued for 3 days after defervescence. Patients are kept in isolation until delousing is accomplished.

Q FEVER

The causative organism, *Rickettsia burnetii,* is hosted by domestic and wild animals. Farm animals, sheep and goats in particular, have been implicated. The west coast states report the highest rates of Q fever in the United States. Human infection occurs by drinking contaminated milk or inhaling infected material. After a 2-4 week incubation, there is an abrupt onset of fever with chills, malaise, and weakness. Respiratory tract symptoms of cough and chest pain grow worse in the next few days. Unlike the other rickettsial illnesses, there is no rash. The disease gradually resolves up to a month after onset. An occasional patient may develop endocarditis.

The diagnosis is most readily made by demonstrating a fourfold rise in complement fixing antibodies.

Chloramphenicol and tetracycline are the drugs of choice depending on the patient's age. Isolation is not necessary.

RICKETTSIALPOX

Rickettsia akari is the organism that causes rickettsialpox. It is transmitted to man by the flea vector, *Allodernanyssus sanguineus,* which lives on domestic mice. The illness is not communicable from man to man. Infections are found most often in urban areas.

After an incubation period of 7-10 days, a papulovesicular lesion occurs at the flea bite site. The patient then experiences a generalized maculopapular rash with fever. The disease is relatively benign without complications and with full recovery as a rule.

Diagnosis is made by a fourfold rise in complement fixing antibodies. However, there may be cross reactivity with Rocky Mountain spotted fever complement fixing antibodies.

Antibiotic therapy is the same as for the other rickettsial diseases and no isolation is necessary.

ROCKY MOUNTAIN SPOTTED FEVER

Rickettsia rickettsii is the causative organism of Rocky Mountain spotted fever. It is transmitted by the common dog tick, *Dermacentor andersoni,* which is found throughout the United States. The disease is most common in the western states during springtime, and during summertime on the east coast. Dogs and rodents are common hosts.

After an incubation period of 1-10 days, the disease is ushered in by a fever, malaise, and headache. Three or four days afterwards, a maculopapular often hemorrhagic rash makes its appearance. The rash is greater on the distal extremities. Complications involve the heart and central nervous system. Recovery is the rule in 2-3 weeks.

The Weil-Felix test is positive with agglutinins against Proteus OX-2 and OX-19 developing as the acute phase subsides. Complement fixation titers rising toward the end of the second week aid in making the diagnosis as does the indirect fluorescent antibody test.

Therapy is identical to that for the other rickettsial diseases. Individuals exposed to tick infested areas should wear protective clothing, use repellents, and examine themselves periodically to remove ticks before they embed themselves in the skin.

RABIES

Rabies is a viral disease transmitted to man by the bite of an infected animal or by inhaling infected material (bat dung). The causative agent is a rhabdovirus that is found in the saliva of infected animals. In this country, the reservoir of infection has been maintained by the wild animal population particularly skunks, raccoons, foxes, coyotes, and bats. Rabies is likely to be a more serious threat when the disease spreads to the domestic animal population (dogs and cats) since human exposure is increased.

The incubation period varies markedly from 10 days to as long as a year in rare cases. The site of inoculation influences the incubation period. Bites on the face and hand tend to shorten incubation periods unlike bites on the trunk or lower extremities.

Clinical manifestations include fever, hyperexcitability, peripheral neuritis, somnolence, dysphagia, convulsions, and death. The mortality rate is extremely high, approaching 100%.

The diagnosis is usually made by identifying rabies virus by fluorescent microscopic techniques in the saliva and brain tissue of the biting animal or in skin from the patient's bite area. Antirabies antibodies can be useful in diagnosing the disease in patients who have not been vaccinated against rabies. In any case, extreme caution should be observed in handling the specimens to avoid infecting laboratory workers. Strict isolation is required and great care taken to avoid exposure to the patient's saliva.

Management consists of vaccinating exposed individuals as soon as possible. The decision is more easily made when the biting animal is captured, observed and, if ill, examined for rabies virus (brain and saliva). When the animal has eluded capture and is a likely animal carrier (skunk, bat, coyote, fox, wolf, raccoon - not rabbit, squirrel or other rodents) then vaccination must be carried out. Domestic animals, such as dogs and cats who have not been immunized to rabies and who have not been provoked to bite, are more likely to be rabid. In these instances, if they cannot be observed vaccination is indicated for the patient. In all cases, the incident should be reported to local health officials who may lend assistance in identifying the animal and in determining the prevalence of rabies in the area.

The vaccine of choice is now the human diploid cell vaccine (HDVC), not the old duck embryo vaccine (DEV). It is safer with far fewer side effects and elicits a greater antibody response.

Therapy then consists of:

1. Thorough cleansing of the bite wound with soap and water-followed by 70% alcohol and, finally, 1% zepharin.
2. Tetanus immunization, if needed.
3. HDVC 1 cc IM as soon as possible then 1 cc at intervals of 3, 7, 14, and 28 days.
4. DEV is an acceptable alternative when HDVC is unavailable. Use 1 cc subcutaneous/day for 21 days, or two 1 cc injections subcutaneous for 7 days, then one 1 cc injections subcutaneous for 7 more days (total of 21 injections). Subsequently, a 1 cc booster dose is given on day 10 and on day 20 after the primary series. Antibody response is measured at the time of the second booster to insure complete immunization. DEV should be used with caution in patients allergic to chicken, duck, or egg protein.
5. Human rabies immune globulin (HRIG) should be used in combination with the first vaccine inoculaton to provide

a measure of immediate protection. Use 20 IU/kg of
body weight. Half the dose is used to infiltrate the bite
wound, the other half is given IM.

Antirabies horse serum, an older preparation, is not advised because of the frequency of allergic reactions (40%)
unless HRIG is not available. Immune globulin may be eliminated if the patient has been previously immunized (veter-
inarians, animal handlers, etc., may have been) and, in the
case of DEV, shown to have produced antibodies.

PARASITE INFESTATION

Among the dozens of varieties of parasite infestation existing in the United States only a few are encountered with
a relative degree of frequency. Pinworms, ascaris, tricuris
or whipworm, tapeworm, hookworm, and *Giardia lamblia* are
the more common parasites implicated as disease-causing
agents.

PINWORM INFESTATION

The predominant symptom is rectal pruritus. Irritability is
also noticeable. Otherwise the child is well and nutrition
does not suffer. Rectal excoriation may be seen on examination, but the worms seldom will be directly observed.
Diagnosis is made by using a piece of scotch tape applied
to the anus either before bedtime or upon awakening. The
Roerig Co. makes a very useful patient handout pack for
this purpose. Ova deposited on the tape can be seen on
microscopic investigation.

Communicability is high and contaminated hand to
mouth transmits the infestation. All family members should
be tested as well as other intimate contacts. Treatment is
90% effective with a single dose of pyrvinium pamoate
(Povan) 5 mg/kg po. Occasionally, a second dose may have
to be repeated 1 or 2 weeks later. Pyrantel pamoate
(Antiminth) 10 mg/kg is also effective and is better in com-
bating concomitant ascariasis infestation. Piperazine
(Antepar) given for 1 week is a useful alternative therapy,
as is a single dose of mebendazole, 100 mg po (65 mg/kg for
7 days).

ASCARIS INFESTATION

Colicky abdominal pain, poor nutrition, irritability, fatigue, and eosinophilia are the common signs and symptoms observed. Many times the worm will be passed in the stool and the diagnosis made by the parent. Three or more stool examinations for ova will establish the diagnosis. Occasionally, the radiologist will make the diagnosis on an abdominal contrast x-ray. Since passage to the gastrointestinal tract includes a pulmonary phase, a chest x-ray is indicated. One of the etiologies of Loffler's syndrome (pneumonia and esoinophilia) is ascariasis.

Treatment is with pyrantel pamoate, a single dose of 11 mg/kg or mebendazole 100 mg bid for 3 days. Piperazine citrate 75 mg/kg for 2 days is an accepted alternative.

TRICHURIS TRICHIURA OR WHIPWORM INFESTATION

These small thread-like worms are sometimes observed in the stool. Symptoms are mild, usually with slight abdominal pain. Nutrition is usually not altered significantly. Eosinophilia and observation of the stool for ova are helpful tests. Treatment consists of mebendazole 100 mg bid for 3 days.

TAPEWORM INFESTATION

The tapeworm imbeds itself in the intestinal mucosa where it grows to great length shedding its eggs in large numbers. Nutrition may be seriously compromised, particularly if more than one worm is present. Abdominal pain and hunger are frequent symptoms. Diagnosis, if not made by passage of the worm, is established with stool examinations. Treatment with niclosamide is effective. A single dose of 1 g is given for children weighing 11-34 kg and 1.5 g for children over 34 kg. Paromomycin is an effective alternative given as 1 g q 15 minutes for four doses.

NECATOR AMERICANUS OR HOOKWORM

Prevalent in the south of the United States. Penetration is through the skin, usually the foot. Initially, symptoms are respiratory (cough). Afterwards, they are gastrointestinal (diarrhea, abdominal pain). Anemia and weight loss may be found. Severe growth retardation and even congestive heart failure have been reported. Diagnosis is by identification of the ova in stool specimens.

Treatment with a single dose of pyrantel pamoate 11 mg/kg or with mebendazole 100 mg bid for 3 days is effective.

GIARDIA LAMBLIA

Currently identified as the most common intestinal parasite in the United States, Giardia is recognized as a cause of gastroenteritis. Symptoms include foul-smelling diarrhea, vomiting, abdominal distention, and cramps. Mucus and blood are usually absent from the stool. Returning travelers are frequently infected particularly from contaminated water and food. Occasionally, a chronic stage is reached characterized by failure to thrive, steatorrhea, and general debility. A stool examination will confirm the diagnosis particularly if three or more specimens are obtained on alternate days. It is more difficult to identify the organism in chronic cases where small intestinal biopsy may be needed. The treatment of choice is quinacrine (Atabrine) 2 mg/kg tid for 7 days below 8 years of age, 100 mg tid for 7 days in older children. Metronidazole (Flagyl) and Fluroxone are effective alternatives; however, the former is unapproved by the FDA as potentially carcinogenic and the latter, while the only liquid preparation available, also has been implicated in the development of mammary tumors in rats. Symptomatic children should be treated but the indication for treating the asymptomatic patient is still debatable.

COMMON SKIN DISEASES

IMPETIGO

Impetigo is a very common occurrence in pediatric practice. Lesions may appear anywhere on the body. Characteristically, they begin as vesicles and progress rapidly to pustules and these become encrusted. Pruritus is present as well as regional lymph adenopathy. Usually several lesions are clustered in one area and affected areas may be widely scattered about the body. Careful scrutiny of the entire child should be undertaken. The etiology is most often group A *Streptococcus* or *S. aureus*. The major complication with streptococcal impetigo is glomerulonephritis.

Helpful Laboratory Tests

1. Bacterial culture of the pustules
2. Urinalysis 2 weeks after the onset of infection to rule out poststreptococcal glomerulonephritis

Therapy

1. Topical — soaking in surgical soap or warm water, three times daily, is helpful in dislodging the crusts that form, so topical antibiotics may reach the bacteria. Soaking is followed by an antibiotic ointment containing bacitracin, neomycin, gramacidin.
2. Systemic—penicillin, or erythromycin in the event of penicillin sensitivity, should be given for 10 full days in the case of streptococcal impetigo. (See Table 7-3.)
3. General — the child's fingernails should be cut closely and scrubbed while the soaking is taking place since organisms may thrive under dirty nails. Scratching the lesions should be discouraged. The temporary use of an antipruritic agent may be useful (Temaril). Whoever touches the infected area (mother) should wash her hands carefully. Relatives and siblings must be observed carefully and cultured since communicability is a possibility.

MONILIA OR INFECTION WITH CANDIDA ALBICANS

Monilian infection is largely confined to infancy. A rare case is encountered in older debilitated children and an association with hypoparathyroidism has been observed.

Infection may occur in three clinical forms: oral, cutaneous, and systemic. Oral moniliasis (thrush) is a benign, self-limited condition. Lesions resembling curdled milk appear on the buccal mucosa and attempts to dislodge the patch will result in bleeding. Spread of organisms throughout the gastrointestinal tract and onto the skin around the diaper area is believed to be the pathogenesis for cutaneous moniliasis. Typical of this form is the appearance of small, red papules, initially around the rectum then spreading to the rest of the diaper area and even beyond (satellite lesions). Excoriation, intense erythema, and pruritus are common associated findings.

Generalized moniliasis is a life threatening form of the disease. It is encountered in very young infants and in debilitated children, usually seen in marasmic states (chronic gastroenteritis) or in children treated with long-term steroids. The clinical manifestations resemble those of sepsis.

Therapy

1. **Prevention:** The source of monilian organisms can be found almost anywhere. Monilia thrives in damp soil, both indoors and outdoors. Maternal vaginal infection and improper formula preparation may be the cause. Cleanliness and particularly care in the preparation of milk formulas can be helpful prophylactically.
2. **Specific therapy:** Oral moniliasis readily responds to 1 or 2 weeks of nystatin 1.0 ml four times daily given po by medicine dropper. Cutaneous moniliasis clears dramatically with ointments containing nystatin (mycostatin ointment applied three times daily. Systemic moniliasis is a difficult illness to treat. The antibiotic of choice is amphotericin B and side effects may be serious and are encountered frequently.

TINEA

Tinea or ringworm is caused by several species of fungi. *Microsporum audouini*, *Microsporum canis*, *Trichophyton tonsurans* and *rubrum* are some of the common types in the United States. Different clinical forms exist and are classified according to the type of lesion and bodily location. The following are the common ones:

1. Tinea capitis — scalp location
2. Tinea corporis — trunk and limbs
3. Tinea cruris — inguinal area
4. Tinea manuum — hands
5. Onychomycosis — finger or toenail

Symptoms are those of pruritus and secondary infection or impetiginization. A stubborn case of impetigo should lead one to suspect an underlying tinea. Occasionally, a generalized maculopapular eruption occurs known as the "id" reaction. The lesions are oval or circular and display central healing and an erythematous slightly raised peripheral margin. On the scalp there will be a path of alopecia. Hair loss unlike other causes of alopecia (alopecia aereata) is partial. Broken hair roots remain. Occasionally, a thickened, large, fungating plaque called a kerion occurs. This is most often due to *Trichophyton* infection. On the finger or toenails marked deformity of the nail takes place and breakage and nail loss occur.

Helpful Laboratory Tests

1. Hairy regions may be fluoresced with a Wood's lamp. The infected hair will fluoresce as a bright green in microsporon infection. *Trichophyton* infections do not cause fluorescence.
2. Skin scrapings prepared with KOH will display mycelial forms.
3. Culture on Sabouraud's media will grow the fungus.

Therapy

Therapy varies according to the site of infection:

1. Tinea capitis
   a) Shave the scalp for 1 or 2 inches around the lesion.
   b) Apply an antifungal ointment. (Desenex, Hydrocortisone-vioform ointment three times a day.)
   c) Give griseofulvin 10 mg/kg/24 hr once a day for 4-8 weeks.
2. Tinea corporis — steps (b) and (c) above are applicable.
3. Tinea cruris and tinea manuum — same as Tinea corporis except therapy may have to be continued for a longer period of time (8-12 weeks). In cases of *Trichophyton rubrum palmaris*, therapy may be needed for as long as 6 months.
4. Onychomycosis — therapy may fail completely despite all measures. A prolonged period of griseofulvin is

indicated: 6 months to 1 year. Topical ointments do not reach the organism unless the nail is removed. Nail removal helps speed the cure.

Practical Points

1. Remember that griseofulvin may cause WBC count depression — usually readily reversible. A weekly WBC count should be done during therapy.
2. Communicability is high. Siblings should be carefully watched. After a week of therapy including the covering of infected sites, little likelihood of transmission exists.
3. Griseofulvin is not an antiinflammatory drug. Local therapy to decrease inflammation is still helpful. In inflammed areas, wet soaks are helpful. When bacterial superinfection occurs an antibiotic ointment should be used; otherwise, keratolytic agents are useful.

MOLLUSCUM CONTAGIOSUM

Molluscum contagiosum is probably caused by a viral agent. The hallmark of this disease is the characteristic appearance of the lesion. Small fleshy, almost warty lesions appear usually in one area of the body. They are umbilicated and somewhat cystic. The lesions are pruritic. The umbilication, pruritus, and lack of induration distinguish them from warts.

Therapy is curative with complete removal by curettage or upon application of canthandin 0.7%.

HERPES SIMPLEX

Herpes simplex may present as an infection of either mucous membranes of the skin (type I), or as a generalized infection occurring infrequently in infants less than 1 month of age (type II), or in sexually active or abused children (type II). Most often mucous membranes are involved, particularly the oral cavity, less often the vaginal or rectal areas, and rarely elsewhere. The causative agent is the herpes simplex virus. The incubation period varies from 2 to 12 days. Lesions appear as neat, round, or oval shaped, punched out, shallow ulcers. These are painful to touch. In children who are experiencing primary infections, numerous lesions may occur accompanied by systemic symptoms of fever, anorexia, and irritability. Lesions in the mouth tend to involve the anterior portion of the oral cavity. Labial, buccal, gingival, and glossal mucosa are frequently involved. Chewing and swallowing may be so painful that the child may actually become dehydrated and require intravenous fluids. Regional lymph nodes are enlarged and tender.

A very serious form of herpes is herpetic conjunctivitis. Delay in therapy can lead to blindness from corneal ulceration (the dendritic ulcer).

Therapy is symptomatic and is supportive for herpes except in the eye and in generalized infections. (See p. 44.) In the eye, iododeoxyuridine (IDU) or vidaribine in the form of drops is instilled hourly until the ulceration is no longer visible on fluorescein staining. An ophthalmologist should be consulted.

Therapy of oral herpes consists of bland, cool liquids. Semisolids like milk, Jello, and ice cream are given to avoid causing pain while maintaining hydration and nutrition orally. Topical anesthetics in a viscous vehicle (viscous xylocaine) can be effective when used prior to meals but it is potentially sensitizing. Aspirin or acetaminophen is effective in controlling both pain and fever.

THERAPY FOR GENITAL HERPES

Painful cervical and vulvar lesions with fever and inguinal lymphadenopathy may be severe and persist for up to 3 weeks. Contiguous spread to adjacent skin is common in both sexes and disseminated infection can occur.

A Papanicolaou smear may permit diagnosis by demonstrating a Tzanck cell, which is a multinucleated giant cell with intranuclear inclusion bodies.

Therapy is generally unsatisfactory. Relief can be achieved by Indian and warm baths. Drying agents cause the lesions to dry up quickly, but no curative therapy is available at this time. Acyclovir is now approved for oral use. It provides symptomatic relief but does not prevent recurrences.

Chapter 8

FLUID AND ELECTROLYTE THERAPY

Significant water and electrolyte disturbances in infants and children, requiring parenteral fluid therapy, are not uncommon in pediatric practice. Loss of body fluid without the loss of supporting tissue is termed dehydration. Dehydration can be *isotonic* when there is proportional loss of water and solute, *hypotonic* when the solute loss is proportionately greater than the water loss, and *hypertonic* when the water loss proportionately exceeds that of solute loss. The characteristics of these three types of dehydration are given in Table 8-1.

The plan of therapy in a clinical situation should provide for (1) the deficits of water and electrolytes, (2) the normal losses from the body and, (3) the abnormal losses that will continue to occur until the illness subsides.

WATER DEFICITS

The deficit is reflected in the weight change before and after start of the illness. Also an educated guess of the existing deficit can be made on the basis of the degree of dehydration clinically observed. In general, the following guide is practical in planning the deficit therapy:

Table 8-1 Characteristics of Different Types of Dehydration

	Isotonic	Hypotonic	Hypertonic
General condition	Apathetic, inactive	Apathetic, inactive coma	Hyperirritable
History	Diarrhea, vomiting, fasting, intestinal fistulas and suctioning	Excessive sweat loss with water ingestion. Untreated salt-losing states, e.g., adrenogenital syndrome, chronic diarrhea, cerebral salt-losing states	Intake of fluids with high solute load, salt poisoning, newborns with renal immaturity
Physical signs: skin	Cold. Loss of skin turgor	Cold, clammy. Loss of skin turgor	Warm or cold. Doughy feeling. Turgor fairly well maintained
Laboratory findings	Serum Na normal	Serum Na less than 130 mEq/L	Serum Na more than 150 mEq/L

Table 8-1 (Cont'd.) Characteristics of Different Types of Dehydration

	Isotonic	Hypotonic	Hypertonic
Fluid for correction	1/3-1/2 isotonic multiple electrolyte maintenance solution (7:2:1 solution with potassium)*	Mild: 1/2 isotonic multiple electrolyte. Severe: calculate NaCl required** to restore normal concentration and use 3-5% hypertonic NaCl for correction. Follow with maintenance therapy with 1/3-1/2 isotonic multiple electrolyte maintenance solution (7:2:1 with K)*	Multiple electrolyte solution with Na about 20-25 mEq/L

*See text for composition.
**mEq/NaCl required = 0.6 x body weight in kg x desired increase in concentration.

Mild dehydration: loss of 3-5% body weight
Moderate dehydration: loss of 6-9% body weight
Severe dehydration: loss of 10-15% body weight

Usually the initial phase of deficit therapy is a medical
emergency as significant losses of water and electrolyte
from the body lead to shock. Probable deficits of water and
electrolytes in different types of dehydration have been
estimated (Table 8-2). Such figures can serve as guidelines
in formulating the deficit therapy in terms of amount of
water and type of electrolytes. However, in practice, except for the initial phase of rapid expansion of extracellular
volume by infusion of isotonic solutions such as normal saline
(20-30 ml/kg), the rest of the deficit therapy is administered
in conjunction with the maintenance therapy using one of
the basic multiple electrolyte solutions (see below) capable
of correcting the deficits over a period of time, in addition
to providing for normal needs.

NORMAL LOSSES

Replacement of normal losses (insensible loss, stool, urine)
constitute the maintenance therapy. Fluid requirement for
maintenance needs may be calculated on the basis of (a)
calories expended or (b) surface area of the body and/or (c)
kg body weight.

EXPENDED CALORIES

Normal losses of water and electrolytes depend on the metabolic turnover of the body. Hence, it is most precise to calculate maintenance needs on the basis of calories expended.
The usual expenditure of water and principal electrolytes
per 100 calories metabolized is as follows:

Water 150 ml
Sodium 2-3 mEq
Potassium 2-3 mEq

Estimations of total number of calories metabolized per 24
hours during parenteral therapy are given in Table 8-3.

Table 8-2 Probable Deficits of Water and Electrolytes in Infants with Severe Dehydration

Condition	H_2O ml	Na mEq per kg of body weight	K* mEq	Cl mEq
Fasting and thirsting	100–200	5–7	1–2	4–6
Diarrhea				
Isotonic	100–120	8–10	8–10	8–10
Hypertonic	100–120	2–4	0–4	–2–6**
Hypotonic	100–120	10–12	8–10	10–12
Pyloric stenosis	100–120	8–10	10–12	10–12
Diabetic acidosis	100–120	8–10	5–7	6–8

*Converted for breakdown of tissue cells: –1 g; N = 3 mEq of K.
**Negative balance of chloride indicates excess at beginning of therapy.

From Cooke, R.E.: Nelson Textbook of Pediatrics, 9th ed., W.B. Saunders Co., Philadelphia, 1969. (Reproduced with publisher's permission.)

SURFACE AREA

With certain exceptions, caloric expenditure, and therefore, the fluid requirement, correlates with body surface area. The advantage of using body surface area for calculation of the fluid requirement lies in the fact that such an estimate can be made for children of all ages and sizes with the aid of a single parameter [square meter (m^2)] instead of multiple values for different weights and ages needed in other calculations. Thus, with the exception of the first few days of life

Table 8-3   Calories Expended per 24 Hours During Fasting

Subject	Calories/kg
Newborn	45-50
3-10 kg	60-80
10-15 kg	45-65
15-25 kg	40-50
25-35 kg	35-40
35-60 kg	30-35
Over 60 kg	25-30

Basis for estimating requirements for parenteral fluids.

From Darrow, D.C.: The physiologic basis for estimating requirements for parenteral fluids, Pediatr Clin North Am 11:823, 1964. (Reproduced with permission of W.B. Saunder Co., Philadelphia.)

the water and electrolyte requirements per square meter of surface are:

Water 1500-2000 ml
Sodium 40 mEq
Potassium 40 mEq

During the first few days of life the requirements are about two-fifths of these amounts. The surface area can be obtained from standard nomograms (see Appendix, p. 528). However, for quick reference the following figures can be memorized:

Approximate average surface area of 10 kg child = 0.5 m^2
Approximate average surface area of 30 kg child = 1 m^2
Approximate average surface area of 60 kg child = 1.5 m^2

BODY WEIGHT

Finally, fluid requirements for maintenance therapy as calculated per kilogram of body weight at different ages will also give figures reasonably satisfactory for fluid therapy.

Approximate requirements per kilogram can be remembered as follows:

> Water: 0-10 days (newborn): 65 ml/kg
> First 10 kg: 100 ml/kg
> Next 10 kg: 50 ml/kg
> Beyond 20 kg: 25 ml/kg
> Na: 3-5 mEq/kg
> K: 3-5 mEq/kg

It must be noted that although the total amounts of water and electrolytes when calculated using any one of the above methods vary, sometimes as much as 50% in a given situation, they all, nevertheless, fall within the range of body tolerance normally provided by homeostatic mechanisms and, there-fore, are well tolerated. The appreciation of this simple fact should impart a good deal of flexibility in managing fluid therapy.

ABNORMAL LOSSES

The quality and quantity of abnormal losses that will con-tinue to occur depend on the nature of the illness. These should be replaced by appropriate solutions, volume for volume. Composition of fluid loss in different situations is given in Table 8-4. In diarrheal disease, usually the losses are hypotonic in nature and do not exceed 10-25 ml/kg/day.

Practical Points

1. The range of tolerance for water and electrolytes be-comes narrowed in certain clinical situations as in renal and adrenal insufficiency states. Extreme care should be taken in fluid management in such instances.
2. Inability of the kidney of the newborn to either concen-trate electrolytes or excrete hydrogen ions to the same extent as seen in older children, makes the newborn particularly susceptible to develop hyperelectrolytemia and acidosis under stressful situations.
3. In practice, once the initial phase of the therapy is under-taken by infusion of normal saline (0.9% sodium chloride) 20-30 ml/kg to expand the extracellular volume rapidly,

Table 8-4   Composition of External Abnormal Losses

Fluid	Na	K	Cl	Protein g%
Gastric	20-80	5-20	100-150	-
Pancreatic	120-140	5-15	90-120	-
Small intestine	100-140	5-15	90-130	-
Bile	120-140	5-15	80-120	-
Ileostomy	45-135	3-15	20-115	-
Diarrheal	10-90	10-80	10-110	-
Sweat: Normal	10-30	3-10	10-35	-
Cystic fibrosis	50-130	5-25	50-110	-
Burns	140	5	110	3-5

From Cooke, R.E.: Textbook of Pediatrics, 9th ed., W.B. Saunders Co., Philadelphia, 1969. (Reproduced with publisher's permission.)

the balance of fluid for repair and fluid maintenance needs may be hypotonic solution (one-third to one-half isotonic containing 5% glucose in water, sodium, potassium, chloride, and lactate). Many such solutions are commercially available. They provide essential electrolytes as required in most clinical situations, with enough free water to enable the homeostatic mechanisms of the body to do the rest in bringing back the equilibrium. Somewhat similar solutions can also be made on the wards by mixing seven parts of 5% glucose in water, two parts of normal saline, one part of 1/6 M lactate and adding potassium chloride to provide 20 mEq of K/L (7:2:1 solution with potassium).

4. Administration of potassium must be done only after making sure that the child is voiding. In general, fluids used for IV therapy should not contain more than 40 mEq of K/L.

5. Renal and adrenal insufficiencies are some of the important contraindications for the use of potassium.

6. Serum potassium levels do not reliably indicate intracellular potassium deficiency. The presence of generalized muscle weakness and ECG findings are a more reliable indication. (See p. 204.)

7. In hypernatremia, the kidneys cannot excrete sodium in enough concentration to correct hypernatremia rapidly.

8. Intracellular potassium deficiency usually accompanies metabolic acidosis and is regularly seen in states of metabolic alkalosis. A low serum sodium level usually is accompanied by a high serum potassium.

9. With body homeostatic mechanisms working optimally, correction of even severe states of acidosis or alkalosis can be accomplished by administration of water alone with a few essential electrolytes like Na and K.

10. A rise in pH may decrease the serum content of ionized calcium thus precipitating tetany. However, the development of hypocalcemia in the postacidotic state following fluid therapy in infantile diarrhea is an infrequent phenomenon.

11. Use of solutions containing excessive amounts of sodium but free of potassium tend to increase the likelihood of hypocalcemia in infants recovering from acidosis and dehydration.

12. Correction of acidosis is difficult in the presence of potassium deficiency.

13. Use of bicarbonate for correction of acidosis is superior to the use of lactate in small infants.

EXAMPLES OF FLUID THERAPY

DIARRHEA AND DEHYDRATION

Dehydration resulting from acute diarrhea is the most common pediatric problem requiring fluid therapy. In the majority of instances the dehydration is isotonic in nature. Metabolic acidosis often accompanies dehydration. The following recommendation is applicable in the management of children with isotonic dehydration with or without metabolic acidosis.

1. Assess the degree of dehydration (see p. 195) and calculate the amount of fluid required to correct the deficit. A rough calculation using the guidelines described previously is all that is necessary.
2. If the child is severely dehydrated, push 20-30 ml/kg of normal saline IV slowly over a period of about 30-60 minutes. Subract this amount from the total amount calculated for deficit therapy. Plasma or blood can be used instead of normal saline when required.
3. Calculate the maintenance requirement of fluid and electrolytes for 24 hours using any of the methods for calculation.
4. Calculate fluid at the rate of 5-20 ml/kg – depending on the severity of diarrhea – to provide for the continued abnormal loss.
5. Add up all the figures obtained.
6. **a)** If there is no significant metabolic acidosis (blood pH greater than 7.1), prepare a solution that is roughly one-third to one-half isotonic by mixing seven parts of 5% glucose water, two parts of normal saline, and one part of 1/6 M lactate (7:2:1). To this add an amount of KCl solution that would provide 20 mEq/L of potassium after assuring that the child is voiding. Alternatively, one of the commercially available multiple electrolyte maintenance solutions (Isolyte P or Pedialyte which is roughly one-third isotonic) may be used.
   b) If there is significant metabolic acidosis (pH less than 7.1), make up a solution by mixing two parts of 5% glucose water and one part of 1/6 M sodium bicarbonate. Also, add potassium chloride as indicated above. Final solution has a tonicity between one-third and one-half of an isotonic solution.
7. Administer half the total amount in the first 8 hours and the remaining half during the next 16 hours of the 24-hour period, adjusting the number of drops per minute as needed.
8. If treating situation 6b, check patient and pH after 6-12 hours and if the acidosis is improved switch over to 7:2:1 solution as in 6a.
9. Periodically, check the clinical condition of the patient, body weight, and specific gravity of the urine and adjust the rate of flow of fluid. Specific gravity of the urine is

a reliable indicator of adequacy of fluid therapy. Normally, the specific gravity of urine is around 1.010, but the kidney can dilute the urine to a specific gravity of 1.001 when there is excess water in the body to be excreted, or concentrate up to 1.030 when the body needs to conserve water. Fluid therapy is inappropriate if the specific gravity of urine is repeatedly close to either one of these two extremes. You may increase or decrease the amount of fluid to achieve a specific gravity close to 1.010.

10. After the first 24 hours, reassess the fluid requirement. Fluid for deficit therapy may be needed at this time. Use clinical judgment, specific gravity of urine, and weight changes as measurements for fluid requirements.

11. If hydration is good and the child is not vomiting after 24-36 hours of IV therapy, start the patient on calculated amounts of oral multiple electrolyte solutions for the next 12 hours. Switch to the regular milk formula soon after this.

Example 1(A): 10-kg Infant with Severe Diarrhea

Percentage of dehydration: 10%
Surface area: 0.5 m^2
Amount (first 24 hours):

For deficit therapy	1000 ml (10% of 10 kg)
For maintnenace therapy	750 ml (1500 ml/m^2)
For abnormal losses	50 ml (5 ml/kg/24 hr)
Normal saline for IV push	300 ml (30 ml/kg)
Balance of IV fluid for 24 hours	1800-300 = 1500 ml

Composition*: 7:2:1 solution with potassium 20 mEq/L

7 parts 5% glucose water	1050 ml
2 parts normal saline	300 ml
1 part 1/6 M lactate	150 ml
Total	1500 ml

KCl (add if patient is voiding or as soon as he voids)   15 ml (30 mEq potassium)

---

*Commercially available multiple electrolyte alternative fluids may also be used.

Administration: "Run" saline 300 ml in 30-60 minutes IV.
Administer 750 ml (half the amount) in the first 8
hours – the remaining half in the next 16 hours.

Example 1(B): 10-kg Infant with Severe Diarrhea and Metabolic Acidosis

Percentage of dehydration: 10%
Surface area: 0.5 m^2
Blood pH less than 7.1
Amount (first 24 hours):

For deficit therapy	1000 ml (10% of 10 kg)
For maintenance therapy	750 ml (1500 ml/m^2)
For abnormal losses	50 ml (5 ml/kg/24 hr)
Total	1800 ml

Normal saline for IV push	300 cc
Balance of IV fluid for 24 hours	1800-300 = 1500 ml

Composition*: 2:1 solution with potassium 20 mEq/L

2 parts 5% glucose water	1000 ml
1 part 1/6 M sodium bicarbonate	500 ml
Total	1500 ml
KCl (add if patient is voiding or as soon as he voids)	15 ml (30 mEq potassium)

Administration: As in example 1(A)

PYLORIC STENOSIS

1. Development of dehydration is more gradual than in children with acute diarrhea so that it is seldom necessary to expand the extracellular volume rapidly.
2. Metabolic alkalosis with intracellular potassium deficiency is a rule as a result of loss of acid gastric contents.

---

*Switch to 7:2:1 solution with potassium or to one of the commercially available multiple electrolyte solutions as the pH shows a steady return to normal value.

3. Although low serum potassium may reflect intracellular potassium deficiency, the ECG is more helpful in making the diagnosis of potassium deficiency. ECG changes of hypopotassemia are: prolonged QT interval, depression and broadening of T wave.
4. More chloride is lost from the body in relation to sodium. Therefore, fluids both for deficit therapy and for maintenance therapy should consist of chloride as the essential anion.
5. A solution containing two parts of 5% glucose in water and one part of normal saline with added KCl providing about 20 mEq/L of K generally provides needed cations and anions to bring back the equilibrium.
6. In an occasional infant, inability of the kidney to concentrate urine because of potassium deficiency may be noted.

Example 2: 5-kg Infant with Pyloric Stenosis and Metabolic Alkalosis

Percentage of dehydration: 10%
Surface area: 0.25 m^2
Amount (first 24 hours):

For deficit therapy	500 ml (10% of kg)
For maintenance therapy	375 ml (1500 ml/m^2)
For abnormal losses	0 ml*
Total	875 ml
Normal saline for IV push	100 ml (20 ml/kg)
Balance of fluid	775 ml
Composition: 2:1 solution with potassium 20 mEq/L	
2 parts 5% glucose water	517 ml
1 part normal saline	258 ml
Total	875 ml
KCl (after voiding)	8 ml (16 mEq of K)

---

*In cases where a significant amount of fluid is obtained by gastric aspiration, it should be replaced volume for volume with fluid having a composition similar to that described above.

Administration: Run saline (100 ml) over a period of 30-60 minutes IV. Administer half the total in the first 8 hours and the remaining half in the next 16 hours.

DIABETIC ACIDOSIS

1. Dehydration results from glucose diuresis to begin with and progresses later with the loss of electrolytes and water. Also there is excessive insensible water loss consequent to hyperpnea and Kussmaul breathing.
2. Ketoacidosis will promptly disappear once the utilization of carbohydrate by the body is established by administration of insulin and glucose. Prompt therapy with insulin is essential to make fluid therapy relatively simple.
3. Significant hyperkalemia is rarely present in children. When present, the ECG shows peaking of T waves.
4. Administration of potassium early in fluid therapy is essential as the potassium level of blood tends to drop rapidly shortly after administration of glucose and insulin.
5. There is a need for larger quantities of potassium than ordinarily present in maintenance solutions. Usually in the first few hours, normal saline and 1/2 normal saline are used. When the blood glucose level reaches about 300 mg/dl, the maintenance solution with glucose is used.

Example 3: 30-kg Child with Diabetic Ketoacidosis

Percentage dehydration: 5%
Surface area: 1 m^2
  Insulin therapy: start immediately (see p. 369)
  Fluid therapy: first 24 hours
Amount:

For deficit therapy	1500 ml (5% of 30 kg)
For maintenance and for abnormal losses	2500 ml (2500 ml/m^2)
Total	4000 ml
Normal saline for push	600 ml (20 ml/kg) first 2 hr
1/2 normal saline with potassium	40 mEq/L = 1400 cc next 6 hr

Balance for 24 hours   2000 ml

Composition: 7:2:1 solution with potassium 30 mEq/L
    7 parts 5% glucose water   1400 ml
    2 parts normal saline   400 ml
    1 part 1/6 M lactate   200 ml
    KCl   50 ml (100 mEq K)

Adjusted total   2050 ml

Administration: Run saline 600 ml in 120 minutes IV. Administer 1400 cc of 1/2 NS with potassium (40 mEq/L during the next 6 hours. Administer the remaining in the next 16 hours. After 24 hours administer maintenance requirement.

HYPERNATREMIC DEHYDRATION
(See Table 8-1)

Practical Points

1. Seen in approximately 20% of all children with diarrhea and dehydration.
2. There is a contraction of the intracellular volume and a relatively well-maintained extracellular volume. This accounts for the lack of classical signs of dehydration seen in other types of dehydrations.
3. Large potassium deficits often are noted in these children.
4. Low calcium levels are frequently noted.
5. Intracranial bleeding and subdural effusions are found in some children.
6. In most instances, there is a slight deficit of total body sodium and a small excess of chloride.
7. Attempts to reduce sodium concentrations by too rapid infusing fluid containing very low concentrations of sodium should be avoided as this would precipitate convulsions by causing cerebral edema and disturbing the newly acquired adjustments of brain cells to the state of hypernatremia. Calculate fluid for 48 hours and administer one-forty-eighth of the volume per hour for 48 hours.
8. Satisfactory results are obtained using solutions containing about 20-25 mEq/L of Na. Maximal safe amount

of potassium (about 40 mEq/L) should be added to the solution to correct potassium deficiency. Similar concentrations of Na are found in many of the commercially available multiple electrolyte solutions. Results using these solutions have been satisfactory.

Chapter 9

COMMON SURGICAL PROBLEMS

APPENDICITIS

The need for an early and an accurate diagnosis of appendicitis cannot be understated if mortality is to be kept to a minimum. Emphasis must be on the early signs and symptoms rather than late ones so that the diagnosis is made as soon as possible.

HISTORY

In older children, symptoms of GI function commonly precede the onset of pain. Flatulence, constipation, diarrhea, and gastric distress following a meal may be elicited. It is important to note the order in which symptoms and signs have occurred. Pain commonly begins in the periumbilical or epigastric area and, only some hours after onset, localizes to the right lower quadrant. Anorexia, often progressing to nausea and vomiting, usually takes place a few hours after the initial pain. Low-grade fever occurs still later in the course of appendicitis but is most often present in the first 24 hours of illness. A fever of 103°F or higher is less likely to be associated with early appendicitis uncomplicated by peritonitis. A temperature that is normal initially and then begins to rise is highly suspicious.

Local tenderness in the iliac fossa, often appearing abruptly, usually occurs just before the fever. Leukocytosis generally begins after the appearance of both fever and local tenderness. Muscular rigidity may be entirely absent in the early stages and is a rather late sign. Perforation may take place without rigidity ever being observed.

When this progression of signs and symptoms is observed, the diagnosis may be made with a high degree of certainty. It must be borne in mind that a retrocecal appendix is characterized by less vomiting, pain, and local rigidity.

PHYSICAL EXAMINATION

The abdomen is observed and percussed for cecal distension. On palpation, local tenderness is sought in the right lower quadrant. Often, but not always, the point of maximum tenderness is over McBurney's point. Rebound tenderness is a reliable sign of peritoneal irritation and may be elicited in a hyperexcitable child even after mild sedation (pentobarbital 2.5 mg/kg by rectal suppository) has been administered. The psoas sign is also a fair indication of peritoneal irritation. Abdominal rigidity may be found. A rectal examination to elicit tenderness or swelling in the right iliac fossa must be performed on all patients suspected of having appendicitis although it may be of limited value in the very young.

HELPFUL LABORATORY TESTS

The white blood cell count is often elevated in the first 24 hours of illness. It becomes elevated after the onset of local pain and fever. The differential shows an increase in polymorphonuclear leukocytes.

An abdominal flat plate may give some supportive evidence of appendicitis by demonstrating a fecalith or cecal distension and air-fluid levels indicating obstruction or ileus, but a negative x-ray does not rule out the diagnosis.

DIFFERENTIAL DIAGNOSIS

Influenza, basilar pneumonia especially with pleurisy, gastroenteritis, colic, gastric upset, urinary tract infection, early rheumatic fever, mesenteric adenitis, and other less common conditions may simulate appendicitis. The lack of association of other "flu" symptoms, such as generalized aches, helps rule out influenza. Rales, cough, and a positive chest x-ray indicates basilar pneumonia.

Borborygmi, lack of pain localizing to the right iliac fossa of rebound tenderness, and diarrhea may distinguish gastroenteritis. Pressure over the abdomen usually relieves the pain of colic and there is no localization even after several hours of observation. Gastritis attacks also do not progress the way appendicitis does and observation alone will rule out the possibility.

The urine must be carefully examined for pyuria and bacteriuria. Occasionally, an inflamed appendix located close to the ureter will lead to pyuria. The presence of bacteria on a truly clean catch specimen is sufficient to exclude appendicitis as a cause of pyuria. Fever of 103°F and chills are more common than in appendicitis. An IVP may be helpful in ruling out a right-sided hydronephrosis and in differentiating a retrocecal appendicitis from an acute renal problem. Early acute rheumatic fever may give rise to abdominal pain only. An antecedent history of sore throat, the presence of an early murmur, and lack of the usual progression of signs help distinguish this entity. The erythrocyte sedimentation rate (ESR) is the most helpful laboratory test in these instances. It is markedly elevated in rheumatic fever and either normal or slightly elevated in appendicitis. Sometimes, the ECG will show PR interval prolongation and the changes compatible with rheumatic fever. Mesenteric adenitis usually does not give rise to increasing right lower quadrant pain and rebound tenderness, nor is the rectal exam positive. In addition, an associated upper respiratory infection often is found.

An occasional child with pharyngitis or tonsillitis may present with a picture closely resembling appendicitis. Finding the throat infection allows the proper diagnosis to be made. In blacks, the abdominal crisis of sickle cell disease should also be included in the differential diagnosis.

Laparoscopy, in experienced hands and doubtful cases, can help in establishing a correct diagnosis without further surgical intervention.

Therapy consists of surgical removal of the appendix as the diagnosis is made.

Practical Points

1. The WBC and differential count serve only to alert the physician to the presence of an acute inflammatory process. They are not to be relied on to either establish or rule out the diagnosis of acute appendicitis.
2. Persistent and frequent vomiting points away from the diagnosis of appendicitis. Vomiting in appendicitis is relatively infrequent.
3. A retrocecal appendix may give relatively mild pain and no tenderness over McBurney's point. Rigidity of the muscle wall may also remain absent. The progression of the other characteristic signs and symptoms may not take place or takes place very rapidly. The clinician can afford no delay in this situation.
4. If sufficient evidence of appendicitis exists so that the diagnosis cannot be dismissed, and if no other diagnosis can be established beyond a reasonable doubt, then surgery is indicated. It is better to remove a normal appendix than to risk perforation and peritonitis.

CRYPTORCHIDISM

Nondescent of the testes into the scrotum is noted in approximately 30% of the premature and 3% of the full-term infants at birth. In most instances, complete descent takes place within 3 months after birth in the former and within 6 weeks in the latter. After infancy, spontaneous descent is extremely rare before puberty. In some children, descent will take place at the time of puberty. Controversy exists concerning the functional status of the testes that descend spontaneously after infancy. The severity of impairment seems to be proportionate to the delay in the descent. Infertility is the rule in those with untreated bilateral cryptorchidism past puberty. Bilateral nondescent occurs in about 20% of cases. When unilateral, it is more common on the right than on the left.

In a small percentage of children, cryptorchidism is associated with significant urinary tract abnormalities. Incidence of torsion and malignancy is more common in the undescended than in the normal testicle. Orchidopexy performed early, may reduce the incidence of malignancy.

Early changes are detectable by electron microscopy at 2
years of age. For this reason, surgical correction should be
undertaken before the age of 2 years.

In the diagnosis of cryptorchidism, care must be taken to
differentiate the condition from retractile testicles. In the
latter situation, the hyperactive cremasteric reflex causes
the testicles that are normally present in the scrotum to
retract into the inguinal canal or within the abdomen. By
careful manipulation, it is possible to bring the testes down
into the scrotum.

The pathogenesis of nondescent is not entirely clear.
Gonadotrophic hormonal deficiencies, anatomical obstruction in the pathway of descent, and genetic factors are all
postulated as possible causative factors. Cryptorchidism
may also be attributed to testicular dysgenesis. Whether or
not the dysgenesis is primary or secondary to maldescent
is difficult to determine.

The treatment of choice is surgical. Orchidopexy is best
carried out before 2 years of age. Controversy exists concerning trial therapy with gonadotropin to stimulate the
testes to descend before resorting to surgery. Chorionic
gonadotropin in a total dosage up to 10,000 U given in single
doses of 1000 U over a period of 3 weeks is recommended
for the trial therapy. Therapy should not be repeated if the
patient fails to respond. Success has been claimed in 20-30%
of children who receive hormone therapy.

HERNIAS

UMBILICAL HERNIA

Umbilical hernias are the result of a failure of the umbilical
ring to close. They are often associated with diastasis recti.
Umbilical hernias occur in all races but are particularly common in blacks. The hernia consists of a soft swelling covered
by skin which may contain omentum or portions of the small
intestines. The hernia may only appear with crying, straining,
or coughing. It is easily reduced by applying gentle pressure.
The fibrous ring outlining the defect may vary from less than
a centimeter to as large as 5 or 6 centimeters.

Practical Points

1. Nearly all umbilical hernias close off during the first 6 years of life.
2. Strangulation is extremely rare.
3. Temporary taping may be indicated when the baby has a cold and cough. Taping does not influence the rate of resolution.
4. When taping is attempted, the hernia should be reduced and the adjacent areas of the abdominal wall brought together and then taped.
5. Avoidance of surgery should be mandatory unless the hernia persists after 5 or 6 years of age, causes symptoms, becomes strangulated (very rare), or becomes progressively larger after the age of 2 years.

EPIGASTRIC HERNIA

These hernias occur in the midline between the lower end of the sternum and the umbilicus. They are not common. When they do occur, they are much the same as umbilical hernias but generally require surgical correction.

CONGENITAL OMPHALOCELE

An omphalocele is a herniation or protrusion of abdominal contents into the base of the umbilical cord. The sac is covered only with peritoneum without overlying skin. This type of hernia occurs in about 1/5000 births. Other less obvious intestinal or abdominal defects may be associated.

Immediate surgical repair before infecton has occurred and before drying of the tissues has taken place is considered essential for survival of the infant.

INGUINAL HERNIA

The vast majority of inguinal hernias are of the indirect rather than the direct type. They occur more frequently in boys than in girls. The hernias may be present at birth or may appear at any age and are found more frequently in children with other birth defects as well as prematures. They are more often seen on the right side (55%) than the left (30%) and, not infrequently, are bilateral (15%).

Although the hernial sacs are present at birth, usually the hernia is not observed until 3-4 months of age. There are no symptoms associated with the empty hernia sac. When peritoneal fluid or an abdominal organ is forced into the sac, it appears as a bulge in the inguinal area extending into the scrotum or the labia. There still may be an absence of symptoms, or there may be symptoms of incomplete intestinal obstruction such as fretfulness, difficult defecation, and poor eating. If a loop of intestine becomes incarcerated in the sac, all the signs and symptoms of intestinal obstruction occur, ultimately leading to strangulation of the bowel and death.

Practical Points

1. In female infants, the ovary may prolapse into the hernial sac, appearing as a 1-2-cm, freely movable, nontender, inguinal mass. Immediate surgical exploration and replacement of the ovary is indicated.
2. In small infants, the history of the intermittent appearance of a bulge may be the only basis for the diagnosis of a hernia.
3. Confirmatory signs of an empty hernia sac are a thickened spermatic cord on the involved side and the "silk glove" sensation which occurs when the two sides of the sac are rubbed together.
4. The hernia sac should be moved as soon as the diagnosis is made to prevent an incarceration at a later time.
5. The hernia can usually be distinguished from a hydrocele by transillumination. A hernia is usually opaque to transmitted light whereas the hydrocele is translucent.
6. The hernia is usually reducible, the hydrocele is usually not.
7. The treatment of inguinal hernia in infants and children is by surgical repair as soon as the defect is diagnosed.
8. Trusses and injection of sclerosing agents are not indicated under any circumstances.
9. Even in the high-risk surgical patient (such as the child with congenital heart disease) hernia repair can be safely carried out with optimal preparation, high-quality anesthesia, and surgery.

10. Incarceration of inguinal hernias is common in infancy, although it is unlikely to occur in hernias that are not immediately detectable on physical examination. Attempts to reduce the hernia under sedation are often successful. Elective hernioorhaphy should then be carried out when the infant is in good condition and the edema of the hernia sac has subsided.
11. In children with hernias, < 2 years, 60–70% have bilateral ones. Some surgeons prefer bilateral repair in this age group even when no obvious hernia is found on physical examination.

HYDROCELE

The common type of noncommunicating hydrocele forms an oval, tense, translucent mass, and the spermatic cord and ring can generally be palpated above it. The fluid gradually absorbs during the first year of life. Surgical correction, therefore, is not indicated.

Communicating hydrocele is difficult to distinguish from an inguinal hernia. Indeed, a hernia is often also present. The appearance of a hydrocele some time after birth is evidence of a persistent processus vaginalis and, therefore, should be extirpated by the inguinal route and the hernia sac removed.

DIAPHRAGMATIC HERNIA

The majority of these hernias are congenital in origin. Herniation of the abdominal contents into the thoracic cavity may result in severe respiratory distress and constitutes a medical-surgical emergency in the neonatal period, especially if symptoms occur within 24 hours of birth (mortality = 40–70%). Other symptoms present shortly after birth or later include vomiting, colicky pain, constipation, and dyspnea.

Practical Points

1. With extensive herniation, the abdomen is small and scaphoid.
2. The infant is cyanotic in such cases and has obvious respiratory distress.

3. Signs and symptoms of intestinal obstruction also may be present.
4. Occasionally, sounds of peristaltic movements can be heard over the chest.
5. The diagnosis is usually established by a plain x-ray of the chest which reveals fluid and air-filled loops of intestine which resemble cysts.

The newborn infant, with a diagnosis of diaphragmatic hernia, who is in respiratory distress should receive oxygen. The infant should be positioned with the head and chest higher than the abdomen to encourage the downward displacement of the abdominal organs. Emergency surgical correction is indicated in most cases.

CUTANEOUS HEMANGIOMAS

1. The vast majority of hemangiomas (98%) involute spontaneously and do not require specific therapy.
2. Parents seek treatment for these lesions and must be skillfully counselled and reassured.
3. The need for treatment is rare and should generally be reserved for:
   a) An alarming rate of growth (triples or quadruples in size within a few weeks)
   b) Giant hemangioma with thrombocytopenia
   c) Encroachment of the hemangioma into vital tissues such as the orbital cavity, eyelids, nares, or the ear
   d) Ulceration and superinfection
4. When therapy is indicated, oral corticosteroids and/or surgery should be considered carefully by an experienced specialist.
5. Irradiation of hemangiomas in children is contraindicated because of the dangers of irradiation and because time alone may resolve the problem.

CIRCUMCISION

1. There is no medical justification for performing circumcision routinely at birth.
2. Extreme phimosis with or without balanoposthitis and the occurrence of paraphimosis constitute indications for circumcision.

3. Although the lowered incident of carcinoma of the penis is noted among men who underwent circumcision in infancy, a direct relationship has not been established.

TONSILLECTOMY AND ADENOIDECTOMY

1. Although morbidity and mortality following tonsillectomy and adenoidectomy are relatively small, it must be remembered that approximately 300 deaths per year are attributed to tonsil and adenoid surgery.
2. Although the indications for tonsillectomy and adenoidectomy have been considerably reduced during the past several years, thousands of children still undergo the procedure needlessly each year.
3. The indications for the removal of tonsils and adenoids are different. Adenoids need not be routinely removed at the time of tonsillectomy and vice versa.
   The five indications for tonsillectomy are:
   a) Chronically enlarged tonsils causing mechanical interference with normal breathing, particularly if cor pulmonale develops
   b) Peritonsillar and retropharyngeal abscess formation
   c) Malignancy of the tonsils
   d) Peripheral sleep apnea syndrome secondary to hypertrophy
   e) Multiple episodes of streptococcal tonsillitis ($\geq$ 7 in 12 months)
4. Repeated attacks of acute otitis media related to infected, hypertrophied adenoids constitute an indication for adenoidectomy.
5. Tonsillectomy should not be performed on children who have not been adequately immunized against poliomyelitis.

TONGUE-TIE

It is only rarely necessary to clip the frenulum in children who are tongue-tied. If sufficient mobility of the tongue exists to permit the child to touch the inner surfaces of his superior central incisors, then speech will not be impaired. If the child has a speech impediment, other causes should be searched for.

MENINGOCELE

1. Newborns with meningoceles that are well covered with skin will need eventual closure of the meningocele sac. This may be delayed until the third month of life when the presence of neurological symptoms and particularly hydrocephalus can be better ascertained.
2. When spinal cord and/or meninges are present in the sac, this is referred to as meningomyelocele. Neurological symptoms are to be expected and an associated hydrocephalus is frequently present. Surgery is generally indicated immediately after birth.

NECK LUMP

Several conditions producing a lump in the neck must be distinguished clearly from each other. Cervical lymphadenopathy, branchial cleft cysts, thyroglossal duct cysts, cystic hygromas, and hemorrhage or fibrosis of the sternocleidomastoid muscle must be differentiated:

1. Branchial cleft cysts are usually located laterally on the neck anywhere from the supraclavicular area to the level of the hyoid bone. They are firm and, unless infected, painless.
2. Cystic hygromas also are located on the side of the neck but they are usually larger and have a soft cystic feel.
3. Thyroglossal duct cysts are found between the thyroid gland and the foramen cecum along the anterior midline of the neck. These cysts may be adherent to the overlying skin, are firm, and tend to move upward when the child swallows. Occasionally, they become infected causing pain and swelling.
4. Hemorrhage and fibrosis of the sternocleidomastoid muscle produce a nodular swelling in the body of the muscle. As the muscle contracts, the location of the mass will be distinguished. Torticollis may result when the fibrotic area contracts, shortening the muscle.
5. Treatment of thyroglossal duct cyst, cystic hygroma, and branchial cleft cyst is elective surgical removal of the cyst and any associated tracts. When infection occurs, appropriate antibiotic therapy, incision and drainage, and later, corrective surgery is indicated.

Chapter 10

EMERGENCY CARE

CARDIAC ARREST

A variety of clinical conditions can lead to cardiac arrest. The usual implication of the term cardiac arrest is that of an unexpected, abrupt cessation of respiratory and circulatory efforts. Unlike the arrest that occurs in a child with a terminal illness for whom everything possible has been done, the child with an abrupt arrest is often salvageable. Abrupt or unexpected cardiac arrest may occur in a variety of circumstances. Table 10-1 lists some common ones.

During cardiac arrest, insufficient oxygen is supplied to the body tissues. As a consequence, anaerobic metabolism occurs leading to a rapid increase in organic acids and the development of metabolic acidosis. One of the effects of this is to displace potassium ions from within the cells to the extracellular compartment giving rise to hyperkalemia. The net effect is a rapidly worsening state of:

Hypoxia (paO_2 decreased)
Metabolic acidosis (pCO_2 increased)
$\qquad\qquad$ (base excess decreased)
$\qquad\qquad$ (blood pH decreased)
Hyperkalemia (serum K increased)

Table 10-1   Conditions Leading to Cardiac Arrest

Anaphylaxis

During anesthesia

During overdose and other types of poisoning

Myocarditis

Increased intracranial pressure (plumbism, meningitis)

Accidental drowning, smoke inhalation

Severe trauma

Electrocution

Cerebrovascular accidents

Transfusion reactions and other hemolytic processes

Sequestration crisis in sickle cell disease

Acute blood loss

Aortic stenosis

Severe respiratory disease

Hyperkalemia, hypocalcemia

The effect of severe acidosis on the heart (particularly the SA node) is to cause it to be refractory to stimulation, thus making it more difficult to reestablish spontaneous heart beats. In addition, an increased serum potassium level will prevent the heart from contracting. The other major organ most affected by this set of circumstances is the brain. Neurons are extremely sensitive to oxygen lack, irreversible damage occurring to them in a matter of a few minutes.

This altered physiology dictates the goals of therapy which are to:

1. Reestablish ventilation (O_2 supply and CO_2 elimination)
2. Reestablish circulation (carry O_2 to the heart and brain and bring away CO_2 and organic acids)

3. Combat metabolic acidosis (reestablish normal myocardial receptivity)
4. Counter hyperkalemia (reestablish normal myocardial contractility)

METHODS (SEE TABLE 10-2)

The immediate steps are:

1. Quickly clear the airway.
2. Insufflate the lungs once or twice.
3. Initiate external cardiac massage.
4. Coordinate cardiac massage with ventilatory assistance (four to five cardiac compressions to every respiration). Both cardiac compression and pulmonary insufflation cannot be allowed to occur simulatneously without damaging vital structures.
5. Establish a rate for cardiac massage at three-fourths the patient's normal heart rate.
6. Obtain assistance, but not by leaving the patient or suspending the resuscitative effort.
7. When assistance is available, start an IV infusion and/or cut down without interrupting the ongoing resuscitation.
8. Administer oxygen.
9. Administer $7\frac{1}{2}$% sodium bicarbonate, 1 mEq/kg IV dose (1 ml = 1 mEq).
10. While this is being done, have an electrocardiographic monitor attached to the patient.
11. Dopamine or isoproterenol can be administered to provide assistance. Each exerts a positive inotropic and chronotropic effect. Dopamine provides an increase in total peripheral resistance, thereby elevating blood pressure. Isoproterenol elevates blood pressure by increasing cardiac output. This effect exceeds the action of both drugs in lowering the total peripheral resistance. Isoproterenol is contraindicated in head trauma.
12. If steps 9 and 11 are unsuccessful, repeat them. Sodium bicarbonate may be repeated every 8 minutes for no more than five doses. More than this will lead to hypernatremia and THAM should be used instead.
13. Treat hyperkalemia if the typical ECG pattern (prolonged PR interval, tall T waves) is seen.

Table 10-2 Life Support Drugs

Oxygen
 Initial dose at onset of CPR is 100%. Afterward as
 dictated clinically and by arterial blood gases

Sodium bicarbonate
 1 mEq/kg IV initially, then q 10-15 minutes or as
 determined by arterial blood gases

Epinephrine
 (1/10,000) 10 mg/kg IV or 1 cc intratracheally

Atropine
 0.01 mg/kg IV, minimum dose 0.20 mg q 5-10 minutes
 to a maximum total of 2.0 mg

Calcium chloride
 10 mg/kg IV

Calcium gluconate
 30 mg/kg IV

Naloxane
 0.01 mg/kg IV

Glucose
 1.0 g/kg IV

Furosemide
 1-2 mg/kg IV

Lidocaine
 1 mg/kg IV q 5 minutes for a total of four times.
 Infusion rate 10-20 mg/kg/min

Dopamine
 2-10 mg/kg/min

Isoproterenol
 0.1 mg/kg/min IV

Table 10–2   (Cont'd.)

Bretylium
  5 mg/kg IV   followed by defibrillation; if unsuccessful,
  10 mg/kg IV   followed by defibrillation

Defibrillation current
  2-4 watt–sec/kg lower dose initially

---

a) Give calcium gluconate to the older adolescent or
adult, 100 mg/kg/dose by slow IV push, monitoring
the heart rate so that bradycardia is avoided. Administer glucose and insulin, 1 g glucose/kg/dose with
1 U of regular insulin added for each 3 g of glucose
(50 ml of a 50% glucose solution with 8 U of regular
insulin should be kept ready in the refrigerator).
14. The young child will correct hyperkalemia with an IV infusion of glucose. If ventricular fibrillation or other arrhythmias occur, be prepared to treat them with defibrillation. Lidocaine as a bolus frequently corrects ventricular ectopic beats or fibrillation. Bretylium prior to
electrical defibrillation is also effective. Defibrillation
current is initially 2 watt–sec/kg and in subsequent dosages is offered at 4 watt–sec/kg. If a spontaneous heart
beat is obtained and remains fairly stable, the child may
be accompanied to an intensive care area where hypothermia, mechanically associated ventilation, and careful monitoring can be established.

BURNS

Adequate immediate treatment of extensive second- and
third-degree burns has been shown to reduce mortality and
disfigurement significantly. As an example, a burn of 50%
of the body surface has an overall mortality of about 50%
but in the better burn centers in this country, the mortality
is as low as 5%. Prognosis and therapy depend on three
basic factors:

Extent and degree of burns
Age and general health of the patient
Cause of the burn injury, i.e., thermal, electrical, or
    chemical

EXTENT AND DEGREE OF BURNS

1. First-degree burns: Erythematous areas without blisters
   or areas of induration. Pain is exquisite. Healing is
   rapid.
2. Second-degree burns: Blistering and peeling occur with
   some induration and pain on touch.
3. Third-degree burns: Indurated and leathery. Not painful
   to light touch (nerve endings are destroyed).
4. The extent of the burned area is estimated by the Rule of
   Nines (See Figure 10-1).

First-degree burns are not associated with significant degree of fluid loss and mortality is not a factor. Second- and
third-degree burns are potentially life-threatening when 20%
or more of the body surface has been burned. The mortality
is 50% when 50-60% of the body is involved.

AGE AND GENERAL STATE OF THE VICTIM

Mortality increases at both ends of the age scale. Children
under 14 years and adults over 50 years have a measurably
higher mortality risk. The state of the patient's health is of
great importance. Where extensive injuries are present, in
addition to the burn, the mortality rate can be expected to
increase.

CHEMICAL AND ELECTRICAL BURNS

1. The outcome of therapy in chemical burns depends on
   immediate treatment. Duration of exposure to the
   chemical is the crucial factor. Adequate washing of the
   exposed area with copious amounts of water is necessary.
   In lye burns of the eyes, for example, washing must begin
   within minutes and 2 or more liters of water used to flush
   each eye if corneal damage is to be minimized.
2. Electrical burns, unlike thermal or chemical burns, may
   affect cerebral centers and the cardiac pacemaker. In

B U R N S

Estimate per cent of body surface involved using the following "Rule of Nines."

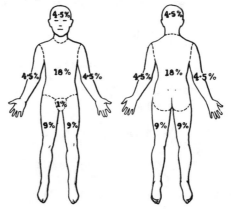

The Rule of Nines

These may have to be modified according to the patient's age in the following manner.

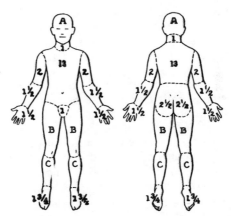

Relative percentage of areas affected by growth (After Lund and Browder.)

Age in years:	0	1	5	10	15	Adult
A=1/2 of head	9-1/2	8-1/2	6-1/2	5-1/2	4-1/2	3-1/2
B=1/2 of thigh	2-3/4	3-1/4	4	4-1/4	4-1/2	4-3/4
C=1/2 of l leg	2-1/2	2-1/2	2-3/4	3	3-1/4	3-1/2

Figure 10-1

the case of cardiac standstill, resuscitative efforts should not be quickly abandoned. Case reports of successful resuscitation after periods of 90 minutes or longer are on record. Estimating the extent of injury in electrical burns is difficult because most of the damage is internal rather than superficial. Forty-eight hours or so after the injury, the underlying muscle should be tested for signs of viability. The patient should be under close supervision for 3 weeks. Electrical burns can cause a gradual necrobiosis extending the burn site and predisposing the patient to sudden hemorrhage.

THERAPY OF BURNS

Second- and third-degree burns may be life-threatening. If more than 10% of the body surface area is involved, the patient should be admitted for hospital care.

1. Immediate therapy includes:
   a) Cold water soaks
   b) Intravenous fluids. Use sodium salt-containing fluid with sufficient base to correct metabolic acidosis. Ringer's lactate is usually adequate. Renal output should be maintained at 40 ml/m^2/hr (1 ml/kg/hr). Ringer's lactate is given at 4 ml/percent burn/kg over 24 hours. Half of the volume is given in the first 8 hours.
   c) Fluid intake by mouth should be no more than small sips since vomiting may occur due to ileus.
   d) Local therapy to the burn area:
      (1) Debridement of dead tissue
      (2) Cleansing - daily with mild surgical soap
      (3) Topical antimicrobial dressing - sulfadiazine cream 1% bid, sulfamylon, and silver nitrate soaks. Sulfadiazine is the drug of choice.
2. Systemic antibiotics initiated if signs of sepsis occur. Early signs of sepsis include:
   a) Tachypnea
   b) Ileus
   c) Disorientation
   d) Fever
   e) Infected appearance to wound
   f) Elevated WBC count
   g) Platelet decrease

3. Penicillin and gentamycin (4 mg/kg/24 hr) are used. The most common infecting organism is streptococcus. Insure a warm environment with radiant heat to prevent chilling from increased heat loss through damaged skin.
4. Maintain the osmotic pressure of blood by keeping the serum albumin at 2 g or more. Albumin may be administered IV, 1 g/kg/24 hr.
5. Maintain the hemoglobin level at 10 g or better with blood transfusions.
6. Maintain nutrition and a stable weight. After the first 2-3 days, ileus is less common and mild feedings between meals may be given as tolerated. Intravenous hyperalimentation is indicated for the child who cannot maintain his weight by an oral intake.
7. Give multivitamins and trace minerals, zinc, etc.
8. Tetanus toxoid booster dose or tetanus antitoxin (human).
9. Tracheostomy for severe pulmonary burns and/or smoke inhalation.
10. Analgesics but not narcotics like morphine and barbiturates because of their antiduretic effect.
11. Splint involved joints to prevent contractures.
12. Pressure dressings to prevent scarring.
13. Later therapy includes:
    a) Skin grafting
    b) Physical therapy
    c) Psychotherapy for depression resulting from disfigurement and/or disability.
14. Complications: Many possible complications may occur. Some of these are:
    a) Infecton - local or systemic, bacterial or fungal
    b) Shock and renal failure
    c) Pulmonary edema, bronchitis, pneumonia
    d) Ileus, Curling's ulcer
    e) Heart failure with fluid overload
    f) Anemia
    g) Contractures and disfigurement

SMOKE INHALATION, ACCIDENTAL DROWNING, CARBON MONOXIDE POISONING

The therapy of accidental drowning, carbon monoxide poisoning, and smoke inhalation is not very different from that of cardiac arrest except that pulmonary function may be seriously compromised. In these instances, oxygen should be employed. In the case of smoke inhalation or carbon monoxide poisoning, Solumedrol, bronchoscopy, and irrigation of the major bronchi with saline solution are indicated. Purulent bronchitis secondary to the irritation caused by carbon particles may be avoided this way. Antibiotics are given for secondary bronchial or pulmonary infecton.

SHOCK

Acute blood loss, sepsis, severe respiratory or cardiac disease, overdosage of medications, severe renal disease such as the hemolytic uremic syndrome, etc. may lead to shock in children. Shock is an unfavorable complication of widely diverse disease processes. The physiological aberration characteristic of shock, regardless of etiology, is poor tissue perfusion and, therefore, failing cellular function. This leads to the following changes:

1. Build-up of organic acids
2. Loss of tone in the precapillary sphincters and splanchnic pooling of blood
3. A vicious cycle of increasingly poor perfusion leading to increasing loss of precapillary sphincter tone, greater splanchnic pooling and, therefore, still worse perfusion

Toxins as found in endotoxic shock are suspected of playing a role in anaphylactic shock.

Clinical manifestations include pallor, cyanosis, cold clammy skin, agitation or lethargy, tachycardia, hypotension, and oliguria. Signs of infection, dehydration, or hemorrhage may be associated findings.

HELPFUL CLINICAL AND LABORATORY TESTS

1. Central venous pressure decreased
2. Arterial pressure decreased
3. Heart rate increased
4. Blood gases – pH decreased
   base excess decreased
   pCO_2 decreased or increased
   pO_2 decreased

5. Urine output decreased
6. Chest x-ray - pulmonary vascular markings increased or frank pulmonary edema
7. Body weight - increased (edema)
8. Cultures - to identify a bacterial pathogen
9. Electrolytes
10. BUN, glucose, CBC, ammonia (Reyes syndrome)
11. Coagulation tests (clotting time, platelet retraction time, fibrinogen, fibrin split products, prothrombin, partial thromboplastin time, and factor V)
12. Cardiac output and plasma volume
13. Serum enzymes (SGOT, SGPT, LDH)

THERAPY OF SHOCK

1. Manage the primary disease.
2. Insure an adequate airway and good ventilation. Tracheal intubation or tracheostomy may be required as well as mechanically assisted ventilation.
3. If central venous pressure is high while inadequate tissue perfusion exists:
   a) Digitalize the patient
   b) Give antiarrhythmic drugs if needed
   c) Administer oxygen
   d) Correct acidosis with sodium bicarbonate or THAM (see p. 201).
   e) Administer cardiac inotropic and chronotropic agents (see p. 221).
4. If decreased venous pressure is present (hypovolemic shock), expand circulating volume. If water and salt alone have been lost, replace with water and electrolyte solution. If bood has been lost acutely, replace with whole blood. If blood loss has occurred over a long period of time, replace with packed red cells. If fluid has been lost because of decreased osmotic pressure, give plasma expanders like albumin, dextran, or plasma.
5. If low urinary output and the threat of renal shutdown occur, but no hypovolemia exists, mannitol may be used.
6. If disseminated intravascular coagulation is present:
   a) Heparin may be useful
   b) Replacement therapy with whole blood or clotting factors, platelets, etc.

Practical Points

1. Steroid levels in patients in shock are generally found to be elevated. The use of a very high dose of steroids in animals has a beneficial effect which is felt to be pharmacological rather than physiological. Although the role of steroids in treating human shock is still not fully understood, some evidence exists that it results in a lower mortality. The recommendation has been made to use dexamethasone 1.5-3.0 mg/kg/24 hr. It should be used with great caution in the presence of bacterial infection. Methylprednisolone 30 mg/kg is an acceptable alternative drug.
2. Vasoconstrictive drugs, formerly enjoying a major role in the therapy of shock, have now been relegated to a secondary position. Their use is restricted to instances of abrupt hypotension to avoid cardiac arrest. They should be used temporarily and never where poor perfusion is suspected.

ANAPHYLAXIS

Anaphylaxis is an immune phenomenon involving an antigen-antibody reaction in a sensitized individual with release of chemical mediators and the abrupt development of severe, life-threatening symptoms. The anaphylactic reaction, unlike the allergic reaction, does not depend on a host with a genetic predisposition to developing allergic symptoms. Anaphylaxis can be provoked in any host with a challenge by a suitable antigen (foreign protein).

   Anaphylactic reactions occur most often with the parenteral administration of medications, particularly penicillin, horse serum antitoxins (tetanus and diphtheria), allergens given in the course of allergy testing or hyposensitization, and anesthetics. Symptoms are immediate within seconds or minutes, but may occur after some hours. Conjunctival itching and tearing, nasal congestion, sneezing, cough, wheezing, and dyspnea characterize the initial symptoms. Within a very short time, increasing dyspnea, tachycardia, vomiting, angioedema, stridor, cyanosis, and cardiovascular collapse may occur. The mortality rate is very high unless therapy is rapidly instituted.

TREATMENT

1. If the antigen has been injected in an extremity, place a tourniquet proximal to the injection site.
2. Inject 1-1000 epinephrine 0.5 ml in one of the other limbs and 0.2 ml in the antigen-injection site distal to the tourniquet.
3. Inject Benadryl 1 mg/kg IM.
4. Begin an IV infusion (preferably a cut down if the patient does not improve quickly).
5. Maintain an adequate airway. If laryngeal edema (stridor) occurs, intubate or perform a tracheostomy.
6. Give oxygen if cyanosis occurs.
7. Support cardiovascular function if hypotension occurs by:
   a) Vasopressors (Aramine 0.5 to 1.0 mg by slow IV drip, or Levophed 1 ml of 0.2% solution in 250 cc of glucose and water by slow IV drip).
   b) Cardiac massage if arrest occurs (see p. 221).
8. Give aminophylline 4 mg/kg/20 min maximum 15 mg/kg/24 hr by slow IV drip.
9. Administer Solu-Cortef 100 mg IM (effective for long-term rather than immediate effect (2-6 hours required for response).
10. Admit patient for further care and/or observation if reaction has been more than mild.
11. Continue glucocorticoids and evaluate renal status over several days to insure adequate function.

SUDDEN INFANT DEATH SYNDROME (SIDS)

These unexpected and unexplainable deaths occurring in infancy have yet to be understood. The problem occurs in 2 infants of every 1000 live births in all socioeconomic groups in the United States although there is a higher incidence reported in lower income populations. Males outnumber females 2:1 and the peak age of incidence is 8-16 weeks. Infants of low birth weight who had perinatal difficulty, particularly respiratory, are at greater risk as are infants of mothers who smoke cigarettes.

Therapy is directed toward the parents. Alleviation of guilt feelings is a cornerstone of management. The physician and possibly a sympathetic nurse or clergyman must spend time reassuring the parents that the death of their child was not through their negligence. Parent groups have been developed in some communities to provide peer support.

An occasional aborted sudden infant death occurs where resuscitative measures are successful. In these instances, long-term ($\geq$ 12 months) infant monitoring at home may be attempted. Cardiac and respiratory monitoring equipment with both visual and auditory alarms is available for purchase and/or rental. The parents will need to be instructed in the use of the equipment and in basic cardiopulmonary resuscitation. It is helpful to alert the local rescue squad to assist whenever needed. It is difficult to know when to terminate home monitoring since SIDS has been reported into the second year of life.

Chapter 11

ACCIDENTAL POISONING

More than 300 preschool children die from poisoning every year in the USA and more than 2,000,000 people are estimated to be poisoned annually. (See Table 11-1).

Table 11-1 Morbidity and Mortality of Acute Poisoning

Estimated 2,000,000 nonfatal poisonings annually in the United States

Number of deaths annually in United States = 2000

Number of deaths annually in children less than 5 years old = 300-400

Peak age incidence for accidental poisoning = 2 years

Most of the research applied to this field has been directed toward determining the effects of the poisoning agent. Relatively little attention has been given to environmental and host factors. Significant environmental factors include the type and quantity of potentially harmful substances kept in the home, the way in which this material is stored, the degree of emotional stress present, and the amount of supervision the child receives. Important host factors include the child's age and personality.

The poisoning agents implicated most often are medications (45%) particularly analgesics, household preparations, bleach, detergents, polishing agents, caustics, cosmetics, and insecticides.

The group at highest risk is the preschool-age child. Boys outnumber girls by 3:2 and an increased incidence is found in the lower socioeconomic group.

The age factor greatly influences the type of poison ingested. Children from 1 to 2 years tend to ingest household preparations stored at an accessibly low level while medications usually kept in higher places are encountered more often in 2-4 year olds capable of climbing. (See Table 11-2.)

Table 11-2 Most Common Poisons

Age	
1 year	Parent-administered items (overdosage of medication-ASA)
1-3 years	Household products stored close to ground (detergents, bleaches, corrosives)
3-5 years	Products stored in cabinet areas (medications)

Diagnosis may be difficult when an adequate history is lacking. Many helpful symptoms and signs exist and particular attention should be paid to odors, the patient's sensorium, the pupils, and the respiratory and circulatory systems. A careful scrutiny should be made of body fluids including the vomitus, urine, and blood for possible clues as to the nature of the poison. The ferric chloride test is a very useful laboratory procedure for this purpose. (See Table 11-3.) Bizarre or not readily explainable symptomatology should cause one to think of the possibillity of poisoning.

BASIC STEPS IN MANAGING THE ACUTE INGESTION

1. Identify the poison
2. Estimate the quantity ingested
3. Remove and/or neutralize the poison
4. Monitor and support life function

IDENTIFICATION OF POISONS

1. If container is available, simply read the label. For a pharmacy-dispensed item, call the pharmacy.
2. If container is unavailable and if at home, send someone for it. If no container exists but tablets or capsules are available, consult the product identification section of the PDR. Call Poison Control Center.
3. If, after identifying the poison, you are unfamiliar with it, call Poison Control Center for advice. Consult one of the recognized references.

Table 11-3 Ferric Chloride Test

	Urine Color
Salicylates	Purple to reddish purple (Resistant to heat)
Ketones	Purple to reddish purple (Disappears with heating)
Phenothiazines	Lilac-violet color (Purple with compazine)
INH	Gray to green
Phenylketones	Green
Imidazolepyruvic acid (histidinemia)	Green – fades within 30 seconds
Maple sugar urine disease	Green – fades within 30 seconds

Table 11-3 (Cont'd.) Ferric Chloride Test

	Urine Color
Homogentisic acid, bile	Green - fades within 1-2 seconds
Catecholamines (pheochromocytoma)	Green
Malignant melanoma	Green

ESTIMATION OF THE QUANTITY INGESTED

1. Pills: add the number used previously and the remaining pills; subtract from the original quantity. Remember to subtract any intact pills recovered from the patient subsequently.
2. Liquids: estimate as for pills. Less reliable. (Average swallow volume is 0.21 ml/kg or approximately 4-5 ml for a 2-year-old.)

REMOVAL AND/OR NEUTRALIZATION OF THE POISON

1. Removal:
   a) Syrup of ipecac
   Dose - 15 ml po repeated in 20 minutes x 1, if no vomiting occurs
   200 ml of saline given by mouth after ipecac
   Efficacy - 90-99%
   Average time emesis - 17-18 minutes
   b) Apomorphine
   Dose - 0.07 mg/lb
   Efficacy - virtually 100%
   Average time emesis - 5 minutes
   Naloxone given afterwards to counteract sedative action 0.01 mg/kg

   c) Gastric lavage
   Less effective recovery of poisons than above two
   methods. Indicated for:
   (1) Unconscious patients
   (2) Ingestion of lethal amounts of petroleum distillates
         only (use cuffed nasogastric tube)
   d) Purgatives and enemas
   Magnesium sulfate
   Milk of magnesia
   Oily purgatives (castor oil, mineral oil) should not be
   used to avoid aspiration pneumonia
   e) Increasing urinary excretion. Urine may be acidified
   or alkalinized to increase excretion of poisons
   f) Peritoneal dialysis (see Table 11-4)
   g) Renal dialysis
   h) Exchange transfusion
2. Neutralization:
   a) Specific antidotes (see Table 11-5)
   b) Activated charcoal (Merck) or Nurit A, Nuchar. (These
   are the best products.) Do not give together with
   ipecac since it will be absorbed. The dose of charcoal
   should be no less than five times the estimated dose
   of the poison. Ten times the dose has been proven to
   be effective. Optimal time of administration is within
   30 minutes of ingestion. Effective up to 2 hours after
   ingestion. Little dissociation is known to occur in the GI
   tract. Not effective for ethyl and methyl alcohol,
   caustic alkalis, mineral acids. Activated charcoal is
   effective for
      Aspirin
      Barbiturates
      Chloroquine
      Chlorpheniramine
      Chlorpromazine (Thorazine)
      Glutethimide (Doriden)
      Kerosene
      Propoxyphene (Darvon)
      Strychnine
      Tylenol (acetaminophen)

Table 11-4   Peritoneal Dialysis

Useful for alcohols	Ethanol	Heavy metals
	Methanol	INH
	Isopropanol	Bromides
	Boric acid	Amphetamines
	Aspirin	

Less useful for barbiturates (poor peritoneal clearance)

Not useful for:

Compounds strongly bound to tissues:

Antidepressants	Most tranquilizers
Most hallucinogens	(phenothiazines)
Most antihistamines	Dibenzodiazepines
	like Librium
	Carbamates like
	Miltown

Useful also to correct:

Severe acid-base imbalance
Electrolyte abnormalities
Fluid deficit or overload
Abnormal renal function

MONITORING AND SUPPORT OF LIFE FUNCTIONS

1. Cardiovascular: Heart rate and rhythm, blood pressure, electrocardiogram, central venous pressure
2. Renal: Urinary output, concentration, glomerular and tubular functions
3. Respiratory: Rate, adequacy of air exchange, intubation, respirator, O_2
4. Multiple systems: Acid-base balance (blood gases, pCO_2, pO_2, blood pH, urine pH), serum electrolytes, hydration, body temperature, pain

5. Hematological: CBC, clotting ability
6. Liver: Liver function tests
7. CNS: Convulsions, coma, hyperactivity

SPECIFIC POISONS

ACUTE SALICYLATE POISONING

1. Symptoms: Anorexia, fever, vomiting
   a) Early (few hours postingestion): Sweating, flushed
      skin, hyperventilation
   b) Dehydration, sensorium changes (delirium, hallucina-
      ations), convulsions, coma, pulmonary edema
2. Laboratory findings: Plasma bicarbonate decreased, negative base excess
   a) Frequent: Plasma pCO_2 decreased, blood pH variable
      (neutral, acid, alkaline, see Table 11-6), reducing sub-
      stances in urine, ketonuria
   b) Occasional: Increased Na (dehydrated patients), gly-
      cosuria, and hyperglycemia
3. Diagnostic study: Serum salicylate level (interpreted by
   Done Nomogram, see Figure 11-1)
4. Toxic dose in acute ingestion: 50 mg/lb of body weight
5. Maximum absorption: 90 minutes
6. Average half-life: 6 hours (90% excreted by kidneys)
7. Management:
   If patient is conscious and alert:
   a) Administer 15 ml syrup of ipecac (effective up to 2
      hours after ingestion, longer if stomach contains food)
   b) Administer 200 ml saline
   c) Administer activated charcoal (10 mg charcoal for
      each 1 mg of salicylate ingested)
   d) Obtain blood for salicylate level

Further therapy depends on severity of poisoning.

1. Asymptomatic patients with serum salicylate level in
   asymptomatic to mild range:
   a) Force fluids by mouth
   b) Observe for 12-24 hours
   c) Counsel parents on poison prevention

Table 11-5 Specific Antidotes

Compound	Antidote
Morphine	Nallorphan
Demerol	Nalline or Naloxone
Methadone, etc.	Levallorphan
Propoxyphene	
Parathion and other organic phosphate esters	Atropine
Parasympathomimetics: philocarpine, muscarine	
Arsenic	BAL
Mercury	Penicillamine
Bismuth	
Antimony	
Gold	
Lead	EDTA and BAL
	Penicillamine
Iron	Deferoxamine
Cyanide	Sodium nitrite
Formaldehyde	Ammonium hydroxide
Methemoglobin	Methylene blue
Iodine	Sodium thiosulfate
Caustic alkali	Weak acids (vinegar, fruit juices)
Strong acids	Weak bases which do not produce CO_2 (MgO, Amphojel, MOM)
Phosphorus	Copper sulfate
Anticoagulants	Vitamin K

Table 11-6   Pathophysiology: Acute Salicylate Poisoning

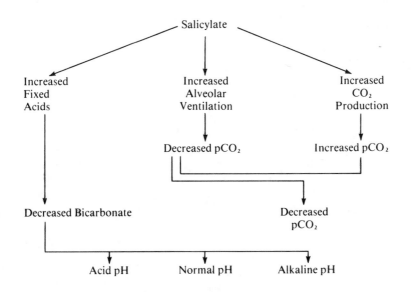

RESULT: Older Children and Adults
            Respiratory pCO_2 decreased
            Alkalosis   Blood pH increased
                                   Serum bicarbonate decreased
                                     (Renal compensation)

            Infants and Younger Children
            Mixed pCO_2 decreased
            Respiratory
            Alkalosis and
            Metabolic   Blood pH variable
            Acidosis   Serum bicarbonate decreased

(Modified from Barnett, H.L.: Pediatrics, 14th ed., Appleton-Century-Crofts, New York, 1968.   Reproduced with publisher's permission.)

POISONING

A. SALICYLATE POISONING

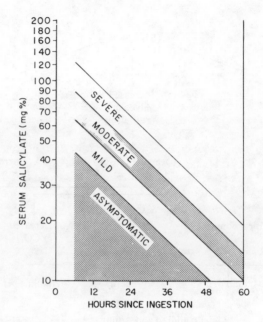

Figure 11-1   Nomogram relating serum salicylate concentration and expected severity of intoxication at varying
intervals following the ingestion of a single dose of
salicylate. (From Done, A.K.: Salicylate intoxication,
Pediatrics 26:800, 1960. Reproduced with permission
of American Academy of Pediatrics, Elk Grove, IL.)

2. Symptomatic patients with serum salicylate level in mild
   to moderate range:
   a) Obtain blood gases and serum electrolytes
   b) Monitor vital signs, intake and output
   c) Start IV fluids and correct dehydration
      (1) Use one-third to one-half isotonic solutions to pro-
          vide extra water for renal excretion.

(2) 3000 ml/m^2 of 5% glucose solution (repletes liver glycogen and provides substrate for Kreb's cycle). Plus KCl 40 mEq/m^2 (after urine flow is established) corrects hypokalemia. Plus sufficient sodium bicarbonate to correct negative base excess.
(3) Acetazolamide (Diamox) 5 mg/kg subcutaneously. Repeat two times at 5-hour intervals to alkalinize the urine. Extreme caution is advised in using Diamox in acidotic or potentially acidotic patients since it does cause an obligatory loss of alkali in the urine and has led to seizures. If acidosis is severe, it is preferable to use sodium bicarbonate.
(4) Monitor urinary pH. Should be 7.5 or greater.
3. Severely symptomatic patients with serum salicylate level in severe range: Patients with:
    Hyperpyrexia
    Poor renal function
    Coma
    Convulsions
    Acute pulmonary edema
    Serum sodium level in severe range
should have exchange transfusion, hemodialysis, or peritoneal dialysis

IRON POISONING

1. Induce emesis
    a) Syrup of ipecac
    b) Apomorphine
2. Partially neutralize ferrous sulfate with sodium bicarbonate given orally (makes ferrous carbonate)
3. Obtain blood for serum iron, TIBC, CO_2, Na, K, Cl, Ca, P, BUN, CBC, type and cross match, pH (if acidotic clinically)
4. Correct acidosis and dehydration if present
5. Combat peripheral vascular collapse
    a) Whole blood transfusion
    b) Plasma or plasma expanders
6. Obtain abdominal flat plate since iron pills are radiopaque
7. Administer deferoxamine for:
    a) Symptomatic patients
    b) Patients known to have ingested dangerous amounts of iron (greater than 500 mg of elemental iron)

c) Serum iron level exceeds TIBC by 50 mg
d) Serum iron level is greater than 500 mg/100 ml
Dose: 90 mg/kg IV in 5% glucose/water over 1-2
hours. Do not exceed a rate of 15 mg/kg/hr.
If urine turns reddish brown give repeat dose in 12
hours by continuous IV. Further doses may be calculated on the basis of serum iron levels. Monitor blood
pressure. Hypotension is chief complication of
deferoxamine therapy
8. Consider peritoneal dialysis if renal function is inadequate
9. Watch for symptoms of gastrointestinal scarring in convalescent period (1-2 months postingestion)

INGESTION OF CAUSTICS

1. Administer weak acid (vinegar acetic acid 2%) or milk
2. Do not induce vomiting or lavage stomach
3. Steroid (methylprednisolone sodium succinate 20 mg, q 12
hr IM, to minimize esophageal scarring)
4. Antibiotic - ampicillin or penicillin to prevent secondary
infection
5. Esophagoscopy to determine extent of esophageal damage.
Must be done as soon as possible, within first 12 hr of ingestion
6. If no esophageal burns are visualized, treatment may be
discontinued
7. Extensive burns may require prolonged therapy (2 weeks)
and esophageal dilation

LEAD POISONING

Lead poisoning is a common manifestation in urban populations in the United States, being particularly prevalent in the
2-5-year-old age group in the lower socioeconomic strata. As
many as 25% of these at-risk children have elevated blood
lead levels. In a child with pica, lead poisoning may be caused
by the ingestion of available lead-containing paint chips and
loose plaster in aging apartments. Inhalation of "lead dust"
and fumes from auto exhaust may also contribute to the lead
burden. The onset of symptoms is insidious. Subtle behavior
changes, irritability, anorexia, and constipation are the symptoms commonly noted. Frequently, no symptoms are manifest until the child is dangerously intoxicated. Then the

presenting picture may consist of convulsions and coma due to lead encephalopathy, even though it usually requires at least 8-12 weeks of continuous intake for the child to have become severely poisoned. The safest way to detect lead poisoning is to screen all at-risk 2-5-year-olds routinely in endemic areas since a history of pica may be absent.

The diagnosis is readily established by laboratory means. the best tests are the blood level and the free erythrocyte protoporphyrin (FEP). Blood lead levels of 0.04 mg% and above are considered abnormally elevated for an urban population. FEP levels > 500 µg/dl are compatible with an increased lead burden and higher than levels found in iron-deficiency anemia. Clinical symptoms may be detected at blood lead levels of 0.06 mg% and above. Considerable variability exists in the correlation of blood lead with symptoms. Children with 0.06 mg% have died while others with levels in excess of 0.1 mg% are symptom-free. Other helpful laboratory tests are:

1. CBC
   a) Normocytic, normochromic anemia
   b) Basophilic stippling
2. Urine - increased coproporphyrins
3. X-ray - radiopaque material in the abdomen and increase in radiodensity at the metaphysis of long bones (may be difficult to interpret)

Treatment consists of the removal of lead from the body and prevention of further poisoning. Prevention requires the avoidance of lead at its source. Houses must be repaired and mothers educated to watch their children for pica.

Specific Therapy

Removal of lead requires therapy with edathamil calcium disodium (EDTA), a chelating agent. After cleansing enemas to remove any lead from the lower intestinal tract, and the assurance from a urinalysis and a BUN that no gross renal impairment exists, EDTA is given IM 50-75 mg/kg/24 hr in four divided doses for 7 days. It is safer and more effective to give BAL 4 mg/kg/dose IM together with EDTA. For levels less than 0.1 mg% one course is usually enough to lower the blood lead level to less than 0.06 mg%. However, higher levels might require two or more courses. In the event a second course is needed, a 2-week period without therapy is observed to minimize the risk of renal toxicity from EDTA. In addition, monitoring the renal function with urinalyses and BUNs is indicated.

Another chelating agent, d-penicillamine, has been shown to be effective as well. It may be used initially in the dose of 100 mg/kg/day orally $1\frac{1}{2}$ hours before meals if there is no evidence of lead in the GI tract and if the blood lead level is 0.8 mg%. This dose should not be continued for more than 5 days. It may then be used on a long-term basis (2-6 months) at a dose of 40 mg/kg/day if the patient can be protected from further lead exposure.

The therapy of lead encephalopathy is aimed at reducing the increased intracranial pressure, controlling seizure activity, and removing lead as safely as possible in addition to supporting life functions.

The method of choice is mannitol 1-2 g/kg of a 20% solution IV at a rate of 1 ml/minute. Before using mannitol, renal output must be reasonably normal. Secondly, hypothermia is induced and the body temperature maintained at 90-92°F. Steroids have been used but may facilitate increased renal damage from the toxic effect of lead. Surgical decompression or removal of spinal fluid to lower CNS pressure is fraught with danger and best avoided. Convulsions are controlled with paraldehyde 0.1 ml/kg IM.

Practical Points

1. Lead can cause renal tubular damage giving rise to a Fanconi-type syndrome of proteinuria and glycosuria. Since EDTA can do likewise, a urinalysis prior to therapy is mandatory. The renal effect of EDTA is usually easily reversible.
2. Cardiac effects of lead poisoning have been described with an altered ECG pattern.
3. Long-term neurological and behavioral sequelae of lead poisoning frequently occur. An inestimable toll of human potential has been exacted in American children from this preventable disease.

ACETAMINOPHEN

The increasing use of acetaminophen preparations has contributed to a rising incidence of overdose with this compound. An essential feature of acetaminophen toxicity is the delay that occurs before signs of serious liver damage become manifest. The saturation of normal conjugation pathways by acetaminophen leads to the gradual accumulation of metabolic intermediaries which combine with liver macromolecules and precipitate liver necrosis.

Clinical Symptoms

Stage I: First 2-24 hours - Gastrointestinal symptoms of anorexia, nausea, and vomiting dominate the early clinical picture. The patient may also appear weak and drowsy, pale, and diaphoretic.

Stage II: 12-36 hours - Improvement may occur to a point of complete recovery. Serum transaminase may rise at this stage.

Stage III: 36 hours to 1 week - Signs and symptoms of liver damage prevail; these include hepatomegaly, liver tenderness, and icterus. The clinical picture may be accompanied by sensorium changes, coma, and clotting disorders. Renal failure also may occur.

Stage IV: 2 days to 3 months - Complete recovery is the rule but it may take many weeks for liver functions to return to normal.

Laboratory Findings

1. The serum transaminase increases at 24 hours and peaks by day 4.
2. Prothrombin time increases (twofold or greater increases indicate a poor prognosis).
3. Serum bilirubin increases (> 4 mg%, also indicates a poor prognosis).
4. Liver biopsy demonstrates focal to complete necrosis.

Prognosis

The prognosis may best be gauged by the amount ingested and the plasma acetaminophen level related to the time of ingestion. Although the minimal toxic amount is not yet known in children, it is approximately 150 mg/kg. In adults, an amount $\geq$ 7.5 g is likely to produce serious liver damage. A plasma acetaminophen level exceeding 200 µg/ml 4 hours after ingestion is indicative of probable future liver damage. Nomograms should be consulted to gauge prognosis.

Treatment

Treatment is still currently being studied. Agents that bind acetaminophen in competition with liver macromolecules are being tried. In the United States, N-acetylcysteine or Mucomyst is the most readily available of the sulfhydryl compounds. Present indications are that early administration (within 10 hours) of Mucomyst may be protective against liver damage. It is best diluted to a 20% solution and then mixed in a 1:4 ratio (Mucomyst to cola) in a cola beverage for oral administration. Use 140 mg/kg as an initial dose; then 70 mg/kg q 4 h for 18 more doses.

In cases identified shortly after ingestion, ipecac-induced gastric emptying followed by the administration of activated charcoal is effective in absorbing acetaminophen within the first 4 or 5 hours. However, if activated charcoal is given, it should be removed before giving oral Mucomyst since it will bind this compound as well.

ACCIDENT PREVENTION

Accidents are the leading cause of death in childhood. Specifically, motor vehicle accidents are, at present, the major cause of childhood and adolescent morbidity and mortality in the United States. (See Table 11-7.)

The nature of accidental injuries is age-related. During the first 1-2 years of life, childhood suffocation and ingestion of foreign objects are the most frequent causes of death. Motor vehicle accidents, burns, and drowning increase in incidence after 1 year of age. Drowning and motor vehicle injuries steadily increase with age while burns decrease.

Table 11-7   Statistics on Some Leading Causes of Accidental Deaths

---

Motor Vehicle Accidents

About 2 million injured each year of which 25% are children

Over 52,000 deaths of which about 4100 are children under 14 years

Prediction is 2 out of every 100 children born today will be in a motor vehicle accident

Burns

Second leading cause of accidental deaths
100,000 are hospitalized
7800 die

30% of these deaths are among children under 15 years of age

Third leading cause of accidental death among children 5-14 years of age

Drowning

About 7000 drowning deaths each year of which 1550 are children under 15 years

Back-yard swimming pools responsible for about 250 deaths per year among children

---

Because of the degree of human wastage involved, anticipatory guidance should begin prior to the birth of the child. Issues to bring up are:

1. In the Home
   a) Smoke detectors should be in place and functional.
   b) Cribs should be safe and free of toxic surface materials.
   c) Thermostat settings for hot tap water in the dwelling should be less than 120° to avoid thermal injury.

    d) New parents should be forewarned not to leave the baby unattended on a bed or bassinet risking a fall, or on the floor where the infant could be stepped on.

    e) Once crawling, the active child can tumble downstairs. Gates should guard the top and bottom step and all windows.

    f) Coffee tables and end tables with sharp edges are often responsible for head lacerations in the "just ambulatory" child and should be removed or modified to protect the child.

    g) Electrical plugs and cords must be covered or out of reach to prevent devastating electrical burns.

    h) Christmas trees should be tied back and placed in a secure stand. Ornaments should be unbreakable and tinsel should not be used to prohibit its ingestion.

2. In the Car

    a) The newborn should leave the hospital in a proper car restraint not in a parent's arms.

    b) Car doors accessible to the child should be locked.

    c) The rear door or window on hatchback or station wagon vehicles should be closed to prevent carbon monoxide poisoning.

    d) Infants should not be left unattended in a vehicle, particularly in hot weather.

3. At the Table

    a) Hard foods risk suffocation or aspiration.

    b) Nuts, bacon, lettuce, and carrot sticks should not be given to toddlers.

    c) Dangerous substances should not be placed in familiar containers, for example, turpentine in a soda bottle.

4. General Measures

    a) Syrup of ipecac should be in every household and renewed yearly.

    b) Poison control numbers and emergency procedures should be verbally rehearsed and placed next to each telephone in the home.

Practical Points

1. Periodic review of environmental and age-related hazards should be an integral part of routine office visits. (See Table 11-8.)

Table 11-8   Early Childhood Safety Counselling Schedule

Preventive Health Visit	Minimal Safety Counselling		
Age	Introduce	Reinforce	Materials
Prenatal/ newborn	Infant car seat Smoke detector Crib safety		
2-4 weeks	Falls	Infant car seat	
2 months	Burns—hot liquids	Infant car seat Falls	Questionnaire 1 Safety sheet 0-6 months
4 months	Choking	Infant car seat Falls Burns—hot liquids	Safety sheet 0-6 months
6 months	Poison Burns—hot surface	Falls Burns—hot liquids	Safety sheet 7-12 months Ipecac syrup Poison center sticker

Table 11-8 (Cont'd.) Early Childhood Safety Counselling Schedule

Preventive Health Visit		Minimal Safety Counselling		
Age	Introduce	Reinforce		Materials
9 months	Water safety Toddler car seat	Poison Falls Burns		Safety sheet 1–2 year
1 year		Poison Falls Burns		Safety sheet 1–2 years
15 months	Specific to need— optional			Questionnaire 2
18 months		Poison Falls Burns		Safety sheet 1–2 years

2 years	Fall—play equipment, tricycles Auto—pedestrian	Auto—restraints Poison burns	Questionnaire 3 Safety sheet 2–4 years
3 years		Auto—restraints, pedestrian Falls Burns	Safety sheet 2–4 years
4 years		Auto—restraints, pedestrian Falls—play equipment Burns	Specific to need

Reproduced with the permission of the American Academy of Pediatrics.

2. Inquiry should be made and appropriate measures taken to safeguard all children from occupational hazards related to adult employment regardless of the location of the place of employment.
3. Safety posters and handouts are available and are valuable in an office, school, or hospital-based safety program.

Chapter 12

CONVULSIVE DISORDERS

Seizure disorders constitute the most frequently encountered neurological problem in pediatric practice. The incidence rate of this disorder among children under 5 years of age is in the range of 5-7%. Seizures may be acute and shortlived or chronic and recurring. The term epilepsy is applied to the latter type. The overall incidence of epilepsy is between 0.3 and 0.7% per year. Causes of seizures are many and varied (Table 12-1), but in every case they result from paroxysmal, uncontrolled electrical discharge from the neurons. Seizures fall into a few recognizable clinical patterns. It is important to recognize these patterns, as it may help identify the etiology of seizures and guide one to select appropriate anticonvulsant medications. The following abbreviated version of the international classification of seizures includes those seizure types most often recognized in infants and children.

1. Partial seizures (focal)
   a) Jacksonian epilepsy, and secondarily generalized seizures, psychomotor epilepsy
2. Generalized seizures (bilaterally symmetrical without local onset)
   a) Tonic-clonic seizures (grand mal)

Table 12-1   Some Causes of Convulsions in Childhood

Fever (febrile convulsions)

Infections, e.g., meningitis, encephalitis, subdural empyema, intracerebral abscess, shigellosis, toxoplasmosis, cytomegalovirus infection

Encephalopathies, e.g., lead encephalopathy, immunization reactions

Space-occupying lesions, e.g., subdural hematoma, neoplasm

Cerebral degenerative diseases, e.g., Tay-Sachs, Schilder's disease, metachromatic leukodystrophy, neurofibromatosis, tuberous sclerosis

Congenital CNS defects, e.g., hydrocephalus, porencephaly

Metabolic disorders, e.g., hypoglycemia, hypocalcemia, hypomagnesemia, hypernatremia

Vascular problems e.g., intracranial bleeding, Sturge-Weber's syndrome

Intracranial injuries, e.g., birth trauma, anoxia

Drugs, e.g., antihistamines, theophylline, phenothiazines

---

    b) Atonic
    c) Absences (petit mal)
    d) Myoclonic seizures
3. Unclassified epileptic seizures (due to incomplete data)

PARTIAL SEIZURES

JACKSONIAN EPILEPSY AND SECONDARILY GENERALIZED SEIZURE

These are partial seizures with or without retention of consciousness. They may stay focal or partial but may become generalized. Jacksonian seizures may be sensory or motor in nature and the clinical expression of the seizure is related to the location of the neurons in the brain with abnormal activity. If the motor cortex is involved, one might see clonic-tonic movements of the parts of the body represented by the involved cortical area. The seizure activity usually begins in a limited area of the brain and then spreads to the adjacent areas. This is expressed clinically by the so-called jacksonian march: seizures beginning in the fingers, spreading to the wrist, to the arm on the same side, and then to the leg on the same side. With the further spread of abnormal neuronal activity, a tonic-clonic type of generalized seizure, indistinguishable from grand mal seizures, may ensue. Focal seizures usually imply the presence of an organic lesion in the brain but occasionally can occur without a detectable lesion.

PSYCHOMOTOR EPILEPSY

These are partial seizures with complex symptoms. The seizure activity usually originates from the temporal area of the brain. Following a brief period of aura marked sometimes by nausea, epigastric discomfort, and shrill cry, the seizure activity is characterized by organized but purposeless actions which are repetitive and often surprisingly complicated, e.g., repeatedly opening and closing a door, pacing the floor, etc. Often patients exhibit automatic movements such as lip smacking, chewing and swallowing motions, and fiddling with the fingers. Sometimes the seizures may consist of gradual loss of muscle tone. Usually there are no tonic-clonic movements. Vasomotor changes with flushing and pallor of skin may be seen in some. Attacks may last from seconds to several minutes. Fatigue, drowsiness, and sleep often follow the seizure episode. EEG changes tend to be localized to the temporal lobe but may be normal during seizure-free periods.

GENERALIZED SEIZURES

TONIC-CLONIC (GRAND MAL)

The clinical symptomatology seen in children with grand mal seizures is indicative of generalized and bilaterally symmetrical involvement of the entire cerebral hemisphere. The seizure usually is preceded by an aura either sensory (headache, irritability) or motor (twitching movements) or occasionally both and is characterized by loss of consciousness with tonic (generalized contractures of muscles) and clonic (rhythmic contractures of muscles) phases. During the tonic phase, cyanosis due to temporary cessation of respiration, tongue biting, and drooling of saliva are often noted. Micturition and less commonly defecation may follow sudden contraction of abdominal muscles. The postictal phase of grand mal seizures is marked by confusion, drowsiness, and sleep. Occasionially automatism and transient paresis may follow an acute attack. EEG tracings show significantly abnormal fast and slow waves. Sometimes generalized seizures are marked only by generalized loss of muscle tone, the atonic seizures. Diagnosis of a seizure disorder in these cases often can be difficult.

ABSENCES (PETIT MAL)

Petit mal seizures usually occur in children after the age of 3 years. They occur many times a day and consist of a brief lapse of consciousness usually lasting for less than 30 seconds. Typically the seizures begin with abrupt interruption of ongoing activity with the child often appearing to stare blankly. Minor motor activities such as rhythmic movements of eyelids, mouth, and hand are often associated with these staring spells. The end of the seizure is as abrupt as the beginning without any postictal manifestations. Petit mal seizures can be precipitated by hyperventilation and by photic stimulation typically. EEG tracings show bilaterally synchronous 3-per-second spike and wave patterns.

MYOCLONIC SEIZURES

These seizures are characterized by sudden jerk-like flexion movements either generalized or focal without apparent loss of consciousness. Flexion movements of the extremities, often prominent in the arms, and sudden dropping of the head are most often associated with the seizures. The attacks occur many times a day, often appearing in clusters alternating with seizure-free intervals. In myoclonic seizures of early infancy appearing before the age of 4 months, congenital or organic cerebral disorders are most likely causes. Tuberous sclerosis is often implicated in many cases. Seizures appearing later in infancy in an otherwise normal infant may be due to an underlying disorder of cerebral metabolism. In many children, the etiology remains obscure. EEG tracings are characteristically abnormal, showing paroxysms of high-voltage slow waves and spikes, a pattern referred to as hypsarrhythmia.

UNCLASSIFIED EPILEPTIC SEIZURES

FEBRILE SEIZURES

A common occurrence in pediatric practice, seizures associated with fever occur in 2-5% of children. In most children, the seizures are benign in nature and do not carry any risk for either recurrence or later development of epilepsy. Febrile seizure usually occurs in children between 6 months and 5 years of age with a peak incidence around 18 months of age. They are generalized in nature and occur soon after the onset of fever. Recurrences are uncommon in a vast majority of children. Certain risk factors are associated with recurrence and subsequent development of afebrile or epileptic seizures. These include:

1. Early onset (before 6 months of age),
2. Presence of neurological or developmental abnormality preceding the first seizure episode,
3. Duration of seizure longer than 15 minutes,
4. Family history of afebrile seizure, and
5. Focal type of seizures.

Most children with febrile seizures will not require any long-term treatment with anticonvulsant medications. Only those whose seizures are associated with two or more risk factors should be considered for treatment with anticonvulsant mediations.

Differential Diagnosis

It is important to differentiate certain emotional and psychiatric problems from seizure disorders. *Syncopal attack* is usually a functional disturbance and occasionally may be due to cardiovascular disorders. Often, differentiation between functional syncopal attack and atonic type of epileptic seizures presents a diagnostic dilemma. A functional syncopal attack in a child usually is preceded by an emotionally disturbing experience, and is not associated either with an aura or postictal symptomatology. The child is usually pale with cold, clammy skin and shallow respiration during an episode. The EEG tracing both during and immediately following recovery from a syncopal attack is normal. *Sleep disorders* (nightmares, night terrors) are often functional disturbances but may very occasionally be of epileptic origin. Familial and environmental circumstances leading to marked emotional disturbances such as fear, anxiety, and depression should make one consider sleep disorders of functional origin. A *breath-holding spell* can end with a convulsive episode. But the sequence of events leading to a convulsion—provocation, cry, breath-holding, cyanosis, and convulsion—usually rules out epilepsy. In addition, the EEG will be entirely normal in children with breath-holding attacks.

Workup of Child with Seizure Disorder

Clinical impressions as to the possible cause of seizures should dictate selection of appropriate laboratory tests. In general, these tests should be directed toward ruling out three important causes of seizures in children: infection, trauma, and electrolyte and metabolic abnormalities. Routine blood counts and urinalysis may give a clue to some underlying systemic illness. Lumbar puncture is almost always indicated in a child with the first seizure to rule out CNS infection and occasionally other pathology such as intracranial bleeding or encephalopathies. A blood sugar estimation at the time of a seizure or a fasting blood level at a later time is indicated to rule out hypoglycemia. Similarly, serum electrolyte determination, when clinically indicated, will rule out hypo- or hypernatremia as cause of seizure. Determination of serum calcium level, particularly in the newborn, and blood urea nitrogen is indicated when parathyroid or renal disease are suspected.

X-ray studies of the skull are indicated to determine the presence of intracranial calcifications associated with certain types of infections, e.g., cytomegalovirus infection and toxoplasmosis. Electroencephalography is helpful to document the presence of abnormal cortical activity, and to determine the seizure pattern. CAT scan of the brain should be carried out whenever an intracranial structural lesion is suspected.

Treatment of Seizure Disorder

Where the cause of seizure is known, treatment should be directed toward eliminating it. However, in a significant number of patients, an etiology cannot be identified. The therapy in these consists of the use of anticonvulsant medication. The most commonly used anticonvulsant medications, their dosage and side effects, and indications for use are given in Table 12-2.

The drugs listed in the table are used either singly or in combination. The choice of drug depends on one's preference based on clinical experience. Generally, it is advisable to start with one drug at the lower end of the dosage range and gradually increase the amount until seizures are controlled or symptoms of overdosage appear. If the regimen is unsuccessful, a second drug should be added after ascertaining that the failure is not related to compliance problems. Changes in drug dosage and withdrawal of a drug should be made gradually. Anticonvulsant blood levels should be checked periodically, particularly in patients showing signs of toxicity or continuing seizure activity. Anticonvulsant therapy can usually be terminated after about 2-3 years of seizure control.

STATUS EPILEPTICUS

Status epilepticus or prolonged repeated tonic-clonic convulsions is a neurological emergency. Significant morbidity and mortality are associated with tonic-clonic status that is allowed to last longer than 6 minutes. The following steps should be considered in the management of a child in status epilepticus.

Table 12-2 Drug Therapy in Seizure Disorders

Seizure Pattern	Drugs Commonly Used	Total Daily Dosage	Therapeutic Range (μg/ml)	Side Effects
Grand mal and focal seizures	Phenobarbital	3-5 mg/kg	15-30	Drowsiness, rash, irritability
	Phenytoin	5-10 mg/kg	10-20	Ataxia, gingival hyperplasia, hirsutism
	Primidone (Mysoline)	12-25 mg/kg	6-12	Anorexia, irritability, ataxia, rash
	Carbamazepine Tegretol	10-20 mg/kg	6-12	Sedation, nausea, nystagmus
Petit mal seizures	Ethosuximide	15-30 mg/kg	40-100	Anorexia, headache, numbness of extremities
	Valproic Acid	Up to 30 mg/kg	50-100	Nausea, vomiting, abdominal pain, alopecia

	Trimethadione	20–30 mg/kg	0.013–0.072	Nausea, dizziness, rash, drowsiness, leukopenia
	Clonazepam (Clonopin)	0.02 mg/kg	6–12	Drowsiness, hypersalivation
Psychomotor seizures	Carbamazepine (Tegretol)	10–20 mg/kg	6–12	Sedation, nausea, nystagmus
	Primidone (Mysoline)	12–25 mg/kg	10–20	Anorexia, irritability, ataxia, rash
	Phenytoin (Dilantin)	5–10 mg/kg	–	Anorexia, irritability, ataxia, rash
Myoclonic seizures	ACTH	20 U IM	–	Salt retention, hypertension, Cushingoid appearance
	Diazepam	0.1–1 mg/kg	0.013–0.072	Drowsiness, ataxia
	Clonazepam (Clonopin)	1–3 mg/kg	15–30	Drowsiness, hypersalivation
Febrile seizures	Phenobarbital	3–5 mg/kg		Drowsiness, rash, irritability

1. Assess cardiopulmonary function, secure the airway, administer oxygen if necessary. Prepare to start intravenous line for administration of fluids. Draw blood for determination of electrolytes, BUN, glucose, and complete blood count.
2. Administer anticonvulsant medications as follows:
   a) Diazepam intravenously at a dosage of 0.3-1 mg/kg no faster than 1 mg/min. Monitor child's respiratory rate, blood pressure, and pulse. Concurrently administer slowly by intravenous route phenytoin 15 mg/kg. Do not administer phenytoin intramuscularly. Monitor cardiac activity.
   b) Alternatively phenobarbital sodium also can be used intravenously in a dose of 10 mg/kg given over several minutes. If seizure persists, a second dose (10 mg/kg) can be given 20-30 minutes after the first dose. Phenobarbital can also be given intramuscularly.
   c) Paraldehyde in a dose of 0.2 to 0.3 cc/kg can be used intravenously or intramuscularly (maximum 5 ml per injection site) as an adjunct to phenobarbital therapy.
   d) In rare instances, when seizures persist despite vigorous therapy with anticonvulsant medications, general anesthesia may be used.

Chapter 13

THE ALLERGIC CHILD

A significant part of clinical practice is concerned with the allergic child. It is estimated that 15% of the pediatric population in the United States has some form of allergy. Since relatively few allergists and pediatric allergists are available, the bulk of these conditions must be treated by primary physicians. This chapter will focus on the basics of office allergy practice. The principles and methods discussed are within reach of the practitioner.

The term allergy is not synonymous with "immune reaction." While most allergic reactons clearly involve immune reactions, so do most viral infections. The difference is that an allergic reaction is an altered or unusual reaction to the presence of an antigen. Allergy means altered reactivity. The clinical manifestations of allergy will vary widely from individual to individual but the pathogenesis is basically the same. There are four classic types of immune reactions. The basic type of reaction discussed in this chapter is type I or immediate hypersensitivity reactions. After an allergic individual has been exposed and finally sensitized to an antigen (or allergen), he develops a characteristic class of antibody to that antigen. This antibody is in the IgE class of immune globulins. The combination of antigen and IgE antibody causes the release of various chemical substances from body tissues. The prototype of these substances is histamine. Others are slow-reacting substance of anaphylaxis (SRS-A), bradykinin, choline, acetylcholine, serotonin, heparin, and eosinophilic chemotactic factors of anaphylaxis (ECF-A).

The effects of these chemical agents are known in clinical practice as the various allergic diseases. The following are the major ones:

1. Bronchial asthma
2. Allergic rhinitis
3. Atopic dermatitis
4. Urticaria and angioedema
5. Gastrointestinal allergy

Host factors are of great importance in the production of symptoms. Asthmatics, for example, have an unusual bronchial response to a variety of nonallergic stimuli. Thus, cold air, strong odors, exertion, emotions, etc., may stimulate bronchial constriction. Respiratory tract infections are important in triggering asthma attacks in as much as 50% of the younger asthmatics.

Many other factors besides host susceptibility are important in the development of allergic disease. Age, climate, season, location, intensity and frequency of exposure (occupation, housing, etc.) all play a vital role.

ALLERGIC MANIFESTATIONS

AGE

Allergic manifestations tend to vary with age. The characteristic forms encountered in the infant and preschool child are cutaneous (eczema) and gastrointestinal allergies. Asthma and allergic rhinitis are more likely to have their onset in the 2- to 10-year-old child. Often, the allergic response will change as a child becomes older so that his eczema will entirely disappear only to be replaced by asthma. Others will be frequently symptomatic but will tend to improve as they get older.

CLIMATE, WEATHER, AND LOCATION

Climatic conditions will have a pronounced effect on allergic manifestations. The effect is both generic in the sense that climate determines which plant antigens will abound, and immediate since weather conditions may trigger symptoms. As an example of the generic effect, a damp wet climate will favor the growth of molds. Each section of the country varies widely in its type of flora. Charts such as the one reproduced here for the Northeast United States may be made up for any location in the world. (See Figure 13-1.) Climate will determine not only the type of antigen being produced but the duration of its production. The ragweed season virtually ends at the first frost; thus, a mild autumn in the Northeast United States will prolong the season. The immediate effect of climate is determined by weather. Sudden change in weather has been known by many allergy sufferers to cause worsening of symptoms. Ragweed sufferers will improve during rainstorms when the air is partially cleared of pollen. Mold sufferers, on the other hand, are made worse because molds thrive on humidity.

INTENSITY AND FREQUENCY OF EXPOSURE

Intensity and frequency of exposure play a large role in the development of allergic manifestations. It is not enough to have a susceptible host (the atopic individual) and a sufficiently sensitizing allergen. The two must be brought together frequently enough for sensitization to occur. Many powerful antigens exist which do not assume clinical importance because few people are sufficiently exposed to them. The allergens that have become important are precisely those that we encounter most often. These are the allergens that abound in the air we breathe outside, at work, or at home. They are substances we come into bodily contact with or ingest.

The principal object of the allergic history is to survey the potential allergens that a given patient is exposed to and with the help of objective tests (skin tests, RAST tests, dietary challenge tests, etc.) to determine the ones that are most likely to be producing clinical symptoms. Four very fertile areas should be investigated: the home environment,

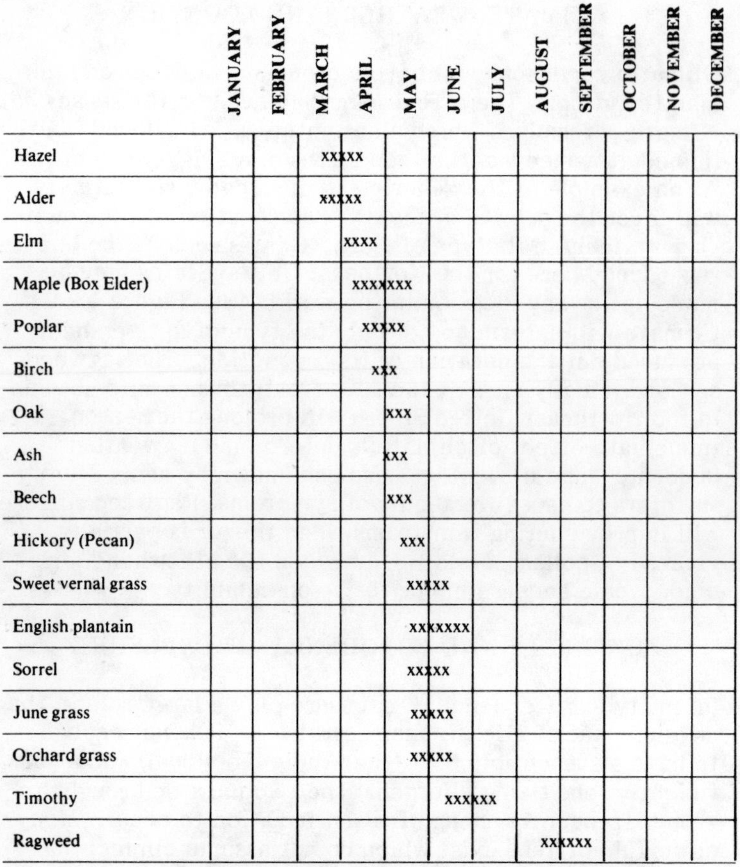

	JANUARY	FEBRUARY	MARCH	APRIL	MAY	JUNE	JULY	AUGUST	SEPTEMBER	OCTOBER	NOVEMBER	DECEMBER
Hazel			xxx	xx								
Alder			xxx	xx								
Elm				xxxx								
Maple (Box Elder)				xxxx	xxx							
Poplar				xxx	xx							
Birch				x	x							
Oak					xxx							
Ash					xxx							
Beech					xxx							
Hickory (Pecan)					xxx							
Sweet vernal grass					xxx	xx						
English plantain					xxx	xxxx						
Sorrel					xxx	xx						
June grass					xxx	xx						
Orchard grass					xxx	xx						
Timothy						xxx	xxx					
Ragweed								xxx	xxx			

Figure 13-1 Pollen season of North America. (From Sherman, W.B.: Hypersensitivity Mechanisms and Management, W.B. Saunders Co., Philadelphia, 1968. Reproduced with publisher's permission.)

school or work environment, the diet, and the circumstances, place and time surrounding the onset of symptoms. Table 13-1 lists the most common allergens found in atopic children and their most likely place of occurrence.

Table 13-1 Allergens of Importance in Pediatric Practice and Their Likely Source

Home	School or Work	Diet	Outdoor or Seasonal
Dust	Dust	Meats pork chicken beef	Local trees
Commercially used animal epithelia goat cattle pig horse rabbit silk wool feathers	Commercially used animal epithelia goat cattle rabbit silk wool fishglue	Dairy egg white cow's milk	Local weeds ragweed platain

Table 13-1 (Cont'd.) Allergens of Importance in Pediatric Practice and Their Likely Source

Home	School or Work	Diet	Outdoor or Seasonal
Pets	Pets	Cereals	Local grasses
cats		wheat	
dogs		corn	
birds		oat	
Commercially used plant fibers	Commercially used plant fibers	Legumes	Certain molds
flaxseed	flaxseed	peas	*Alternaria*
cottonseed	tobacco	lima beans	*Hormodendrum*
orris	kapok	kidney beans	
tobacco	pyrethrum	peanuts	
kapok			
pyrethrum			
Molds	Molds	Vegetables	
Alternaria	*Alternaria*	tomatoes	
Hormodendrum	*Hormodendrum*	onions	
Aspergillus	*Aspergillus*		

Fruits
  peaches
  pineapple
  pears
  plums
  apricots
  strawberries
  oranges

Spices
  mustard
  black pepper

Beverages
  chocolate
  cocoa

All fish and shellfish

All nuts

Many other sub-
stances varying
with occupation

ALLERGY TESTING

Four common modes of allergy testing may be easily undertaken by the nonallergist practitioner:

1. Skin tests, scratch and intradermal
2. Patch tests
3. Diet challenge tests
4. Radioallergosorbent test (RAST)

Of these, the only one with an appreciable risk to the patient is the intradermal skin test. Table 13-2 lists the advantages, disadvantages, and clinical application for each of these tests. Included are the various mucosal challenge tests and passive transfer testing.

Methods of testing, like bronchial challenge testing, passive transfer technique, etc., require rather more complicated techniques than are usually available to the practitioner.

COMMON ALLERGIC SYNDROMES
(See Table 13-3)

ASTHMA

Onset may be as early as the first weeks of life but is most common between 2 and 10 years of age. Often, it is confused with bronchiolitis in preschool age children. In others, it may mimic a pneumonic process. The most common cause of repeated "pneumonias" in childhood is asthma. This is true because patchy atelectasis and the hilar streaking seen so commonly in the chest x-ray may lead to overreading the film. Also, infection is frequently associated and may act as a triggering mechanism for asthma.

Symptoms are predominantly respiratory. Dyspnea and hyperpnea with audible wheezing and a prolonged expiration are characteristic. Fever may be present. On physical exam one may encounter a distended thorax (barrel chest), retractions, and hear bilateral expiratory wheezing and ronchi. Associated fine rales may indicate the presence of pneumonia. Areas of dullness indicate atelectasis. In about 5% of asthmatics subcutaneous emphysema is palpated over the

Table 13-2 The Advantages, Disadvantages, and the Clinical Application of the Major Varieties of Allergy Testing

Type of Test	Advantages	Disadvantages	Clinical Uses
Scratch Test	No limit on number of test performed at one sitting Relatively painless Very safe Simple to store and administer No syringes needed	Difficult to interpret Relatively insensitive with many false negatives Concentration of allergen cannot be varied readily Reliability decreased in infancy because of lessened skin reactivity	To identify strongly positive reacting allergens and eliminate the need to test them intradermally
Intradermal Test	Most sensitive and reliable method of skin testing Relatively safe, but less so than scratch testing. Anaphylactic reactions can occur	No more than 12 tests at any one sitting Relatively painful for small children Requires more storage space than scratch test allergens. Syringes are needed	May be used as definitive testing method for almost all types of allergic disease Least effective for allergy due to foods, physical stimuli, and contact allergens. Highly effective

Table 13-2 (Cont'd.) The Advantages, Disadvantages, and the Clinical Application of the Major Varieties of Allergy Testing

Type of Test	Advantages	Disadvantages	Clinical Uses
Intradermal Test (Cont'd)	Concentration of allergens easily varied to test degree of skin reactivity	Reliability decreased in infant	for inhalants, pollens, and molds
Patch Test	Simple to perform and painless Inexpensive Very safe Sensitive and reliable	Restricted to use in contact allergy	Contact allergy
Dietary Challenge Test	Relatively safe Painless Requires no expensive testing	Dietary restrictions may be unobserved Objectivity depends on parent Relatively long testing period	Food allergy Allergic dermatitis Allergic disease of any kind in children under 2 years

	Advantages	Disadvantages	Indications
RAST Test	Safe, no side effects Relatively painless Not affected by medication	Expensive Restricted to relatively few allergens	May be used as definitive testing method for almost all types of allergic disease
Total serum IGE	Safe, no side effects Relatively painless Not affected by medication	Nonspecific	Useful but not pathognomonic as adjunctive evidence of allergic disease May predict allergic potential expecially in very young patients
Passive Transfer Test (PK)	Absolutely safe for allergic patients As sensitive and reliable as intradermal test	May be dangerous for inadequately screened human volunteer. Serum hepatitis may also be transmitted Expensive	For infants where skin reactivity is poor Children who have widespread skin lesions prohibiting skin testing Children who react positively to all tests (dermatographism)

Table 13-2 (Cont'd.) The Advantages, Disadvantages, and the Clinical Application of the Major Varieties of Allergy Testing

Type of Test	Advantages	Disadvantages	Clinical Uses
Mucosal Challenge Tests (Nasal, Conjunctival, Bronchial)	Sensitive and very reliable	May produce severe symptoms Patient's full cooperation needed Restricted to older children and adults Few tests may be done at one sitting Sophisticated and expensive equipment, facilities, and personnel needed for bronchial challenge testing	Useful for respiratory tract allergy Not as useful for gastrointestinal and contact allergy Main use is to test the sensitivity of a patient to a respiratory allergen suggested by the history but not confirmed by skin testing

Table 13-3 Common Allergic Diseases and Methods of Testing

Specific Allergic Disease	Type of Testing Indicated	Comments
Allergic Rhinitis and Asthma	Scratch Intradermal* Dietary challenge Mucosal challenge* Total serum IgE RAST*	Seasonal allergens, like ragweed, need not be tested below 2 years of age because it is unlikely that sensitization will take place before this time. Intradermal testing with foods is relatively unreliable and carries an appreciable risk. Testing, therefore, is with nonseasonal inhalants and dietary challenge below 2 years. Remember, infant skin reacts less strongly to scratch and intradermal tests so interpretation is made on different criteria. The seasonal inhalants and foods may be tested above 2 years of age. Mucosal challenge tests may be used on older children where full cooperation is assured.

* = Tests of choice

Table 13-3 (Cont'd.) Common Allergic Diseases and Methods of Testing

Specific Allergic Disease	Type of Testing Indicated	Comments
Allergic Dermatitis	Dietary challenge* Patch testing Scratch Intradermal Total serum IgE RAST	Food allergens are the most common cause of allergic dermatitis in children under the age of 4 years. Dietary challenge is the best initial approach. Contactants may prove to be important too and can be tested by patch testing. Scratch and intradermals are used when dietary challenge and patch testing are not helpful and when the child is older than 2 years.
Urticaria Angioedema	Dietary challenge* Scratch Intradermal Total serum IgE RAST	A single episode of urticaria does not constitute sufficient indication for testing. Chronic or recurrent forms may be controlled by dietary restriction. If this fails, scratch or intradermal may be used.

Hymenoptera (Bee, Wasp Stings)	Scratch Intradermal*	Reserved for those patients with systemic symptoms to Hymenoptera stings. Testing is used to gauge sensitivity as well as to identify species.
Gastrointestional Allergy	Dietary challenge* Scratch Intradermal RAST	Dietary challenge is the most useful test. Scratch and intradermal can be helpful but are less reliable.

* = Tests of choice

sternum and upper thorax. Cyanosis is infrequent. Signs of dehydration may be observed. A most ominous finding is the "quiet chest" where neither marked wheezing nor clear alveolar breath sounds are heard. Poor air exchange due to mucous plugs or widespread atelectasis is responsible for this finding and respiratory failure is imminent.

Helpful Laboratory Tests

1. Chest x-ray: commonly shows a flat, lowered diaphragm, small cardiovascular silhouette and increased radiolucency of the lungs, or streaky hilar densities simulating hilar pneumonia, atelectasis, and/or pneumonia.
2. Nasal smear for eosinophils.
3. Peripheral blood for eosinophils or a white cell response indicating infection.
4. Blood gases for the severe persistent attack, pCO_2, sodium bicarbonate, base excess, paO_2. Differential diagnosis includes foreign bodies in the bronchial tree, vascular rings, cystic fibrosis, right middle lobe syndrome, immune globulin deficiencies, pulmonary tuberculosis, hilar adenopathy from various causes, and bronchiolitis in younger children.

Treatment

1. Immediate
   a) Aqueous epinephrine (1:1000) 0.01 ml/kg/dose subcutaneously (maximum 0.3 ml) and repeated at 20-minute intervals when needed for no more than three times. Isuprel may be used in place of epinephrine. If this is unsuccessful, an intravenous infusion is initiated and 4 mg/kg of aminophylline is administered over a 20-minute period by IV drip. This may be repeated at 8-hour intervals. The total 24-hour dose should not exceed 15 mg/kg.

   If epinephrine (or Isuprel) is successful, then long-term bronchodilation with one of the xanthine derivatives (theophylline, or oxtriphylline) is indicated. The dose of theophylline is 15 mg/kg/24 hr. Many asthma medications contain ephedrine as well. While not as potent a bronchodilator as the xanthines, its action

lasts longer. However, recent evidence suggests that ephedrine together with a xanthine may potentiate toxic effects rather than therapeutic effects.
  b) Force fluids orally or give 2000 ml/m^2 if IV infusion is needed.
  c) Mild sedation for the markedly agitated child (phenobarbital). Caution: do not induce respiratory depression.
  d) Oxygen for the cyanotic child.
  e) Assisted ventilation for the child in respiratory failure.
  f) Expectorants—glyceryl guaiacolate, potassium iodide.
  g) Correction of acid-base imbalance (usually respiratory acidosis).
2. Long-term therapy
  a) A careful search for causative allergens must be undertaken. This includes utilizing skin testing and dietary challenge testing.
  b) In those children whose asthma is due to an environmental allergen that can be avoided, every attempt should be made to do so. Thus, cat sensitivity is treated by eliminating the cat.
  c) Where allergens are not avoidable (pollens, some molds) or are only able to be minimized (house dust), hyposensitization therapy is indicated.
  d) Long-term bronchodilators may be required for children with persistent wheezing. Some of the newer xanthine derivative formulations have an advantage over the older preparations by providing a more constant serum level. Theo-Dur, available in 100 mg, 200 mg, and 300 mg capsules is one such product. Slophyllin Gyrocaps can be opened up and the contents sprinkled onto a buttered cracker for administration to younger children unable to swallow capsules. Properly titrated blood theophylline levels may be needed. These newer formulations can provide 8- to 12-hour bronchodilator effect for persistent wheezers.

  The newer β-adrenergic receptor site stimulators like terbutaline, salbutamol, and metaproterenol are also effective bronchodilators with decreased effect on the heart. They come in a variety of forms suitable for oral or inhalation use.

e) Cromolyn sodium has added a welcome new chapter in the therapy of the chronic asthmatic. Evidence has accumulated showing its effectiveness as a prophylactic agent (it should not be used to relieve an acute attack of bronchospasm). Side effects are few. Its chief limitation is the difficulty encountered in teaching younger children to inhale it, therefore it is reserved for children older than 4 years. It should be borne in mind when evaluating its efficacy that a full therapeutic effect may not be observed until 2-6 weeks or more of therapy. Cromolyn sodium is provided in 20-mg capsules that are inserted in an inhaler. Parents must be carefully instructed in the proper use and cleansing of the inhaler. The contents of one capsule are inhaled four times daily and continued over an indefinite period of time. It appears to exert its therapeutic action by inhibiting degranulation of sensitized mast cells and, therefore, the release of the chemical mediators of bronchospasm.

f) Despite all measures a few severe, chronic asthmatics require long-term steroid therapy. This is indicated only after all other measures have proved fruitless. There appears to be an advantage in using topical rather than systemic steroids for asthmatics resistant to other forms of therapy. The British experience with beclomethasone diproprionate by inhalation would indicate that results similar to those achieved with systemic steroids can be obtained with far less adrenal suppression and other steroid side effects. The long-term sequelae are not completely known although there is no evidence to suggest that chronic lung changes occur. Children seem less prone to fungal infections of the mouth than adults. In general, aerosol steroid should not be used to treat the acute asthmatic episode. Short-term oral steroids are better for this purpose, in addition to bronchodilators and other measures described under immediate therapy for the acute asthmatic patient. Inhalation steroid is better reserved for the chronic persistent asthmatic who requires long-term medication and in whom continuous bronchodilation therapy and cromolyn sodium are not effective. It is also indicated for a trial in those children already on long-term systemic steroids.

Initial dosage is two puffs three times a day with in-
dividualization by trial and error and in accordance
with day-to-day need.
g) Psychiatric therapy is helpful when the emotional
component appears to be significant.
Table 13-4 lists the common allergens and where
they are found.
Figure 13-2 lists the steps to be taken in desensi-
tizing a room.

ALLERGIC RHINITIS

A history of frequent "colds" is frequently given by the
parents. On closer questioning the "cold" does not act like
a viral infection. Its course is markedly different. Instead
of a few days of sneezing, tearing, and rhinorrhea progressing from clear to mucopurulent nasal discharge, one finds
that periods of rhinorrhea alternate with periods where
symptoms are absent. Also, the persistence and frequency
of nasal symptoms are very suggestive of allergy. Concomitant sinusitis may confuse the picture, but this is rather
uncommon in childhood. The diagnosis is usually suspected
from the history, the presence of allergy in family members,
and the pale, boggy, bluish, nasal mucosa so often observed.
It is confirmed by a nasal smear showing eosinophils. A
negative smear, however, does not rule out allergic rhinitis.
In this instance, one or more smears should be taken.

Treatment

Antihistamines and decongestants such as pseudophedrine
are helpful for immediate therapy. Cromolyn sodium in
nasal spray from as well as topical steroids 0.025% fluni-
solide (Nasalide) can be very effective in controlling symptoms without many side effects. Long-term management
is designed to discover the causative allergens and eliminate
them. Where elimination is not feasible, then hyposensitization is undertaken. Substantial evidence exists that hyposensitization for allergic rhinitis can prevent the subsequent
development of asthma.

Table 13-4 Common Allergens and Where They are Found

Class	Commonly Found In	Comments
Dust	Home, school	
Cat	Pets (leading cause), covering for toy animals, bedding, furniture stuffing, carriage robes, linings for: caps, coats, gloves, slippers. Furs of other cat families (leopard) may cause symptoms.	+ Skin tests to other members of cat family are frequent. Uncleansed hair is allergenic, properly cleansed hair is not.
Dogs	Furs, robes, rugs, coat lining. Pets (leading cause). Mixed with wool in Chinese rugs.	Uncleansed hair is allergenic: properly cleansed hair is not.
Cattle	Direct animal contact, brushes, coarse blankets, rugs (chenille), toy animals, plushes, rope, upholstery.	Uncleansed hair is allergenic: properly cleansed hair is not.
Goat	Coats and suits of mohair or alpaca, sweaters (angora or cashmere). Oriental rugs. Direct contact is rare cause.	Uncleansed hair is allergenic: properly cleansed hair is not.

Horse	Sofa, floor pads, direct contact with animals.	Cross reactivity to horse serum exists.
Rabbit	Felt cloth, old bedding, old upholstery (no longer widely used), pets.	
Hog	Direct animal contact, padding for rugs.	
Rat	Hair not used commercially, direct animal contact.	
Mouse	Hair not used commercially, direct animal contact.	
Feathers	Pillows, cushions, upholstery, artificial flowers, quilts, toys, dolls, muffs, dress trimmings, plumes.	+ Skin tests among members of the fowl family are frequent.
Wool	Direct contact rare. Except in coarse fabric, wool clothing in nonallergenic. Raw wool is allergenic. May have nonspecific irritating effect on skin of eczema patient.	Raw wool is allergenic; the more it is refined the less allergenic it is. Irritating effect–important in eczema.

Table 13-4   (Cont'd.) Common Allergens and Where They are Found

Class	Commonly Found In	Comments
Orris	Cosmetics	Allercreme, Almay, Ar-ex, and Marcelle manufacture nonallergenic cosmetics.
Cotton-seed	Allergy to seed only not to fiber. Cottonseed oil, cotton linters (used in upholstery, cushions, mattress), fertilizers, animal feed as cottonseed flour.	
Flax-seed	Allergy to seed only, not to fiber. Linseed meal or oil, paint, leather, breakfast foods, flaxseed tea, hair setting lotions. As flaxstraw in couches, car seats, refrigerating insulation.	Cross-reactivity is frequent. Cross-reactivity may also exist with mustard seed, legumes, and nuts.
Kapok	Allergy to seed only, not to fiber. Upholstery, cushions, mattress, toys, life preservers.	

Pyre-thrum	Insecticides (Flit, Blackflag).	Cross reactivity with ragweed.
Silk	Silk floss (stuffing), clothing, fabrics: broadcloth, brocade, chiffon, satin, taffeta, georgette, plush, jersey, pongee, poplin, tulle, velvet.	
Fishglue	Labels, stickers, books, paper boxes, furniture.	Many fatalities to intradermal testing reported.

How to "desensitize" a room

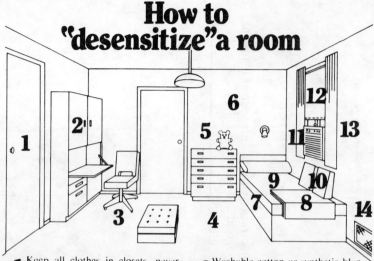

1 Keep all clothes in closets, never lying about room. Keep closet and all other doors closed.

2 No ornately carved furniture—plain, simple designs catch less dust. Avoid books or bookshelves—they are great dust catchers.

3 Replace fabric upholstered chair and hassock with ones covered by rubberized canvas or plastic.

4 Wood or linoleum flooring. No rugs of any kind.

5 No toys or stuffed animals in room. If they must be included, they should be made of wood, plastic, or metal, never fabric.

6 No pennants, pictures, or other dust catchers on wall.

7 Allergen-proof encasings are far superior to plastic for pillows, mattress, and box springs. Vacuum mattress and pillow covers frequently.

8 Washable cotton or synthetic blankets instead of fuzzy-surfaced ones.

9 Use easily laundered cotton bedspread instead of chenille.

10 No kapok, feather, or foam rubber pillows. Use dacron or other synthetics. Foam rubber grows mold, especially in damp areas.

11 Install air conditioning window unit, or central air conditioning. Keep windows closed, especially in summer. No electric fans.

12 Install roll-up washable cotton or synthetic window shades. No venetian blinds.

13 Use easily washed cotton or fiber glass curtains. No draperies.

14 In houses with forced air heat, cost of centrally installed electrostatic air filter may be justified. In any case, filter or damp cheesecloth over air inlet helps reduce dust circulation. Change filters at least every two weeks.

Figure 13-2 Reprinted through the courtesy of the A.H. Robins Co.

ATOPIC DERMATITIS

A papular, erythematous lesion in its initial stages, atopic dermatitis has several different forms. The acute form may become exudative, crusted, and superinfected with staphylococcal or streptococcal organisms. The chronic form may become lichenified and thickened (mummular eczema). The condition is common and largely affects the younger, preschool age group. The distribution of the rash is characteristic. It involves the intertriginous or skin fold areas (popliteal, antecubital, and axillary areas), and the face, particularly the cheeks, buttocks, and exterior surfaces of the extremities. At times it is severe enough to involve the entire body, making skin testing impossible.

The course of atopic dermatitis is one of frequent exacerbations alternating with incomplete remissions. However, the majority of children recover completely, usually by 4 years of age. A small percentage of children have atopic dermatitis that persists into adult life. About half of the children with atopic dermatitis can be expected to develop another allergic disease later in life.

Treatment

The treatment of atopic dermatitis is outlined in Table 13-5.

URTICARIA AND ANGIOEDEMA

Several forms of urticarial disease are found. The acute or simple papular urticaria due to a variety of excitants is the most common type. In this form papules may appear in a localized area or extensively over the body and pruritus is a distressing symptom. Most often, one episode occurs lasting a few hours to 1 week. Occasionally, a second type of urticaria occurs, characterized by chronicity or recurrence of the rash. A third type is angioedema with more deep seated lesions that become considerably swollen and involve lips, periorbital areas and at times the larynx and other internal organs.

The causes of each of these types are multiple. Allergens, particularly foods, play an important role. Drugs (penicillin, aspirin), physical stimuli (cold, light, etc.), insect

Table 13-5   Therapy of Atopic Dermatitis (Eczema)

1. Trial Diet

2. Topical
   a) Steroids-creams, Kenalog, Valisone, Synalar. Apply thinly 3-15 times/day.
   b) Wet lesions-Burow's soaks—1 tablet/pint cool water. Dip cheesecloth in solution and apply over eczema. Wrap towel around and cover with plastic. Keep on as long as possible (20-25 minutes) 6 times/day but not at night—use creams only.
   c) Aveeno baths + Neutragena or Lowila soaps.
   d) Lichenified lesion—coal tar, Tarbonis, Cortarquin 1/4% 6-10 times/day.
   e) Chronic or subacute lesions. Occlusive dressings. Steps:
      (1) Rub in steroid cream.
      (2) Cover area with saran wrap, a plastic "baggie," or plastic glove.
      (3) Seal with 3M Blenderm to make airtight.
      (4) Apply at bedtime, remove in morning. Alternate method: apply Cordran cream to 3M Blenderm and tape over affected areas.
   f) Infected lesions—Burow's soaks plus topical antibiotics (Bacitracin, Garamycin, Vioform). No penicillin or sulfa.
   g) Pruritic lesions—antihistamines.
      (1) Nighttime—Benadryl Elixir (5 mg/kg/24 hr) (10 mg/teaspoon) usual dose 1-3 years three teaspoons (30 mg) at bedtime. Phenergan Fortis (25 mg/teaspoon) 1-3 years one-half teaspoon at bedtime.
      (2) Daytime—Periactin 1 teaspoon tid 2-6 years (2 mg/teaspoon). Actifed 1 teaspoon tid 4 months—6 years. Chlor-Trimeton 1/2 teaspoon tid to 12 years (2 mg/teaspoon). Dimetane 4 mg/kg/24 hr (2 mg/teaspoon). Pyribenazmine 30 mg tid (30 mg/teaspoon).

Table 13-5 (Cont'd.)

    h) Skin softeners—Alpha Keri, Dormol, Ar-Ex bath oil—
       2 cupfuls per tub of water. Apply to skin—Keri lotion,
       Allercreme lotion, or Ar-Ex body lotion.
    i) Wear white cotton pajamas, cover skin with bandages.
       Bathe infrequently, once a week, no more.

---

bites, parasites; and, in the case of hereditary angioedema,
an enzyme inhibitor deficiency (an esterase inhibitor) are
numbered among the various etiologies. Collagen disease
may present with urticarial lesions and this possibility
should be excluded.

Treatment

Symptomatic treatment consists of aqueous epinephrine
(1-1000) subcutaneously. Long-acting epinephrine (Susphrine
1-200) 0.005 mg/kg may also be used when lesions tend to
recur. Ephedrine is useful but requires high doses. Antihistamines (Benadryl 3 mg/kg/24 hr) are also helpful.
Emergency tracheostomy may be required in cases of laryngeal or epiglottal edema.

    A careful search for the cause should be made. In cases
of the self-limited, acute form, dietary challenge testing
and skin testing need not usually be undertaken. In cases
where the urticaria is recurrent, persistent, or causes life-
threatening symptoms, complete testing is indicated.

GASTROINTESTINAL ALLERGY

Usually found in infants and younger children, the most
characteristic symptoms are diarrhea, abdominal cramps,
vomiting, and fretfulness. The most common cause is a
food allergen, particularly cow's milk, nuts, eggs, chocolate,
and pork. Avoidance of the allergen is the cure and may be
readily effected by a hypoallergic diet including a hypoallergic milk substitute.

FOOD ALLERGY

Allergy to foods reaches a peak incidence in early childhood
and can be responsible for a variety of clinical allergic

syndromes including respiratory, cutaneous or gastrointestinal symptoms. It can mimic a number of other clinical entities as well, causing, at times, malabsorptive states, pneumonic infiltrates, and altered behavior. The most frequently implicated foods in infancy are milk, wheat, corn, egg white, and cane sugar. Symptoms may be immediate or delayed. The diagnosis may be assisted by measuring eosinophils in the blood or various bodily secretions. A diet diary may give important clues as to the specific food(s) involved but often does not since the interval between ingestion and onset of symptoms is frequently delayed by 1-3 days. Intradermal skin testing is not too reliable and carries the risk of provoking constitutional reactions. Prick and RAST testing may be helpful. The simplest, safest way of establishing a specific diagnosis is by using an elimination diet and challenge test. The child is placed on a diet free of the more common and likely food allergens. (See Table 13-6.) Improvement, occurring after 1-2 weeks of the diet, implies that one or more of the eliminated foods is responsible for the disease. The clinician watches for the return of symptoms while adding back each food at 4-day intervals. If this occurs, the most recently added food is dropped from the diet and another tested. At the end of the process the child may be challenged a second time with those foods believed to cause symptoms. In this way, a cause and effect relationship can be established. Foods found to be allergenic should be eliminated from the diet for 6 months or more. If they are considered important or desirable, they may be added again afterwards. Many children will not develop allergic symptoms to previous food allergens after a prolonged period of elimination.

Table 13-6   Allergy Trial Diet

Boiled rice or puffed rice (use juice instead of milk)

Ry-Krisp

Lamb

Cooked carrots, lettuce, spinach, string beans

Lemon
Grapefruit
Apricots
Peaches   } Cooked or canned
Pears
Plums
Prunes

Tea with lemon or sugar; lemonade

Salt, sugar, and olive oil is permitted. No other flavoring or seasoning or dressing

Any amount of food in any combination may be served if it is listed above

Chapter 14

COMMON HEMATOLOGICAL PROBLEMS

IRON DEFICIENCY ANEMIA

This is the most common type of anemia in early childhood. Although the incidence is most common between 6 and 24 months of age and in economically deprived populations, it occurs not infrequently in preschool children, and among higher socioeconomic groups.

Approximately 300 mg of iron is present at birth in a normal full-term baby. Iron stores are derived transplacentally from the mother and are primarily contained in the hemoglobin complex. Because of the decreased rate of erythropoiesis in early infancy, the excess iron released from the destruction of the red blood cells is stored in the body for future use. Around 6-8 weeks of postnatal life, when the infant registers its lowest number of red blood cells and hemoglobin levels (physiological anemia), the rate of erythropoiesis gradually accelerates resulting in increased demand for iron. This is met by previously stored iron which is generally sufficient to prevent anemia until about 6 months of age. After this period, supplemental dietary iron is essential to provide adequate requirements of iron.

The causes of iron deficiency anemia can be inadequate availability of iron, or depletion of iron from blood loss.

1. Inadequate availability of iron can be observed under the following circumstances:
   a) Low levels of iron storage at birth, observed in premature and low birth weight infants, and also in infants born to mothers with iron deficiency. Feto-maternal transfusion and placental hemorrhage also will result in low storage.
   b) Rapid growth of the infant resulting in larger demands than are available as seen in premature and low birth weight infants.
   c) Iron deficient diet (e.g., excessive milk intake during infancy).
   d) Malabsorption syndromes resulting in inadequate absorption of iron.
2. Loss of iron from the blood may be due to acute or chronic hemorrhage and parasitic infestations (i.e., hookworm). (Dietary iron deficiency anemia itself can cause fecal blood loss thus compounding the problem. Correction of deficiency stops the fecal loss. Also, enteric loss of blood in infants with iron deficiency anemia resulting from ingestion of whole milk has been reported.)

Clinical manifestations include pallor, irritability, apathy, and loss of appetite. Enlargement of the spleen is occasionally noted. Cardiac enlargement and failure may be noted in children with severe anemia.

HEMATOLOGICAL AND OTHER LABORATORY FINDINGS

1. Hemoglobin <11 g%.
2. Peripheral blood smear: Microcytic and hypochromic erythrocytes with typical central pallor, target cells and poikilocytes.
3. Serum iron less than 50 µg/100 ml.
4. Serum iron binding capacity greater than 350 µg/100 ml.
5. Transferrin saturation less than 16%

Other conditions associated with hypochromic microcytic anemias that should be distinguished from iron deficiency anemia are thalassemia syndromes and lead poisoning. Hypochromia of erythrocytes is also noted in pyridoxine deficiency and in anemias due to copper or transferrin deficiencies.

TREATMENT OF IRON DEFICIENCY ANEMIA

1. Correct the basic etiological factor causing anemia, such as deficiency diet, blood loss, or intestinal malabsorption.
2. Correction of anemia can be successfully done in most cases with oral iron therapy. Dose 5-6 mg, elemental iron/kg divided in three daily doses. Ferrous sulfate is the drug of choice and contains 20% elemental iron. Response to therapy is seen within 3 to 4 weeks. Therapy should continue 4 to 6 weeks after the blood values are normal.
3. Parenteral iron preparations (iron-dextran) may be used in some instances where a child cannot tolerate oral iron or intestinal absorption of iron is severely limited. (See p. 482.)
4. Occasionally, a combination of severe iron deficiency anemia and recurrent infections may require blood transfusion. Rapid correction of anemia in these instances is dangerous. Infusion of 5 ml/kg of packed cells followed by iron therapy constitutes the management of these cases.

The Committee on Nutrition of the American Academy of Pediatrics has recommended the use of iron-fortified formula for all infants until 12 months of age to prevent iron deficiency anemia.

SICKLE CELL HEMOGLOBINOPATHY

In this genetically determined disorder, the individual red blood cells contain varying proportions of an abnormal hemoglobin, hemoglobin S (HbS). The basic defect in the structure of hemoglobin S is the presence of an abnormal amino acid, valine, instead of the normal glutamic acid at the sixth position of the beta chain.

Sickle cell trait (SA) represents the heterozygous occurrence of the sickle cell gene. Approximately 10% of all

American blacks have this trait. The trait is also found in other countries including Africa, Italy, Greece, and India. The proportion of HbS in the RBCs varies between 24 and 45%. The affected children are usually asymptomatic with normal hemoglobin and hematocrit levels. Under severe hypoxic conditions or during high altitude flights, sickling and vascular occlusion resulting in splenic infarction has been noted. Other manifestations include hyposthenuria, priapism, and an increased incidence of pyelonephritis.

Sickle cell disease (SS) represents the homozygous occurrence of sickle cell gene. The incidence has been estimated as ranging between 0.3 and 1.3% of the black population in the United States. The proportion of HbS in the RBCs of the affected individual varies between 80 and 100%.

CLINICAL MANIFESTATIONS

Affected children are usually asymptomatic in the first 6 months of life. Principal features of the disease are hemolytic anemia and the occurrence of intermittent "crises."

1. The sickling of red blood cells and the increased viscosity of its contents are thought to damage the cell wall resulting in hemolysis. The symptoms of chronic hemolytic anemia include pallor, weakness, and easy fatigability.
2. Intermittent crises include:
   a) Vasoocclusive crisis
   b) Aplastic crisis
   c) Hyperhemolytic crisis
   d) Splenic sequestration crisis
      (1) Vasoocclusive crisis is the most common type. Masses of sickled cells block the blood vessels causing ischemic damage in various parts of the body. Vasospasm accompanies the blockage. The phenomenon is usually marked by pain and fever. There are no detectable changes in the hematological profile during the crises. Hand-foot syndrome, usually occurring around 2 years of age and characterized by painful swelling of hands and feet, is a result of circulatory impairment to the metacarpal and metatarsal bones. Beyond

the age of 2 years, painful episodes similarly involving other joints and extremities begin to occur. Abdominal pain, often severe, accompanies infarction of the abdominal organs such as liver and spleen. Severe intrahepatic sickling causes hepatic necrosis and obstructive jaundice characterized by elevated direct bilirubin levels. Blockage of vessels supplying the central nervous system may result in monoplegia or hemiplegia.

(2) Aplastic crisis: Occurs as a result of erythroid aplasia, presumably on the basis of infection, in a child who is constantly hemolyzing. Anemia can be severe with a sharp decrease in reticulocyte count.

(3) Hyperhemolytic crisis: This is marked by the aggravation of hemolysis causing a fall in hematocrit and a rise in the reticulocyte count.
Splenic enlargement may accompany the crises.

(4) Splenic sequestration crisis: May be acute or chronic. In the acute type there is a sudden drop in the hemoglobin level as a result of significant pooling of blood in the spleen. Hypovolemic shock may ensue with marked enlargement of the spleen. This type of crisis usually occurs during the first few years of life. The chronic type results in functional asplenia. These children show increased susceptibility to infection, particularly to pneumococcal and salmonella infections (similar to children who have undergone splenectomy).

HEMATOLOGICAL PICTURE

The affected children usually have a hemoglobin range between 6 and 10 g/100 ml. Reticulocyte and white blood cell counts are increased.

The sickle cell preparation (performed by mixing a drop of blood with sodium metabisulfite) is positive in both the trait and the disease. Peripheral blood smears show sickling of RBCs in cases of sickle cell disease. Note: a few other hemoglobinopathies are known to cause sickling such as HbC Harlem and homozygous alpha thalassemia. These disorders can be differentiated from HbS syndrome by electrophoretic studies.

Differential diagnosis includes: acute rheumatic fever, septic arthritis, osteomyelitis, rheumatoid arthritis, acute abdominal conditions, biliary obstruction, and pulmonary infections. Osteomyelitis, generally caused by *Staphylococcus aureus* and *Salmonella* is often difficult to differentiate from acute vasoocclusive crisis. An absolute band count of greater than $1000/mm^3$ and an ESR of 20 mm or greater are suggestive of osteomyelitis. In many cases, however, the diagnosis of osteomyelitis can only be established by needle aspiration of the suspected area of the bone and isolating the offending organisms in the culture media. Occasionally bone scans may be of some help.

TREATMENT

Supportive in nature and varies according to the clinical picture. Urea administration once thought to be promising in the prevention of sickling is pretty much discounted as a beneficial therapeutic agent.

1. Treat infection with antibiotics promptly. Administer penicillin or ampicillin for significant, unexplained fever.
2. Administer appropriate amounts and types of fluids to combat and prevent dehydration and acidosis, both of which can cause sickling. (See p. 200.)
3. Administer oxygen for anoxia and dyspnea. Remember prolonged use of oxygen may cause suppression of erythropoiesis.
4. Prescribe analgesics (aspirin, acetaminophen, propoxyphene hydrochloride) for pain.
5. Give fresh packed cell transfusions in aplastic and hyperhemolytic crises and whole blood transfusions in sequestration crisis to combat hypovolemia and shock. Also consider blood transfusion in severe venoocclusive crisis associated with Hb less than 5 g and/or serious complications such as meningitis and pneumonia. Partial exchange transfusion followed by packed cell maintenance transfusions at 3- to 4-week intervals may be considered in those children with (a) recurrent cerebrovascular episodes (b) severe recurrent priapism, and (c) resistant leg ulcers.
6. Consider splenectomy after one or two episodes of sequestration crisis.

7. Steroids are generally not recommended in the management of crises. But you may consider its short term use in infants with hand-foot syndrome and in patients with severe crisis with extreme debility and/or shock.

THE THALASSEMIA SYNDROMES

These are a group of disorders in which there is suppression of production of normal hemoglobin, HbA, due to defective synthesis of either alpha (alpha thalassemia) or beta (beta thalassemia) chains in the globin molecule of hemoglobin.

COOLEY'S ANEMIA
(Homozygous Beta Thalassemia)

Also called thalassemia major, Cooley's anemia represents the homozygous occurrence of a gene responsible for defective synthesis of beta chains of hemoglobin. Hemolysis of RBCs and the deficient production of hemoglobin contribute to chronic anemia seen in the affected children. The diagnosis is usually not made until about 4 months of age (because of the presence of large amounts of fetal hemoglobin). However, diagnosis is possible in the newborn period.

Clinical manifestations include pallor, anorexia, easy fatigability, massively enlarged spleen, hepatomegaly, pigmented skin (deposition and melanin and hemosiderin due to repeated transfusions), and characteristic facies, (enlarged head with frontal and parietal bossings, prominent maxilla with protruding and maloccluded teeth, and flattened base of the nose caused by severe bone marrow hyperplasia). The heart is frequently enlarged although cardiac failure is uncommon during early childhood.

Hematological Picture

Peripheral smear: microcytic, hypochromic erythrocytes, anisocytosis, basophilic stippling of RBCs, target cells, and large numbers of normoblasts. Bony changes include osteoporosis of long bones and "hair standing on end" appearance on skull x-ray.

Hemoglobin electrophoretic findings of elevated levels of Hgb F, absent or severely reduced Hgb A and variable amounts of Hgb A$_2$ are characteristic.

Treatment

1. Periodic transfusion of packed red cells to keep the hemoglobin level above 8-9 g/100 ml, to allow a normal range of activities.
2. The use of chelating agents such as deferoxamine is essential to treat iron overload resulting from repeated transfusions.
3. Massive enlargement of the spleen and increasing need for blood transfusions may indicate a need for splenectomy. Production of red cell antibodies can also increase the need for blood transfusions. Identifying these specific antibodies, and transfusion of compatible blood free from the offending antigen, should be tried, if possible, before considering splenectomy.
4. Following splenectomy, prophylactic therapy with oral penicillin for a year or two is recommended to prevent overwhelming infection.
5. Folic acid administration (5 mg/day) may be indicated in some cases.
6. Administration of iron is strictly contraindicated.

SOME INHERITED BLEEDING DISORDERS

Hemophilias are the most common of all the inherited bleeding disorders.

1. Hemophilia A is caused by the deficiency of factor VIII. This is a sex-linked recessive disorder in which asymptomatic female carriers transmit the disease to their male offsprings.
2. Hemophilia B is characterized by the deficiency of factor IX and is transmitted as a sex-linked recessive trait.
3. Hemophilia C is caused by the deficiency of factor XI and is transmitted as an autosomal dominant trait. Both sexes are affected. Some of the salient characteristics of these three disorders are outlined in Table 14-1.

Table 14-1 The Hemophilias

Clinical Manifestations	Laboratory Findings	Management (Acute Episode)	
		General	Specific
Factor VIII deficiency (hemophilia A)			
X-linked recessive trait: carried & transmitted by un-affected female to affected sons. Severity depends on the plasma level of factor VIII. In severe cases these levels may be less than 1-2% of the normal values. Easy bruising, persistent bleeding after trauma or surgery. Hemarthrosis is characteristic. CNS bleeding is serious.	Bleeding time: normal clotting time: abnormal* PTT** and TGT:*** abnormal	Immobilization of the affected joint for 24-48 hours. Application of ice pack over the affected area. Avoid, if possible, suturing, and injections. Do venipuncture, if you have to, only on the extremities, never on the jugular or femoral veins.	a. Fresh frozen plasma 10-15 ml/kg every 12 hours or, b. Factor VIII concentrate: initial dose: 20 U/kg. Maintenance dose: 2/3 initial dose every 12 hours. For minor superficial lesions, local pressure and application of hemostatic agents may be useful.

Factor IX deficiency (hemophilia B)	X-linked recessive trait: severity depends on the plasma level of factor IX. Signs and symptoms indistinguishable from hemophilia A.	Same as above.	Same as above.	a. Fresh or fresh frozen plasma 10–15 ml/kg q 12 to 24 hr b. Factor IX concentrate: Initial dose: 50 U/kg. Maintenance dose: 25 U/kg 24 hours.
Factor XI deficiency (hemophilia C)	Autosomal dominant trait: both sexes can be affected. Usually mild. Posttraumatic or postsurgical excessive bleeding. Nose bleeds.	Same as above.	Same as above.	Fresh or fresh frozen plasma 10–15 ml/kg q 24–36 hr. No concentrates are available.

*May be normal in moderate deficiencies.
**Partial thromboplastin time.
***Thromboplastic generation test.

PURPURAS

Purpuras are disorders characterized by minute petechial or more extensive extravasation (ecchymosis) of blood under the skin. They can be associated with a low platelet count (thrombocytopenic) or normal platelet counts (nonthrombo-cytopenic). The normal platelet count is 150,000–400,000/mm^3.

IDIOPATHIC THROMBOCYTOPENIC PURPURA

This is the most common of the thrombocytopenic purpuras. Autoimmune pathogenesis is postulated. Viral infections usually precede the onset of illness by 1–4 weeks. Generlized petechial hemorrhages of the skin, bleeding from the gums and nose, and occasionally more serious intracranial bleeding are some of the manifestations. The children do not appear sick. Symptoms generally subside within a week or two. Thrombocytopenia (platelet count usually below 60,000/mm^3) is the most significant laboratory finding. Bleeding time is prolonged, the tourniquet test is positive, and clot retraction is poor. Prognosis is usually excellent. No specific therapy is indicated for mild cases. For more severe cases: prednisone 1–2 mg/kg/day (maximum 40–60 mg/24 hr) for 2 weeks. Taper and discontinue steroids over a 3- to 5-day period. The efficacy of plasma and gamma globulin infusions to elevate platelet levels is presently being evaluated.

Other causes of thrombocytopenic purpuras include those induced by drugs (e.g., Quinidine, Sedormid) and Wiskott-Aldrich syndrome (associated with eczema and an increased susceptibility to infections).

Secondary purpuras occur in the course of other diseases such as leukemia, aplastic anemia, and splenic hyperfunction state.

HENOCH-SCHÖNLEIN OR ANAPHYLACTOID PURPURA

This entity is the most common of the nonthrombocytopenic purpuras. The syndrome is characterized by petechial rashes principally over the buttocks and lower extremities. The petechiae usually start as maculopapular erythematous lesions. Other features include arthritis (knees and ankles most commonly involved), gastrointestinal manifestations such as abdominal pain with GI bleeding, intussusception, and perforation. Renal involvement is not infrequent. Central nervous system hemorrhage is seen occasionally. Lymphadenopathy and hepatosplenomegaly are present during the acute phase of the disease. Edema of the eyelids and dorsum of the hands and lips are common. A bleeding workup reveals normal bleeding and clotting times. Platelets are adequate and clot retraction is normal. Occult blood may be demonstrated in the stool. Urinalysis may show RBCs, WBCs, and albumin.

Septicemia, blood dyscrasias, acute abdominal conditions, acute glomerulonephritis, and arthritic disorders should be considered in the differential diagnosis. The prognosis in general is good although 25% of children continue to have findings consistent with renal involvement.

Treatment is symptomatic with analgesics for pain, and antihypertensive agents for the occasional child developing hypertension with renal involvement. Appropriate antibiotic therapy is indicated in children showing evidence of infection. Steroid therapy (prednisone 1-2 mg/kg/day) is beneficial in the acute phase of the illness. Steroids do not influence the course of the renal involvement.

Other causes of nonthrombocytopenic purpuras are congenital vascular defects (Von Willebrand's disease, Ehlers-Danlos syndrome) infections such as meningococcemia, drugs and chemical agents, scurvy, and thrombasthenia (defective platelet function).

LEUKEMIAS

The leukemias are classified under three major categories: (1) acute lymphocytic leukemia (ALL); (2) acute nonlymphocytic leukemia (ANLL); and (3) chronic myolocytic leukemia (CML). Acute lymphocytic leukemia constitutes nearly 75% of all cases of leukemia. Generally four subgroups are identified in this category: (1) the common form; (2) T-cell form; (3) B-cell form; and (4) null cell form. Principal features of acute leukemia are:

1. Normocytic and normochromic anemia with a low reticulocyte count.

2. Bleeding episodes (epistaxis, hematuria, petechiae, ecchymosis with significant thrombocytopenia).
3. Bone and joint manifestations with areas of bone destruction and periosteal elevation as demonstrated by x-ray.
4. Hepatosplenomegaly.
5. Nontender, generalized lymphadenopathy with enlargement of mediastinal lymph nodes.
6. Frequently, leukopenia or leukocytosis (may have normal count) with the blast cell being the predominant circulating cell.
7. Fever is commonly present with or without pyogenic infection. Differential diagnostic conditions include aplastic anemia, infectious mononucleosis, idiopathic thrombocytopenic purpura. Other malignant processes may mimic leukemia. Bone marrow studies are mandatory before a diagnosis of acute leukemia can be established.
8. Survival rates among affected children have improved significantly with the advent of newer chemotherapeutic agents. The specific chemotherapeutic agents include corticosteroids, vincristine, 6-mercaptopurine, methotrexate, cyclophosphamide, and daunorubicin. Because the management can often be complex, it is best that leukemic children are treated in specialized centers where an agreed upon protocol for treatment can be reasonably followed. General supportive treatment consists of blood transfusions and antibiotic therapy for infections.
9. Clinical and laboratory features at the time of diagnosis that offer poor prognosis include, age less than 2 years or more than 12 years, initial white count greater than $50,000/mm^3$, platelet count less than $100,000/mm^3$, presence of mediastinal mass and organomegaly, involvement of central nervous system, and decreased immunoglobulins. Also black children tend to have a poorer prognosis than a white children.

Chapter 15

COMMON CARDIAC PROBLEMS

DIAGNOSTIC TOOLS

HISTORY

The medical history is the physician's first step in establishing a diagnosis. Its importance is not so much in helping to differentiate one congenital lesion from another as it is to assess the severity of the patient's condition.

Practical Points

1. Familial factors:
   a) Family history of cardiac diseases
   b) Gestational history (particularly to rule out teratogenic agents, rubella, etc.)
2. Past history of patient:
   a) To gauge presence of previous symptoms or signs
   b) The progress of these signs and symptoms
   c) Parental knowledge of cardiac illness
   d) Prenatal history. Prenatal history must include maternal disease, medication, trauma, nutrition, and genetic history of disease in both parents' families.

A positive history should result in a more detailed
evaluation of and/or referral for an auscultatory sign
than would be necessitated by an unrevealing medical
history; for example, atrial septal deficit, asymmetric
septal hypertrophy, Noonan's syndrome, and mitral
valve prolapse (Barlow's syndrome may occur as a
mendelian autosomal inheritance).
   e) Perinatal history for signs of cardiac difficulty -
cyanosis, poor feeding, etc. Perinatal history is
equally important in detecting occult disease. Fetal-
fetal or fetal-maternal transfusion, ABO incompati-
bility, jaundice, cyanosis, asphyxia, or RDS are examples of hematological and/or cardiovascular disease
which would cause an anemia or shunt to present as
a murmur; late sequela of an apparently resolved
problem.
3. Present history:
   a) Respiratory tract: Grunting in infancy, tachypnea
and dyspnea, wheezing, frequent lower respiratory
tract infection.
   b) Circulatory: Cyanosis, constant or intermittent,
central or peripheral; syncope (aortic stenosis);
squatting (tetralogy of Fallot).
   c) General: Easy fatigability, e.g., protracted feeding
accompanied by poor suck, restlessness, irritability,
sweating, tachypnea, etc.—indicate easy fatigability
in infants; poor growth rate; chest pain; edema.
   d) Diet: An iron-poor diet, pica, toxin exposure, or fad
diets may present as a hemic murmur.

PHYSICAL DIAGNOSIS

Practical Points

The physical examination plays an exceedingly important
role in the diagnosis of cardiac lesions. It is one of the few
instances where frequently more information can be gathered
than from the medical history.

It is essential that the physical examination not be
limited to the heart alone but include all other systems. In
a systematic fashion the following 10 steps must be accomplished:

1. Estimation of body size and build
2. Present state of activity (particularly for infants)
3. Blood pressure in upper and lower extremities: heart and respiratory rates and cardiac rhythm
4. Color of skin and mucous membranes in all parts of the body (cyanotic heart disease)
5. Funduscopic examination (hypertensive, diabetic, or rubella heart disease)
6. Palpation of peripheral pulses (aortic coarctation). See Table 15-1 for normal pulse rates
7. Inspection and palpation of all extremities for clubbing, edema, abnormal pulsations (Quincke's sign), bruits, (AV communications), and venous engorgement (epigastric veins)
8. Examination of the abdomen (hepatomegaly, bruits, masses)
9. Thorough examination of respiratory function
10. Thorough examination of the heart

Particular attention must be paid to the examination of the heart itself. The following points may be essential for proper diagnosis and management.

1. Point of maximal impulse (PMI): Normally this is found in the fourth left intercostal space just to the left to the midclavicular line in younger children (less than 7 years). In older children (more than 7 years) it is generally at the fifth left intercostal space and inside the midclavicular line. A PMI that is displaced laterally tends to indicate right ventricular enlargement. A PMI that is displaced laterally and downward indicates left ventricular enlargement. A heaving, diffuse impulse is suggestive of left ventricular enlargement while a sharp, tapping impulse suggests right ventricular enlargement. The position of the PMI should be measured with a tape measure, recorded, and checked serially.
2. Heart sounds: Many important diagnostic clues are rendered by changes in heart sounds. There are two heart sounds normally and a third heart sound in approximately one-third of children. Each of the two major heart sounds has two components of valvular origin. The first heart sound is better heard at the apex with the bell

Table 15-1   Pulse Rate Per Minute

Birth	70-170
First weeks	120-140
1 year	80-140
2 years	80-130
3 years	80-120
Over 3 years	70-115

Resting pulse greater than 90-100 is suspicous in a child older than 6-7 years; 8-10 beats/minute must be added for each Fahrenheit degree of temperature rise.

portion of the stethoscope; the second at the base with the diaphragm. Normally, the first sound is louder at the apex than the second sound and, conversely, the second sound is louder than the first sound at the base. When the first sound is markedly increased at the apex, mitral stenosis must be considered.

The two components (aortic and pulmonic) of the second sound should be compared. Except in newborns and young children, the aortic component is the louder. A decreased or absent sound over the pulmonic area (left side of the sternum) indicates pulmonic stenosis just as a decreased second sound over the aortic area (right side of the sternum) is consistent with aortic stenosis. An increase in the second sound's intensity over the aortic area may indicate aortic insufficiency or systemic hypertension. A decrease in the intensity of heart sounds may indicate acute myocarditis or large pericardial effusion. Splitting of the second heart sound at the base may be normal and is useful in ruling out the absence of one of the two valves that contribute to the second sound. If it is heard, the diagnosis of truncus arteriosus is effectively ruled out. Splitting normally becomes wider during inspiration. If it remains wide and unchanging (fixed), atrial septal defect must be considered. Paradoxical splitting may indicate aortic stenosis.

3. The venus hum is a continuous, low pitched sound over the neck and upper sternal areas that can be distinguished from a cardiac murmur because it can be abolished by applying pressure over the internal jugular vein or by turning the head to face toward the side of the body on which the sound was heard.
4. Innocent murmurs. Characteristics are:
   a) Short in duration (not holosystolic)
   b) Heard in systole, not diastole
   c) Usually heard over pulmonary area
   d) Generally (but not always) soft, blowing, or musical in quality
   e) Poorly transmitted as a rule and tending to radiate downward rather than laterally
   f) Tend to vary in intensity with change of position
   g) May change characteristics on subsequent office visits
   h) May vary with respirations and change in physical state (fever, excitement, and exercise)

Growing attention has been paid to prolapse of the mitral valve. In this condition one of the valve leaflets prolapses under the pressure of ventricular systole leading to a state of mitral regurgitation. Patients are usually asymptomatic but are at an, as yet, undetermined risk for developing rhythm disturbances, decompensating mitral insufficiency, and subacute bacterial endocarditis. To prepare for these possibilities, it is important to distinguish mitral valve prolapse from purely functional murmurs. In the typical case (not all are), there is a late systolic murmur and a nonejection midsystolic or late systolic click at the apex. Chest pain may be present in some patients. The diagnosis can usually be confirmed by echocardiography which is safe and noninvasive. Patients need not be restricted in any way unless signs of decompensation or rhythm disturbances are present. Valve replacement has been recommended for the former and propranolol for the latter. Prophylactic antibiotics should be administered on the same indications for any organic heart disease, i.e., dental procedures. Long-term follow-up will be necessary.

ECG

The ECG is an essential diagnostic tool. It is particularly important in establishing the existence of chamber hypertrophy, abnormal rhythms, and pressure overloads. It is also important in gauging the effect of drug therapy and in following the patient's progress in the postdiagnostic period. It is important to remember that most ECG machines allow recordings to be taken at two speeds marked 25 and 50. This means 25 mm/sec and 50 mm/sec. The standard ECG is taken at 25 mm/sec, not 50 mm/sec. When the standard speed is used, each small box on the ECG paper represents 0.04 seconds in duration (moving horizontally) and five of the small boxes (one large box) thus represents 0.2 seconds. Using this, one can calculate the heart rate by measuring the duration (number of boxes) between two R waves or two P waves. If the atrial and ventricular rates are different each may be calculated separately. The 50 mm/sec speed is used only for more detailed visualization and measurement of various components of the electrocardiographic complex.

When the vertical range of the recording needle is calibrated to 2 large boxes (10 small ones) then 10 mm = 1 mV and standard voltage measurements may be made for each positive and negative deflection of the needle. Each small box is exactly 1 mm so voltage may be expressed in the number of millimeters that the tracing extends above and below the isoelectric line.

The standard pediatric ECG must include a recording from either V_{3R}, V_{4R}, or V_E to be complete. Because of the greater preponderance of right ventricular forces in early childhood, leads taken farther to the right than V_1 are necessary to establish the progression of R and S waves from various positions on the thorax.

Figure 15-1 depicts the normal waves of the ECG tracing. Figure 15-2 illustrates the hexaxial system.

X-RAY

Cardiac x-ray studies range from the simple PA view of the chest to cineangiography. Several points must be borne in mind. The PA chest view, if it is to yield maximum information, must be standard and must eliminate distortion. This entails proper alignment of the patient and the x-ray cone.

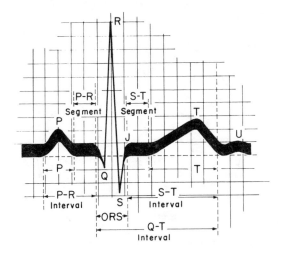

Figure 15-1   The waves of the normal electrocardiogram.
(From Nadas, A.S.: Pediatric Cardiology, 3rd ed.,
W.B. Saunders Co., Philadelphia, 1973. Reproduced
with publisher's permission.)

The child is positioned so that his anterior chest wall is perpendicular to the direction of the x-rays. Younger children
who may not be able to cooperate are better off being
strapped into a restraining device. The cone of the x-ray
machine should be far enough away from the patient so that
the rays are essentially parallel and undue magnification of
the heart shadow is avoided (distance of 6 feet). As a rough
index of normality the maximum transverse diameter of the
heart on such a standard PA film should not exceed 55% of
the thoracic diameter measured at the level of the right
hemidiaphragm from the inner surface of the right ribs to
that of the left ribs. Cardiac configuration, pulmonary vas-
culative, and the course of the great vessels should be observed. Lateral 6-foot films and left anterior and right
anterior oblique views after a barium swallow are also essential in judging heart size and the enlargement of specific
chambers. (See Figures 15-3A, 15-3B, and 15-3C.)

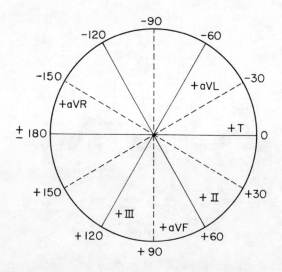

Figure 15-2 The hexaxial system. (Nadas, A.S.: Pediatric Cardiology, 3rd ed., W.B. Saunders Co., Philadelphia, 1973. Reproduced with publisher's permission.)

Angiography is essential for the differential diagnosis of cyanotic heart disease but not so important for acyanotic left to right shunts. X-rays are more useful for volume overload than pressure overload.

Practical Points

1. It is helpful to think of two basic types of congenital cardiac lesions when interpreting x-rays: obstructive and shunting.
   a) Obstructive lesions (pulmonary stenosis, aortic stenosis, aortic coarctation) normally do not alter pulmonary vascular markings. Occasionally, these markings may be decreased as in pulmonic stenosis but they are not increased. Also, the cardiac silhouette is usually altered significantly (exception is aortic coarctation).
   b) Left to right shunting lesions (ASD, VSD, PDA) usually do alter pulmonary vascular markings causing an increase in both the markings and the pulmonary artery

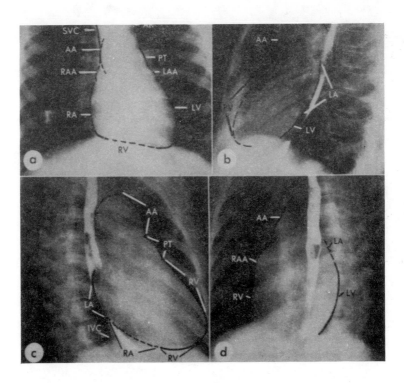

Figure 15-3A Cardiac structures forming the normal cardiovascular silhouette in the four conventional views.
(a) Posteroanterior view. (b) Lateral view. (c) Right
anterior oblique view. (d) Left anterior oblique view.
Key: SVC—superior vena cava, AA—ascending aorta,
RAA—right atrial appendate, RA- right atrium, RV—
right ventricle, LV—left ventricle, LAA—left atrial
appendage, PT—pulmonary trunk, AK—aortic knob,
LA—left atrium, IVC—inferior vena cava. (From
Elliott, L.P. and Schiebler, G.L.: Postgrad Med.
37:A89, Jan. 1965. Reproduced with permission of
McGraw-Hill, New York.)

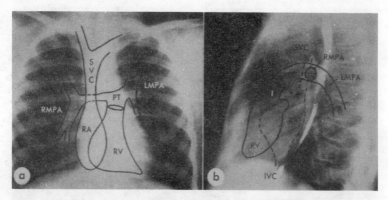

Figure 15–3B Schematic drawing of the right–sided cardiac
chambers and vessels superimposed on normal thoracic
roentgenogram. (a) Posteroanterior view. (b) Lateral
view. Key: SVC—superior vena cava, RA—right
atrium, PT—pulmonary trunk, RV—right ventricle,
RMPA—right main pulmonary artery, LMPA—left
main pulmonary artery, I—right ventricular infundi-
bulum, IVC—inferior vena cava. (From Elliott, L.P.
and Schiebler, G.L.: Postgrad Med. 37:A89, Jan. 1965.
Reproduced with permission of McGraw-Hill, New York.)

area of the cardiac silhouette on a PA view (see Figure 15–4). Significant cardiac enlargement occurs but
usually becomes marked only in the more severe lesions.
Pulmonary artery prominence is seen as a bulge in the
left upper cardiac border best seen on PA and RAO
views.

2. When the pulmonic area is prominent on x-ray and there
   is also increased peripheral pulmonary vascular markings,
   PDA, ASD, or VSD are likely diagnoses. When peripheral
   pulmonary vascular markings are decreased, pulmonic
   stenosis is likely. See Table 15–2.
3. Aortic enlargement is best seen on PA and LAO views as
   a bulge in the upper right cardiac silhouette. Think of
   two possibilities: PDA (since blood is shunted into the
   ascending aorta) and aortic stenosis with poststenotic
   dilation. Aortic aneurysm is rarely encountered in children. See Table 15–3.

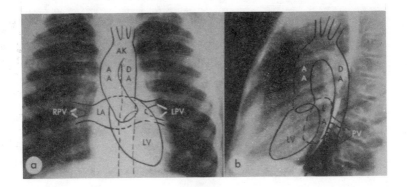

Figure 15-3C Schematic drawing of the left-sided cardiac
chambers and vessels superimposed on the normal
thoracic roentgenogram. (a) Posteroanterior view.
(b) Lateral view. Key: AK—aortic knob, AA—ascending aorta, DA—descending aorta, LA—left atrium,
RPV—right pulmonary veins, LV—left ventricles,
LPV—left pulmonary veins, PV—pulmonary veins.
(From Elliott, L.P., and Schiebler, G.L.: Postgrad
Med. 37:A89, Jan. 1965. Reproduced with permission
of McGraw-Hill, New York.)

Another helpful point, when a left to right shunt is
present, with its accompanying increase in pulmonary
vascular markings, an enlarged aorta indicates an extra-
cardiac shunt such as PDA rather than an intracardiac
one such as ASD or VSD.

Remember to look for right-sided aortas on the PA
film.

4. Right atrium—best views: PA and LAO. Enlargement is
seen as an increased convexity of the right heart border.
ASD is a common cause.

5. Left atrium—best views: PA, lateral, RAO. Left atrium
forms the upper part of the cardiac silhouette on lateral
and RAO views. A double density in the midcardiac area,
elevation of the left main stem bronchus, and posterior
deviation of the barium-filled esophagus on a lateral film
are indicative of left atrial enlargement. VSD and PDA
are common causes.

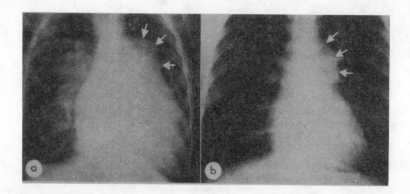

Figure 15-4 Abnormal pulmonary artery. (a) Posteroanterior view. Prominent pulmonary trunk and central and peripheral pulmonary arterial vessels in L-R shunt. (b) Posteroanterior view. Isolated prominence of pulmonary trunk (arrows) but normal peripheral pulmonary vessels in obstructive lesion (pulmonary valvular stenosis). (From Elliott, L.P. and Schiebler, G.L.: Postgrad Med. 37:A89, Jan. 1965. Reproduced with permission of McGraw-Hill, New York.)

6. In left to right shunts at the atrial level, the left atrium is normal in size (ASD). In left to right shunts at the ventricular level (VSD) or extra cardiac shunts (PDA), the left atrium enlarges because of excess blood flow from the overloaded pulmonary circulation.
7. Right ventricular enlargement—best views: PA, lateral, and LAO. On the PA view the apex is displaced toward the left and tends to be uplifted. On the LAO view the anterior heart border shows increased convexity. On the lateral view, the anterior heart shadow merges with the sternal shadow throughout its entire length. Normally, the upper portion of the cardiac shadow has separated from the sternum after infancy.
8. Left ventricular enlargement—best views: PA and LAO. On the PA view, the apex is displaced toward the left and downward. On the LAO view, the posterior wall of the heart projects over the spine. Phonocardiography, vectorcardiography, and cardiac catheterization may be employed by the cardiologist in making the final diagnosis. See Table 15-4.

Table 15-2   Summary of X-Ray Findings

No cyanosis:	Heart size normal Normal pulmonary-vascular markings		Coarctation of the aorta Aortic stenosis Pulmonic stenosis
	Large heart Prominent pulmonary vascular markings	LVH:	PDA VSD AV canal Endocardial sclerosis
		RVH:	ASD Tetralogy of Fallot
Cyanosis:	Heart size normal Decreased pulmonary-vascular markings		
	Large heart Prominent pulmonary-vascular markings		Complete transposition of the great vessels Total anomalous pulmonary drainage

CARDIAC ARRHYTHMIAS

The following three basic types of arrhythmia exist: defective formation of the cardiac impulse, defective conduction of the cardiac impulse, and continuous or cyclic conduction of the cardiac impulse. See Table 15-5.

The treatment of these arrhythmias depends on drugs that primarily affect conduction velocity, depolarization rate, duration of the refractory period, and the automaticity or rate of spontaneous discharge of cardiac cells. The key to treating any arrhythmia is the accurate assessment of its basic pathogenesis. If, for example, an arrhythmia is due to increased conduction velocity, a drug that decreases conduction velocity is chosen. It must be said, too, that knowledge

Table 15-3 Summary of Congenital Heart Disease in Children

	History and Course	Physical Findings
Pulmonic stenosis	Varies from asymptomatic to dyspnea, easy tiring, cyanosis, and heart failure.	Loud ejection systolic murmur maximum at upper left sternal border.
	Endocarditis	Transmission—back and neck P2 decreased
	X-ray	ECG
	Mild cases Normal	Mild cases Normal
	Severe cases Dilatation of pulmonary artery	Severe cases Strain, wide QRS-T angle P pulmonale
	RVH RAH Decreased pulm. flow Angiography indicated to demonstrate lesion	

Condition	Symptoms	Physical Signs
Aortic stenosis	Asymptomatic to fatigue and dyspnea. Chest pain and syncope (important, serious symptoms); rarely sudden death and occasionally left-sided heart failure. Arrhythmia Endocarditis	Narrow pulse pressure (sometimes absent). Loud systolic ejection murmur maximum right base. Transmission: neck, along left sternal border. A_2 decreased Sometimes associated AI murmur. Ejection click present with aortic dilatation.

X-ray

Mild cases	Normal
Moderate to severe	LV enlargement

ECG

Mild cases	Normal
Severe cases	LVH, strain pattern

Angiography indicated dilated ascending aorta

Condition	Symptoms	Physical Signs
Coarctation of the aorta	Asymptomatic in young patients Leg pains, headache Rupture of aorta, left-sided heart failure in adulthood Dissectible aortic aneurysm Hypertension Endocarditis CVA	BP in arms increased Femoral pulses decreased Systolic murmur maximum upper back, especially left side

Table 15-3 (Cont'd.) Summary of Congenital Heart Disease in Children

	History and Course	Physical Findings
	X-ray	ECG
	Heart size usually normal	May be normal
	Occasionally LVH	LVH
	LAO and PA films may show co-arctated segment	
	Rib notching in older patients	
Patent ductus arteriosus	Frequently asymptomatic, exertional dyspnea, fatigability. Frequent lower respiratory infection. Occasional cyanosis with OPVD. Failure occasionally.	Bounding pulses Wide pulse pressure Machinery murmur; crescendo-decrescendo, may be continuous especially in older children, maximum at left base.
	X-ray	ECG
	Endocarditis	May be normal
	Small ductus Normal	LVH
	Large ductus LV, LA and aortic enlargement.	OPVD—RVH

		X-ray	ECG
	With OPVD Large RA, RV Pulm. flow decreased Angiography not indicated in clear-cut cases, required in atypical cases.		Systolic murmur, maximum upper left sternal border. Middiastolic murmur at left lower sternal border. Widely split and fixed second sound.
Atrial septal defect Secundum type	Asymptomatic in childhood Later: easy tiring, dyspnea, and heart failure.	Right-sided enlargement Pulm. flow increased Angiography not necessary. May demonstrate abnormal pulmonary veins.	Right axis deviation Right bundle branch block RVH with larger defects
Ventricular septal defect	Asymptomatic or dyspnea, easy tiring, repiratory infections. Heart failure and OPVD can occur. Endocarditis		Loud, harsh pansystolic murmur; maximum left lower sternal border. Transmitted over precordium. Occasional apical diastolic rumble. P_2 may be loud.

Table 15-3 (Cont'd.) Summary of Congenital Heart Disease in Children

	History and Course	Physical Findings
	X-ray	ECG
	Small defect Normal Large defect LAH, LVH Pulm. flow increased (With OPVD: pulm. flow decreased) Angiography not usually necessary. Aortography done if OPVD is present to rule out PDA and aortic abnor- malities.	Small defects Normal Large defects LVH combined ventricular enlarge- ment. RVH with OPVD
Endocardial cushion defect	Dyspnea, tiring, pulmonary infection, and failure. Complete form: early death. OPVD.	Mild or no cyanosis. Harsh holosys- tolic murmur at apex. P2 increased with splitting. No splitting with OPVD.

	X-ray	ECG
	RVH,LAH,LVH with mitral insufficiency. Pulm. flow increased. Angiography indicated.	Superior electrical axis. Counterclockwise vector, loop in frontal plane. Combined ventricular hypertrophy.
Transposition of pulmonary veins	Mild to moderate cyanosis. Failure in infancy and early death. Dyspnea, fatigability, infections. OPVD.	Systolic murmur along left sternal border. P2 split. Third heart sound. Sometimes a fourth heart sound. Occasional presystolic murmur and a continuous murmur at base.

X-ray	ECG
Supracardiac type: figure 8 configuration. RAH,RVH Pulm. flow increased	Right axis deviation, RAH, and RVH
Infradiaphragmatic type: small heart, pulm. flow increased	
Angiography indicated plus pulmonary artery injection	

Table 15-3 (Cont'd.) Summary of Congenital Heart Disease in Children

	History and Course	Physical Findings
Tetralogy of Fallot	Early cyanosis, polycythemia, dyspnea, squatting. Occasional acyanosis and mild symptoms. Brain abscess. Embolism, thrombosis, etc. Endocarditis.	Cyanosis, clubbing P2 decreased. Loud systolic murmur at left sternal border
	X-ray	ECG
	Normal size heart. Pulm. flow decreased. Boot-shaped heart. Right aortic arch sometimes seen.	Cyanotic form—right axis deviation, RVH Acyanotic form—combined ventricular hypertrophy
	Angiography indicated	
Transposition of the great vessels	Cyanosis, dyspnea. Early and progressive failure. Death in first 6 months usual.	Cyanosis- systolic murmur frequent but not always

	X-ray	ECG
	Cardiac enlargement. Increased pulm. flow (occasional pulm. flow decreased with pulm. stenosis). Narrow supra-cardiac stalk.	RVH or combined ventricular hypertrophy
	Angiography indicated.	Occasionally LVH alone
Tricuspid atresia	Early cyanosis and dyspnea. Hypoxic spells, CVA. Death in first year usual.	Cyanosis. Systolic murmur left sternal border.
	Normal-sized heart. Pulm. flow decreased (increased pulm. flow in transposition).	Left axis deviation
		LVH
	Angiography indicated.	P pulmonale

Legend

LAH   Left atrial hypertrophy
LVH   Left ventricular hypertrophy

Table 15-3   (Cont'd.)   Summary of Congenital Heart Disease in Children

Legend (Cont'd.)

RAH	Right atrial hypertrophy
RVH	Right ventricular hypertrophy
OPVD	Obstructive pulmonary vascular disease
Pulm. flow	Pulmonary artery blood flow
BP	Blood pressure
LA	Left atrium
RA	Right atrium
LV	Left ventricle
RV	Right ventricle
LAO	Left anterior oblique
RAO	Right anterior oblique
CVA	Cerebrovascular accident
PA	Posteroanterior x-ray view
AI	Aortic insufficiency

**Table 15-4   Surgical Therapy for Congenital Cardiac
Lesions**

Cardiac Lesion	Surgical Therapy
Aortic stenosis	Good results with valvular, supraval-vular, and subaortic types
Pulmonary stenosis	Brock procedure or valvulotomy may be corrective
Aortic coarctation	Corrective surgery best at 4-12 years of age with end-to-end anastomosis or bridging grafts
Patent ductus arteriosus	Surgery best between 3 and 10 years of age when risk is under 2%. Ligature or division of the ductus can be done.
Atrial septal defect— Secundum type	Defect can be closed by suturing during childhood. Risk is less than 5%.
Ventricular septal defect	Optimal repair is at 4 years of age or a body weight of 11-40 kg. Pulmonary artery banding in children too small for corrective surgery can forestall obstructive pulmonary disease. Definative repair is procedure of choice.
Endocardial cushion defect	Incomplete form is correctable with a 2-5% mortality rate; the complete form with a 15-50% rate. Pulmonary artery banding may be helpful for ventricular level shunts.
Total anomalous pulmonary drainage	Atrial balloon septostomy can be help-ful. Corrective surgery is associated with a significant mortality rate.

Table 15-4   (Cont'd.) Surgical Therapy for Congenital Cardiac Lesions

Cardiac Lesion	Surgical Therapy
Tetralogy of Fallot	Blalock, Potts, and other procedures can be used. The risk is fairly low.
Transposition of the great vessels	Palliative surgery to permit blood flow between the arterial and venous system carries high risk but may help. Total correction carries an even higher risk.
Tricuspid atresia	Blalock or Glenn procedures may help. Newer procedures are being tried and evaluated.
Truncus arteriosus	Pulmonary artery banding is palliative. Corrective surgery is now possible but has a high mortality rate.

of all the effects of the cardiopharmaceuticals is essential in order to avoid undesirable side effects in treating the arrhythmias.

Table 15-6 lists the principal effects of the six most commonly used cardiopharmaceuticals other than digitalis.

Table 15-7 lists the major arrhythmias, the treatment of choice (listed as number one), and alternate treatments.

DEFIBRILLATION

Defibrillation is a valuable, at times, lifesaving procedure. Electrical conversion of the fibrillating heat is quick, easy to perform and relatively safe. In an emergency it is the procedure of choice for these reasons.

Table 15-5 The Types of Cardiac Arrthymias

Defective Impulse Formation	Defective Conduction	Cyclic Conduction (circus movement)
Bradycardia due to depressed SA node	Bundle branch block	Ventricular flutter Ventricular fibrillation
Ectopic pacemaker	Complete and incomplete	Atrial flutter
Atrial premature beats Ventricular premature beats	Heart block	Atrial fibrillation
	Wenckebach phenomenon	
Supraventricular tachycardia	Wolff-Parkinson-White syndrome	
Wandering pacemaker		
Ventricular tachycardia		

Defibrillators are commercially available in a variety of forms and should be a part of every pediatric service where cardiac emergencies could conceivably arise. Ventricular fibrillation may be encountered in children during anesthesia, the course of acute myocardial disease, arrhythmias, as a result of therapy with cardiopharmaceuticals, especially digitalis, Isuprel, and epinephrine, and during almost any illness known to cause hypoxia and acidosis.

Table 15-6   Cardiopharmaceuticals Other than Digitalis

Drug	Conduction Velocity	Depolarization Rate	Duration of Refractory Period	Automaticity or Rate of Spontaneous Depolarization	Clinical Uses	Adverse Effects	Comments
Quinidine	Decreased	Decreased	Increased especially in atria, slightly in ventricles. Decreased in AV node.	Decreased but no effect on SA node.	Atrial and ventricular ectopic beats. Supraventricular tachycardia, atrial flutter and fibrillation.	Potassium enhances quinidine's actions. Hypokalemia decreases it. Contraindicated in complete heart block. May induce bundle branch block, AV	Electrical cardioversion safer and more effective than quinidine for atrial flutter or fibrillation. Digitalization should precede quinidine's use in atrial

flutter and
fibrillation
to decrease
conduction
through AV
node. May be
given po,
IM, IV.
Dose: 3 mg/
lb q 3 h x
5

block,
cardiac ar-
rest. Use
with care
in hepatic
disease (ex-
creted by
liver).
Nausea,
vomiting,
visual dis-
turbances,
etc. may
occur.
Peripheral
dilatation
and nega-
tive ino-
tropic ef-
fect may
occur.

Table 15-6 (Cont'd.) Cardiopharmaceuticals Other than Digitalis

Drug	Conduction Velocity	Depolarization Rate	Duration of Refractory Period	Automaticity or Rate of Spontaneous Depolarization	Clinical Uses	Adverse Effects	Comments
Procainamide (Pronestyl)	Decreased	Decreased	Increased	Decreased	Similar to quinidine	Use with care in renal disease (excreted by kidney). May induce AV block when used to counter digitalis-induced arrhythmias. Hypotension and failure	Very similar action to quinidine. The two drugs are additive. Preferred over quinidine when rapid onset is desired. May be given po, IM, IV.

					Comments	Dose
					occur with higher doses. Similar cardiac side effects to quinidine. Drug-induced lupus may occur, especially on high dosage. Causes peripheral dilatation and negative inotropic effect.	Dose: 7 mg/lb q 6 h, po 3 mg/lb q 4–6 h, IM
Lidocaine	No effect	De-creased	Decreased	Decreased	Ventricular arrhythmias, particularly when quinidine or procainamide	Use with care in liver disease (excreted by liver). CNS symptoms	May be given IV. Dose: 0.5 mg/lb

Table 15-6 (Cont'd.) Cardiopharmaceuticals Other than Digitalis

Drug	Conduction Velocity	Depolarization Rate	Duration of Refractory Period	Automaticity or Rate of Spontaneous Depolarization	Clinical Uses	Adverse Effects	Comments
					fail. Good for digitalis-induced ventricular arrhythmias.	can occur: paresthesias, convulsions. Large doses can cause negative inotropic effect and peripheral dilatation but less than procainamide and quinidine.	

Dilantin	Increased AV node conduction may be accelerated	Increased especially on atria. SA node not affected	Decreased	Decreased	Arrhythmias due to ectopic pacemakers, cyclic arrhythmias, useful in digitalis-induced arrhythmias.	Negative inotropic effect. Peripheral dilatation may induce AV block, bradycardia, cardiac arrest, nausea, vomiting, rash, ataxia. Rare blood dyscrasia may occur.	Counters AV node depression induced by quinidine or procainamide. Counters cardiac side effects of digitalis without negating its therapeutic effect. Do not use in atrial flutter or fibrillation or AV block. May be given IV, or po. Dose: 3-10 mg/kg/24 hr

Table 15-6 (Cont'd.) Cardiopharmaceuticals Other than Digitalis

Drug	Conduction Velocity	Depolarization Rate	Duration of Refractory Period	Automaticity or Rate of Spontaneous Depolarization	Clinical Uses	Adverse Effects	Comments
Propranolol (Inderal)	Decreased	Decreased	Increased	Decreased	Digitalis-induced arrhythmias, premature ventricular contractions. Also good in nondigitalis-induced arrhythmias: paroxysmal atrial tachycardia,	Contraindicated in bronchial asthma, obstructive airway diseases, cor pulmonale. Do not use when AV block is present; reduces cardiac output.	Beta adrenergic blocking agent. Inhibits adrenergic effect. Also has direct cardiac action. Used with digitalis in atrial flutter and fibrillation because

| supraventricular tachycardia with Wolff-Parkinson-White syndrome. Atrial flutter and fibrillation | Inotropic negative effect. May cause hypertension and cardiac failure (can be countered by digitalis). Use cautiously in diabetics. Side effects include vomiting, diarrhea, rash, fever, laryngospasm. | actions are additive and superior to digitalis alone. May be given IV or po. Dose: IV 0.5-1 mg. IV slowly, not to exceed 0.1 mg/kg. po: 10 mg qid |

Table 15-6 (Cont'd.) Cardiopharmaceuticals Other than Digitalis

Drug	Conduction Velocity	Depolarization Rate	Duration of Refractory Period	Automaticity or Rate of Spontaneous Depolarization	Clinical Uses	Adverse Effects	Comments
Potassium	Decreased in AV node and ventricles.		Decreased	Decreased	Digitalis-induced arrhythmias precipitated by hypokalemia	AV block with serum K levels of 7 mEq or more. Rapid infusion may depress myocardial contractility. Use with great caution in renal disease.	Monitor administration with ECG. Use is virtually restricted to arrhythmias complicated by hypokalemia. May be given IV or po. Dose: 40 mEq/500 ml of 5% dextrose/water, no faster than 0.5 mEq/min

Table 15-7 Treatment of Major Arrhythmias (See Table 15-6 for Doses of Medications)

Atrial Arrhythmias
  Atrial premature beats
    Digitalis
    Quinidine
    Procainamide
  Wenckebach's phenomenon
    Treat underlying disorder
  Wolff-Parkinson-White syndrome
  No treatment unless paroxysmal tachycardia is present, then use:
    Quinidine
    Propranolol
  Wandering pacemaker
  No treatment
  Sinus tachycardia or bradycardia
  No treatment
  Supraventricular tachycardia
    Digitalis or electrical cardioversion
    Propranolol
    Quinidine
    Procainamide
    Lidocaine
  Atrial flutter
    Digitalis or electrical cardioversion
    Propranolol
    Quinidine in addition to digitalis
    Procainamide
    Lidocaine
  Atrial fibrillation
    Electrical cardioversion
    Digitalis or digitalis with propranolol
    Quinidine in addition to digitalis
  SA node block
  No treatment if asymptomatic, otherwise:
    Ephedrine
    Atropine
    Isuprel

Table 15-7   (Cont'd.)   Treatment of Major Arrhythmias

Conduction System Arrhythmias
  Nodal rhythm (AV node)
  Similar to supraventricular tachycardia (see supra)
  AV dissociation
  No treatment
  First and second degree heart block
  No treatment
  Complete (third degree) heart block
  No treatment, if asymptomatic, otherwise:
    Isuprel
    Epinephrine (may induce ventricular fibrillation)
    Ephedrine
  Bundle branch block
  No treatment

Ventricular Arrhythmias
  Ventricular premature beats
  No treatment unless severe, then:
    Procainamide
    Propranolol
    Lidocaine
    Quinidine
      Do not use digitalis unless failure is present
  Ventricular tachycardia
    Quinidine
    Procainamide
    Lidocaine
  Ventricular fibrillation
    Electrical cardioversion or digitalis

The diagnosis of ventricular fibrillation is made electrocardiographically. Early ECG signs are ventricular premature beats and ventricular tachycardia.

A diagnosis of ventricular fibrillation calls for immediate corrective action if death is to be avoided.

DEFIBRILLATION PROCEDURE

1. Choose electrode paddles that are adapted to the size of the patient. Electrodes must not be touching nor should they cover a major part of the precordium.
2. Make sure the electrodes are free of corrosion and apply electrode jelly to their surfaces.
3. To deliver an electrical stimulus through the long axis of the heart, place one electrode over the suprasternal notch and one on the midclavicular line at the level of the xyphoid process.
4. Disconnect the ECG leads from the patient to avoid damage to the ECG machine. (Not necessary for newer models).
5. Set the dosage dial to the appropriate dose. (See Table 15-8)
6. Make sure that no one, including yourself, is in physical contact with the patient or the conductive part of the electrode and that the electrodes are not touching. It is safest to have an assistant hold one of the two electrode paddles.
7. Discharge the electrical stimulus.

If anoxia has contributed to causing the patient's ventricular fibrillation, acidosis is likely to coexist. Cardiac receptivity to electrical stimuli is depressed in acidotic states. It is wise, therefore, to make an attempt to correct acidosis before stimulating the heart. An IV push of sodium bicarbonate in the dose of 3 mEq (3 ml of 8.4% solution)/kg body weight should be given prior to defibrillating. In the event the defibrillation procedure fails on the initial attempt, a second dose of sodium bicarbonate may be given and the procedure repeated. The electrical dosage used for the second attempt or for each subsequent try should be increased by 10 watt seconds.

Table 15-8 Watt Second Dosage for Pediatric Defibrillation

Weight in Pounds	Watt Seconds
0-5	10
5-20	20
20-50	30
50-100	50
>100	100-200

Practical Points

1. Indications for early cardiac consultation:
   a) Cardiac failure, especially in first year of life
   b) Cyanosis or other signs of hypoxia (hyperpnea)
   c) Failure to grow at a normal rate
   d) Syncopal attacks
   e) Chest pain of cardiac origin
   f) Squatting
   g) Repeated pulmonary infections suspected to be secondary to heart disease
   h) Newborn with a murmur or other signs of CHD
2. Chest Pain: May occur with aortic or pulmonic stenosis of more than mild degree, acute pericarditis, or mitral valve prolapse. If x-ray and ECG studies are normal and no cardiac abnormalities are discovered on physical examination, the heart is a very unlikely source of the pain.
3. Arrhythmias: Ectopic beats of either atrial, nodal, or ventricular origin may be normal in childhood or may reflect underlying heart disease. A simple way to distinguish a benign from a serious condition is to have the patient exercise. If the ectopic beats increase in frequency with exercise, it indicates an underlying heart disease. Conversely, if the ectopic beats decrease with exercise, they may be considered benign.
4. Exercise: Restriction need not be maintained for all cardiac patients. Children with impending failure and chronic hypoxia tend to limit their own activities without

having to be told to do so. Children with aortic or pulmonic stenosis should be restricted from the most strenuous forms of physical activity if they have symptoms or other evidence of a significant degree of abnormality.
5. Bacterial endocarditis: Is one of the major complications of children with congenital heart disease. Whenever unexplained fever exists or an acute infection is present, the physician must be on the alert for this possibility. Prevention includes adequate antibiotic therapy for all acute infections of possible bacterial etiology and for situations likely to result in transient bacteremia such as a tooth extraction.
6. Pediatric cardiology: Is no different than the rest of pediatrics in that it must deal with that extra dimension introduced by growth and developmental changes. Normal findings at one age may be entirely abnormal at another. The charts on pp. 509 and 310 records the norms for blood pressure and resting heart rate for various ages. If one recalls that in fetal life the right ventricle performs a greater share of the heart's workload, then it is easier to understand why an infant's right ventricle is relatively more potent than an adult's. This explains the increased intensity of the pulmonic second heart sound and the greater prominence of the right ventricle in electrocardiograms.

With growth of the heart (and particularly the left ventricle) and the thorax, the point of maximum cardiac impulse begins to shift downward and laterally.

The growth rate of the patient is also a valuable gauge of the severity of the heart lesion, more severe lesions being associated with growth retardation.

HEART FAILURE

Practical Points

1. Heart failure in children differs from that ordinarily encountered in adults by being primarily a failure of the right ventricle. The following signs and symptoms may be observed.
   a) Poor feeding and easy fatigability
   b) Weak cry
   c) Sweating

d) Tachypnea
e) Tachycardia
f) Hepatomegaly
g) Cardiomegaly
h) Edema and weight gain
   Usually little is heard in the chest, rales being an accompaniment of left ventricular failure.
2. Lanoxin (digoxin) is the best form of digitalis because:
   a) Rapid action (1 hour)
   b) Rapid maximum effect (7-8 hours)
   c) Rapid excretion
   d) Administered by mouth, IM, or IV
   e) Can be used in all age groups
   See Tables 15-9 and 15-10 for the dosage schedule and other characteristics of digoxin.
3. Remember to monitor each digoxin dose electrocardiographically.
   Signs of digoxin toxicity are:
   a) Arrhythmias
   b) Extrasystoles
   c) Heart block
   d) Vomiting
   e) Diarrhea
   f) Increasing heart failure
4. Antidote for digitalis toxicity:
   Potassium chloride:
   po route 1 g q 8 h
   IV route — 40 mEq/500 ml of 5% glucose in water and monitored by ECG
   Do not exceed 0.5 mEq/kg/24 hr
   Peritoneal dialysis may be used if potassium therapy fails.
5. In addition to digitalis the following measures may be taken to control cardiac failure:
   a) Diuretics (see Table 15-11)
   b) Bed rest
   c) Restrict fluids and sodium
   d) Oxygen as needed
   e) Orthopneic position
   f) Cardiotonic drugs: epinephrine 1 µg/kg or isoproterenol 0.05 µg/kg for unresponsive hearts
   g) Watch for pulmonary edema — give morphine sulfate 0.1 mg/kg

Table 15-9 Digoxin (Lanoxin)

How Supplied	Age	*Estimated Total Digitalizing Dose (Oral or Intramuscular)	Maintenance Proportion of Total Digitalizing Dose
Elixir: 0.05 mg/ml Tablets: (scored) 0.25 and 0.5 mg: (unscored) 0.125 mg	Premature infant (> 2500 g)	0.04 mg/kg	1/4 to 1/3 in two divided doses per 24 hours
	Newborn infant (1–14 days)	0.05 mg/kg	1/4 to 1/3 in two divided doses per 24 hours
Ampules: 0.1 and 0.25 mg/ml	Infant (14 days to 2 years)	0.06–0.075 mg/kg	1/4 to 1/3 in two divided doses per 24 hours
	Child (>2 years)	0.03–0.05 mg/kg (maximal total dose of 1.5 mg)	1/4 to 1/3 in two divided doses per 24 hours

*For intravenous administration, use 75% of the dose shown.
From Fink, B.W.: Chapter 5, pp. 150–151. In Gellis, S.S. and B.M. Kagan, Eds.: Current Pediatric Therapy, 5th ed. W.B. Saunders Co., Philadelphia. (Reproduced with publisher's permission).

Table 15-10   Characteristics of Digoxin (Lanoxin) Related to Route of Administration

Route of Administration	Onset of Action	Peak Action	Excretion
Oral	1-2 hours	4-8 hours	4-7 days
Intramuscular	15-60 minutes	2-5 hours	4-7 days
Intravenous	5-30 minutes	2-5 hours	4-7 days

From Fink, B.W.: Chapter 5, pp. 150-151. In Gellis, S.S. and B.M. Kagan, Eds.: Current Pediatric Therapy, 5th ed., W.B. Saunders Co., Philadelphia. (Reproduced with publisher's permission.)

MYOCARDITIS

Inflammation of the myocardium of the heart may be a specific pathologic entity or may be part of a process involving other areas of the heart (pericardium, endocardium) or be secondary to systemic disease processes. The most common known causes of myocarditis are connective tissue disorders and infections with various bacterial, viral, and rickettsial agents.

Practical Points

Clinical findings, apart from those arising from the primary illness, include:

1. Sudden onset of fever
2. Dyspnea
3. Chest pain
4. Muffled heart sounds
5. Tachycardia out of proportion to the body temperature (add ten beats per minute for each Fahrenheit degree of temperature elevation to the normal resting heart beat)
6. Occasional arrhythmias. Most often tic tac rhythm where the diastolic and systolic phases are equal.

Table 15-11   Diuretic Agents

Preparation	Dosage	Route
Potent natriuretics		
Ethacrynic acid*	1 mg/kg/dose	Intravenously only
	2-3 mg/kg/day	Orally
Furosemide	1 mg/kg/dose	Intravenously or intra-muscularly
	2-3 mg/kg/day	Orally
Thiazides		
Chlorothiazide	20-40 mg/kg/day	Orally
Hydrochloro-thiazide	2-5 mg/kg/day	Orally
Aldosterone antagonists		
Spironolactone	1-2 mg/kg/day	Orally

*Manufacturer's note: Until further experience in infants is accumulated, therapy with oral or parenteral ethacrynic acid is contraindicated.

From Gellis, S.S. and Kagan,B.M., Eds.: Current Pediatric Therapy, 8th ed., p. 137, W.B. Saunders, Philadelphia. Reproduced with publisher's permission.)

7. Signs of congestive heart failure
8. Most helpful tests for diagnosis of myocarditis:
   a) X-ray—shows cardiac dilatation
   b) ECG—nonspecific changes. ST-segment and T-wave abnormalities and AV conductive defects
   c) Cultures and serological tests to isolate a pathogen
9. Prognosis in primary myocarditis is generally good, but serious arrhythmias may occur and sudden death is a possibility. In the secondary forms the prognosis will vary according to the systemic disease.

10. Treatment: treat the underlying disease.
   a) For rheumatic fever and the collagen diseases, steroids are helpful in suppressing the inflammatory response. (See Chapter 16)
   b) For bacterial and rickettsial infections appropriate antibiotic therapy is indicated.
   c) For viral infection there is no specific therapy.
   d) Children must be watched carefully. Strenuous exercise should be avoided during the active phase of the illness and probably well into the convalescent period. In cardiac failure the usual treatment as described above is applicable.

Chapter 16

COMMON LONG-TERM
MANAGEMENT PROBLEMS

RHEUMATIC FEVER

Rheumatic fever is an inflammatory, systemic disease
bearing an etiological relationship with certain rheumato-
genic strains of group A streptococci. The exact pathogenesis in the development of rheumatic fever is not clear.
Host and genetic factors, hypersensitivity, and autoimmune
phenomena are all considered in postulating the possible
pathogenesis of acute rheumatic fever. Only a small percentage of children who suffer from streptococcal infection
develop the illness. It occurs most frequently among children between 5 and 15 years of age with a peak incidence of
first attacks between 6 and 8 years of age. It is extremely
uncommon under 3 years of age. The attack rate of the
disease following an epidemic of streptococcal infection is
approximately 3%.

Clinical manifestations: The clinical picture usually
begins to appear 1-5 weeks after an upper respiratory illness. In about half of the patients the history of this preceding illness can be elicited.

ARTHRITIS

Arthritis is one of the important features of the disease. The large joints of the extremities are the ones most frequently affected. The arthritis migrates from one joint to another gradually involving several joints over a period of several days. Occasionally, the temporomandibular joints are affected. Involvement of small joints of the hands and feet is seldom seen. Swelling, redness, tenderness, and limitation of normal movements characterize the arthritis.

CARDITIS

Symptomatology referable to carditis may be absent in many children with cardiac involvement. Occasionally, the affected children may present themselves with cardiac failure or pericarditis with or without a friction rub. More often diagnosis of carditis is based on the following criteria:

1. Tachycardia that persists during sleep and afebrile periods
2. Prolongation of the PR interval on ECG
3. Cardiomegaly with or without congestive cardiac failure
4. Significant cardiac murmurs: These are present in the vast majority of children with carditis. Both the appearance of characteristic new murmurs and change in the quality of a murmur that was previously present are significant. The characteristic murmurs are an apical pansystolic murmur, occasionally accompanied by an apical middiastolic murmur, suggesting mitral regurgitation; and an early diastolic murmur best heard along the left sternal border at the base of the heart, suggesting aortic regurgitation. The presystolic murmur of mitral stenosis and systolic murmur of aortic stenosis are later manifestations.
5. Pericardial rub or effusion:
   a) Subcutaneous nodules: These are pea-sized nodules usually found along the extensor surfaces of hands, feet, and knees. Association of these nodules with the presence of carditis is frequently noted. Subcutaneous nodules may be present in other disorders such as rheumatoid arthritis and systemic lupus erythematosus.

b) Erythema marginatum: Is characterized by erythematous rash with serpiginous borders with a clear center usually distributed over the covered part of the body such as the trunk and proximal part of the extremities. These may appear intermittently throughout the course of the active disease.

c) Chorea: Consists of awkward, purposeless, involuntary movements, principally of the extremities and face, often bilateral, and usually associated with muscle weakness. Chorea occasionally may be the only manifestation of rheumatic fever or may appear when other manifestations have disappeared. The preceding streptococcal infection may have occurred several months previously in these instances. The onset of awkward movements is usually gradual, and the intensity varies from child to child. Emotional disturbance in the affected child is common. Some of the characteristic signs that can be elicited in these children are: choreic hand (hyperextension of metacarpophalangeal joints and flexion of the wrist in the outstretched arms), pronator sign (pronation of the hands when the arm is raised above the head), and sustained patellar reflex.

OTHER MANIFESTATIONS OF RHEUMATIC FEVER

1. Fever, either low grade or as high as 104°F
2. Arthralgia, mild pain in one or several joints without swelling or tenderness or limitation of movements
3. Epistaxis, appearing repeatedly in a small number of patients as an early sign of rheumatic fever
4. Rheumatic pneumonia, occurring rarely and usually associated with severe cardiac manifestations

LABORATORY FINDINGS

1. Elevated ESR (may be decreased in cardiac failure)
2. Positive C-reactive protein (CRP) test
3. Leukocytosis and anemia
4. Isolation of group A streptococci (on repeated throat cultures in a small number of patients)

5. Elevation of ASO titers: Titers equal to or greater than 500 Todd units are clearly significant. Titers between 250 and 320 are highly suspicious. Note: ASO titers may not be elevated in children showing manifestations of the disease such as chorea, occasionally carditis, long after the original streptococcal infection. These titers usually decline about 2 months after the onset of streptococcal infection.
6. Elevation of the streptococcal antibodies such as antistreptokinase (ASK), antihyaluronidase (AH), antideoxyribonucleotidase B (Anti-DNase B), and antinicotinamide adenine dinucleotidase (Anti-NADase), are useful determinations in those children in whom the ASO is borderline.
7. Roentgen examination of the chest may demonstrate cardiac enlargement.
8. ECG tracings reveal prolongation of the PR interval and other findings consistent with carditis and pericarditis.

Presence of two major or one major and two minor criteria supported by evidence of recent streptococcal infection indicates a high probability of acute rheumatic fever. Absence of this supporting evidence should raise doubts concerning a diagnosis of rheumatic fever. Strict adherence to these guidelines should enable the physician to avoid overdiagnosis of the disease with its long-term implications. See Table 16-1.

DIFFERENTIAL DIAGNOSIS

1. Suppurative arthritis, osteomyelitis
2. Rheumatoid arthritis, systemic lupus erythematosus
3. Sickle cell anemia, Henoch-Schönlein purpura
4. Drug-sensitivity reactions associated with polyarthritis, fever, and skin rash
5. Myocarditis and pericarditis of viral origin

Practical Points

1. Avoid initiating therapy with salicylates or steroids until unmistakable signs and symptoms of the disease develop.
2. Disappearance of acute symptoms is the best parameter indicating adequacy of treatment.

Table 16-1   Jones Criteria (Modified) for Diagnosis of Rheumatic Fever (Recommendations of the Committee of the American Heart Association)

Major Manifestations	Minor Manifestations	Supporting Evidence of Streptococcal Infection
Carditis	Arthralgia	Recent scarlet fever
Polyarthritis	Fever	Positive throat culture for group A streptococci
Chorea	Rheumatic fever or rheumatic heart disease in the past	Increased ASO or other streptococcal antibodies
Erythema marginatum	Increased ESR Positive CRP	
Subcutaneous nodules	Leukocytosis Prolonged PR interval	

3. After the initial dosage schedule with antiinflammatory drugs has been established, and if there are no cardiac complications, further treatment may be continued at home.
4. Strict bed rest, in the absence of carditis or acute pain of arthritis or disabling movements of chorea, is of no recognized medical value.
5. Even though no evidence of active streptococcal infection exists at the time of the diagnosis of rheumatic fever, it is desirable to administer a therapeutic course of penicillin to assure complete eradication of the organisms.

6. Salicylates and steroids are the antiinflammatory drugs used in the symptomatic management of the illness. Except in cases of rheumatic carditis, the drug of choice is salicylate. Even in children with **carditis** the superiority **of** steroids is not clearly **established** in terms of reducing the subsequent damage to the heart. Post-therapeutic rebounds are more frequent after steroid therapy than after salicylate therapy. The starting dose of salicylate (aspirin) is 100 mg/kg/day in four divided doses. The dose may be gradually increased up to 200 mg/kg (maximum not to exceed 10 g/day) until therapeutic results are achieved. For steroid therapy, prednisone between 50 and 75 mg/day in divided doses is recommended. Higher doses of up to 120-160 mg/day may be given to children showing no response to the lower dose.

7. The duration of therapy depends on the severity of the disease. Abatement or disappearance of symptoms indicates the adequacy of the dosage while the ESR and C-reactive protein tests are good indices of therapeutic progress. Therapy with salicylates can be discontinued in children with arthritis but without carditis as soon as the ESR shows a significant fall. This period may vary between 2 and 6 weeks. Therapy with steroids in children with carditis may have to be maintained up to 4-6 weeks or even longer depending on the severity of carditis. The steroid therapy should be tapered gradually, with salicylate substitution as the dosage of steroid is gradually cut, to avoid rebound phenomena. The salicylate therapy is then continued for an additional 2-3 weeks.

8. Phenobarbital and tranquilizers such as chlorpromazine may be used to control the movements in chorea. In addition, adequate reassurance to the patient and his family as to the nature of the problem must be given. The disease usually subsides spontaneously after a period of a month or two.

9. No restriction of physical activity is indicated after complete recovery from an attack unless the child has cardiac enlargement. Children with cardiac enlargement who are asymptomatic can usually tolerate moderate exercise and should be encouraged to do so, but should be cautioned to avoid strenuous, competitive sports.

10. Continuous prophylaxis against recurrent streptococcal
    infection with an antimicrobial agent constitutes the
    most effective method of preventing recurrences of
    rheumatic fever. Monthly benzathine penicillin, 1.2
    million U given intramuscularly is the most effective
    method. Oral penicillin 200,000-250,000 U once or
    twice daily or sulfadiazine 1 g daily have also been
    used with satisfactory results. Recommendations as
    to the duration of prophylactic therapy vary. The con-
    sensus at the present time is that prophylaxis be main-
    tained for several years after an attack and at least un-
    til the child has completed his school years. Lifetime
    prophylaxis is recommended for those with significant
    cardiac damage.

JUVENILE RHEUMATOID ARTHRITIS

Rheumatoid arthritis is a systemic disease of unknown etiology characterized by chronic (JRA) synovitis and destructive arthritis. The clinical course varies in its severity,
manifestations, and duration. Three clinical subgroups have
been described.

1. System-Onset Type
   a) Mode of onset is more often insidious than sudden.
      Arthritic manifestations may or may not accompany
      the general systemic symptoms at the onset of the
      disease. Boys and girls are equally affected.
   b) Arthritis: Monoarticular involvement marks the be-
      ginning of the illness in a significant number of chil-
      dren. However, within a short time many more
      joints are usually involved in the majority of the pa-
      tients. The joints are usually affected symmetri-
      cally. Swelling is the predominant finding. Severe
      limitation of movement, erythema, and tenderness
      are not frequent. Hip, shoulders, knees, elbows,
      wrists, ankles, feet, and fingers are most often af-
      fected. Involvement of the cervical spine causes early
      limitation of motion. The fingers assume the char-
      acteristic spindle shape because of the early involve-
      ment of proximal interphalangeal joints.
   c) Fever: Intermittent, high fever is characteristic.
      In some cases fever may precede the appearance of

other manifestations making diagnosis especially difficult. Low-grade fever with temperature falling to normal at times may also be seen.

d) Lymphadenopathy: Axillary, cervical, inguinal, and epitrochlear glands are most often involved. The nodes are nontender and circumscribed. Lymphadenopathy occurs in the majority of children.

e) Hepatosplenomegaly occurs in 80-85% of all children affected. (Splenomegaly more often than hepatomegaly).

f) Subcutaneous nodules occur in about 10% of all children. They are nontender and are usually felt as discrete, cystic-like nodules, near the area of the wrist, over the olecranon process of the elbow, and on the fingers and toes. Subcutaneous nodules are also observed in rheumatic fever and in other related conditions.

g) Rash: Evanescent in nature, the lesions are erythematous or violaceous in appearance, macular and circumscribed, and tend to become confluent. Usual sites of rash are the chest, axilla, thighs, and arms.

h) Growth disturbances: Significant generalized growth failure is usually not seen in mild cases but is common in the more severe cases even when these children are not on steroids. Localized alteration in the bone growth produces localized growth disturbances.

i) Other manifestations include morning stiffness that disappears after a brief period of activity, pericarditis, myocarditis, occasionally with valvulitis, and nonspecific attacks of abdominal pain.

2. Polyarticular Type
   a) Occurs in about 25-35% of children; more often in girls than boys.
   b) Multiple, fairly symmetrical joint involvement, especially of the distal smaller joints. Onset of arthritis is often insidious. Hip and temporomandibular joints are often involved.
   c) Low-grade fever, rheumatoid nodules, hepatosplenomegaly, lymphadenopathy, and mild degrees of anemia may be seen in some. In general, systemic symptoms are mild.

d) Some children in the group are positive for rheumatoid factor and others are not. Prognosis is worse in
the former group.
3. Pauciarticular Type
a) Occurs in about 40-45% of children. Girls are more
often affected than boys. Systemic manifestations
if any are minimal.
b) Only a few joints, usually less than five, are involved.
Knee, ankles, and elbows are often involved. Less
commonly, other smaller joints may be affected.
c) Iridocyclitis, often severe in nature, occurs in a significant number of children.

RADIOLOGICAL AND LABORATORY FINDINGS

1. Radiological findings: Soft tissue swelling, juxtaarticu-
lar osteoporosis, destruction of joint cartilages with
narrowing joint spaces, and occasionally periosteal new
bone formation. Bony ankylosis of cervical vertebrae
may also be seen as an early x-ray sign.
2. Normochromic, normocytic anemia.
3. Leukocytosis with increased polymorphonuclear WBCs
and occasionally eosinophilia. Leukemoid reactions may
be seen in some.
4. Elevated ESR except in very mild cases.
5. Presence of rhumatoid factor: Positive in a very small
percentage (5%) of affected children.
6. Presence of LE cells and antinuclear antibodies: Positive
in a very small percentage of the children with polyarticular and pauciarticular types.

DIFFERENTIAL DIAGNOSIS

Rheumatic fever, lupus erythematosus, suppurative arthritis,
osteomyelitis, tuberculous arthritis, and arthritis accompanying acute infectious illnesses should be considered in the
differential diagnosis.

MANAGEMENT

The overall goal is to enable the child to lead as nearly a
normal life as possible, physically, emotionally and socially.
The child and his family should be educated concerning the
nature of the illness.

Management of Systemic and Arthritic Problems

Aspirin 100 mg/kg/day in four divided doses. Obtain serum salicylate levels periodically. Attempt to keep the blood salicylate levels between 20 and 30 mg/100 ml. Treat for at least 6 months after clinical remission. Gold therapy may supplement aspirin therapy if acute symptoms persist. Careful monitoring of children is important because of the toxicity of gold therapy. Tolectin (tolmetin), a nonsteroidal antiinflammatory drug in a dose of 20-30 mg/kg/24 hr, has been found to be effective in some children.

Use of indomethacin in children who have failed to respond to salicylate therapy is being extensively evaluated. In a dose of 2-3 mg/kg/day, it has been found effective in adolescent patients. Its use in children under 14 years of age is unapproved by the FDA. The use of D-penicillamine in the treatment is currently being investigated. Steroid therapy is indicated in children:

1. Who continue to run high fever with or without severe joint manifestations in spite of adequate therapy with other medications.
2. Who have severe pericarditis and myocarditis, with or without congestive cardiac failure.
3. Who develop iridocyclitis or uveitis (both systemic and topical steroids are indicated).
4. Who begin to manifest severely disabling articular disease in spite of adequate therapy with salicylates and other medications.

The ideal daily dose of steroids is the least amount of drug that gives clinical results. Although 1 mg of prednisone/kg/day is often given, a lesser dose may be sufficient. Some contraindications for steroid therapy are:

1. Mild forms of rheumatoid arthritis
2. Children in whom other antirheumatoid agents were not adequately tried
3. Other coexisting conditions that would be adversely affected by steroid therapy: e.g., peptic ulcer, diabetes mellitus, etc.

Long-Term Chronic Care

1. Orthopedic management involving orthopedists and physical therapists especially trained in the field of rheumatology
2. Home care programs
3. Guidance by physicians and psychologists to enable the child and his family to cope with the emotional aspects of this chronic disease

ACUTE GLOMERULONEPHRITIS

Acute poststreptococcal glomerulonephritis is the most common form of acute glomerulonephritis. In this immune complex disease there appears to be an antigen-antibody reaction following an infection caused by group A beta hemolytic streptococci. The nephritogenic strains of streptococci are types 12 and 49 and, less frequently, types 1, 4, 23, 25, 45, 55, and 57. The peak incidence occurs between 6 and 7 years of age and is extremely rare under 1 year of age. Boys are affected more often than girls.

CLINICAL MANIFESTATIONS

The onset: An episode of upper respiratory infection such as pharyngitis or tonsillitis usually precedes the onset of symptoms by about 1-3 weeks. Less commonly, streptococcal infection of the skin may precede the onset of symptoms. In most instances, the manifestations are mild and only very occasionally the onset may be abrupt and severe.

The usual manifestations in an average case are marked by abnormal urinary findings, edema, and hypertension.

1. Urinary findings: Hematuria is the most common presenting complaint. The urine is smoky in appearance. Further examination of the urine reveals proteinuria and cylindruria. Very often, red blood cell casts and increased numbers of white blood cells are noted. Rarely, children may have acute glomerulonephritis without any of these urinary abnormalities.

2. Edema: Usually mild and mainly manifested as puffiness around the eyelids. Posture determines the edema elsewhere in the body.
3. Hypertension: Present in about 60-70% of all affected children. Elevated systolic pressure may range from 160 to 200 mmHg and diastolic from 100 to 120 mmHg. Hypertension most often is present during the first few days of the acute stage and the pressure returns to normal by the end of the first week. Hypertension is attributed to expanded plasma volume and generalized vasospasm. Symptoms of hypertensive encephalopathy (drowsiness, headache, convulsions, vomiting, visual disturbances, restlessness) may occur in children with hypertension. The symptoms usually disappear within a day or two with the fall in blood pressure.
4. Other manifestations include a mild degree of anemia and hypoalbuminuria as a result of expanded plasma volume and cardiovascular disturbances often marked by congestive cardiac failure. The latter manifestations may occasionally be the presenting picture of acute glomerulonephritis. The roentgenogram of the chest in these instances will show increased pulmonary markings and cardiac enlargement.

Laboratory findings may include:

1. Characteristic urinary findings (see above)
2. Usually elevated ASO, anti-DPNase, anti-DNase B titers, marked depression of serum C3
3. Hypoalbuminemia and mild hypercholesterolemia
4. Mild degrees of anemia and elevated ESR
5. ECG findings: Flattening or inversion of T waves and prolongation of the PR interval
6. Abnormal renal function values, e.g., elevated blood urea nitrogen and serum creatine levels.

DIFFERENTIAL DIAGNOSIS

The most frequently confused condition is acute urinary tract infection. The presence in the urine of a larger number of WBCs in comparison with RBCs, bacteria, and significantly elevated bacterial colony counts should differentiate this condition from acute nephritis. Other conditions associated with hematuria, such as blood dyscrasias, renal tumors and tuberculosis of the urinary tract, should also be differentiated. Nephritic findings associated with conditions such as the Henoch-Schönlein syndrome and systemic lupus erythematosus can be differentiated on the basis of other clinical manifestations present in these conditions. Severe renal function impairment and a past history of renal disease usually help to identify children in whom acute exacerbation of their chronic nephritis mimics acute glomerulonephritis. The nephrotic syndrome with gross hematuria, and other conditions associated with proteinuria (orthostatic proteinuria and other benign proteinurias) are additional conditions considered in the differential diagnosis.

MANAGEMENT

Prompt diagnosis and treatment of streptococcal infections constitute the major step in the prevention of the illness. Once nephritis is established the treatment is symptomatic.

1. Bed rest until the major manifestations of the disease—edema, hematuria, and hypertension—subside. This period usually lasts for 3-4 weeks.
2. Dietary management in terms of protein restriction is necessary only in children with severe oliguria. Similarly, salt restriction is limited to children who develop excessive edema and hypertension.
3. Appropriate antibiotic therapy is indicated for positive nasopharyngeal cultures for streptococci. Penicillin for 10 days is the usual regimen. Prophylactic penicillin therapy following recovery from the illness is not necessary.
4. When administering fluids during the oliguric or anuric phase of the disease, care must be taken to avoid overhydration. An average amount for insensible loss of about 300-500 ml/m^2/day plus the amount equal to urine output should be administered. Use of potassium-containing solutions is strictly contraindicated.
5. Salt restriction, administration of diuretics (ethacrynic acid, chlorothiazide), and digitalis are some of the measures that should be instituted in children who develop severe edema and/or congestive cardiac failure. It should

be remembered that diuretics are usually ineffective in clearing the edema and that the beneficial value of digitalis is clearly not established.

6. Antihypertensive medications are indicated in children developing a diastolic pressure of 90 mmHg or more. The following regimen may be followed:

   a) Children with very mild hypertension: Bed rest, salt restriction, and phenobarbital, 2-3 mg/kg/day, orally. A single dose of phenobarbital may be all that is necessary.

   b) Children with moderate to severe hypertension: Combination of reserpine 0.07 mg/kg and hydralazine hydrochloride (Aspresoline), 0.1 mg/kg administered intramuscularly. Often a single dose is sufficient. The combined therapy may be repeated in 12 hours if necessary.

   c) In those children who do not respond to combined hydralazine and reserpine therapy, the use of alpha-methyldopa (Aldomet) may be considered. The dose is 4-15 mg/kg IV administered over a 5-to-10-minute period and repeated at 6-hour intervals as necessary. Other drugs used in the treatment of hypertensive crisis are guanethidine and diazoxide.

7. Management of children developing hyperkalemia (serum potassium 6.5 mEq/L or higher) with renal insufficiency consists of:

   a) Avoidance of all potassium-containing dietary foods or fluids.

   b) Administration of Kayexalate 1000 mg/kg either orally or rectally as a 20-30% solution. The dose may be repeated after 6 to 12 hours if necessary. Periodically, serum calcium concentration must be checked while the child is being treated. An alternative to Kayexalate therapy consists of administration of insulin and glucose (1 U insulin to 3 g of glucose).

   c) Peritoneal dialysis or hemodialysis for persistent hyperkalemia.

8. Use of steroids or immunosuppressive agents is justified only as investigational drugs in established pediatric renal centers at the present time.

THE NEPHROTIC SYNDROME

The nephrotic syndrome is characterized by proteinuria resulting in hypoproteinemia, edema, hypovolemia, ascites, and hyperlipemia. Hypertension, hematuria, azotemia, and hypocomplementemia occasionally may be seen. The cause of the nephrotic syndrome is unknown although it is generally considered as a disease of hypersensitivity. The syndrome can be grouped into three categories: congenital, secondary and idiopathic.

The congenital nephrotic syndrome is inherited as an autosomal recessive trait. The affected children do not respond to treatment and die within the first year or two of life.

Secondary nephrotic syndrome occurs in association with a specific disease such as collagen disorders (systemic lupus erythematosus, anaphylactoid purpura), parasitic infection (Quarten malaria), and other conditions (amyloidosis, renal vein thrombosis, sickle cell disease, syphilis, chronic glomerulonephritis, diabetes mellitus, etc.). The nephrotic syndrome may also result following administration of drugs (trimethadione, paradione, and heavy metal preparations, e.g., gold, salts, mercury). Bee stings and poison oak are associated in some cases.

IDIOPATHIC NEPHROTIC SYNDROME
(Minimal Change Nephrotic Syndrome)

Idiopathic nephrotic syndrome (minimal change nephrotic syndrome): The vast majority of children with nephrosis fall into this category. The peak incidence is around 2-3 years of age with the incidence of onset relatively rare after 8 years of age.

Clinical Manifestations

Edema is the hallmark of the disease entity and is insidious in onset. The early periorbital edema gradually becomes generalized, producing ascites, scrotal edema, and occasionally pleural effusion. In some untreated children the initial edema may disappear only to come back again after a week or two. Increased susceptibility to infection, peritonitis in particular, has been noted in edematous children. Diarrheal episodes seen frequently in the acute stage are presumably due to edema of the gastrointestinal mucosa. Anorexia and excessive loss of protein in the urine may result in malnutrition. Respiratory embarrassment due to marked ascites may be present.

Laboratory findings include:

1. Proteinuria (more than 2 g/m^2/24 hr)
2. Hypoproteinemia and hypoalbuminemia (average total protein around 4 g/100 ml. Serum albumin is decreased, alpha-2 and beta globulins are increased.)
3. Hyperlipidemia (cholesterol greater than 220 mg/100 ml)
4. Slightly decreased serum sodium values
5. Elevated ESR
6. Normal serum C$_3$ levels
7. Variable renal function values

The various glomerulopathies included under secondary nephrotic syndrome should be considered in the differential diagnosis. Other entities include membranoproliferative glomerulonephritis, focal glomerulosclerosis, and idiopathic membranous glomerulopathy. A lack of good response to steroid therapy and characteristic renal biopsy changes usually distinguish these from idiopathic nephrotic syndrome.

Practical Points

1. A high protein (3-4 g/kg/day) and low salt diet (40-80 mEq/day) should be recommended.
2. Prompt therapy with antimicrobial agents for infections. Antimicrobial prophylaxis is not effective or necessary.
3. Diuretic agents are usually not required since diuresis occurs in most children satisfactorily after the start of steroid therapy. In cases where there are contraindications for the use of steroids or immediate relief from edema is desired, a diuretic such as hydrochlorothiazide (2-4 mg/kg/day) may be used.
4. Corticosteroid therapy is the mainstay in the management. The International Cooperative Study of Kidney Disease recommends the following schedule:
   a) Prednisone 60 mg/m^2/day (maximum 80 mg/day) for 4 weeks. Follow with 40 mg/m^2/day (maximum

60 mg/day) 3 consecutive days in a week for 4 more weeks. If the patient responds during the last 4 weeks, continue intermittent (3 days a week) therapy for 4 more weeks and discontinue the drug.
  b) Children showing relapse after responding to steroid therapy as above are again treated with steroids; first, continuously for 4 weeks, and then intermittently for 4 more weeks, as outlined above.
5. Cytotoxic therapy is considered for steroid nonresponsive children as well as for children who show frequent relapses while on steroids. Drugs such as chlorambucil and cyclophosphamide have been successfully used.

ESSENTIAL HYPERTENSION

A recently assembled body of information has changed the previously held view that the cause of hypertension in children in the majority of instances is secondary in nature. More attention being paid now to routine blood pressure screening has identified a number of children with unexplained or essential hypertension (see table of normal values, Appendix F, p. 509). Blood pressure norms related to height and weight rather than to age and sex appear to be more useful in separating the normal from the abnormal child. Long-term disease relating to this has not been clearly defined and awaits further basic research.

For this reason, therapy is conservative consisting of weight control, dietary restriction of salt and excess sugar, and careful follow-up. Drug therapy, since it is by nature long-term, fraught with possible side effects, and of still doubtful effectiveness, should be reserved only for those children with extreme elevations. It would seem reasonable, until more information is forthcoming, to adopt a clinical goal of reducing persistently elevated blood pressures to within two standard deviations of the norm for height and weight for young children or at least to 90 mmHg for adolescents. Drug therapy includes diuretics, adrenergic nervous system agents, and vasodilators. Prior to therapy, other disease states known to cause hypertension should be carefully ruled out.

DIABETES MELLITUS

Diabetes mellitus is an inheritable, complex, metabolic disorder affecting carbohydrate as well as fat and protein metabolism. The incidence of childhood diabetes is said to be 1.3/1000 children. Three types can be recognized among children with the disease: (1) type I or insulin-dependent diabetes (juvenile-onset diabetes); (2) type II or noninsulin-dependent diabetes (maturity onset or adult-onset diabetes mellitus); and (3) other types, e.g., transient diabetes mellitus of the newborn.

INSULIN-DEPENDENT TYPE I

There is an association with histocompatible antigens, particularly HLA-B8, HLA-BW15, BW3 and DW4. Insufficient insulin activity is the primary factor. Average age at onset is 10-11 years. In one-fourth of the children the onset is before 5 years of age. The remaining three-fourths of children will have their onset between 5 and 15 years of age. Two peaks of incidence occur at approximately 6 and 12 years of age. Usually the onset of symptoms is sudden although the precipitous development of symptoms is not always characteristic. The signs and symptoms that should alert the physician to the diagnosis are polyuria, polydypsia, polyphagia, weight loss, enuresis, pruritis vulvae, irritability, lassitude, and visual difficulties. A significant number of children (10-20%) may be in a state of ketoacidosis when the diagnosis is first established.

Because of the nature of the symptomatology, such conditions as urinary tract infections or emotional problems may be confused with the proper diagnosis. Characteristically, in about 20-30% of children, the initial insulin-dependent phase (2 weeks to 3 months) is followed by a remission phase (2-6 months) when the insulin requirement will drop dramatically. The final phase of total diabetes follows the second phase, and is most commonly triggered by an intercurrent illness.

Diagnosis

1. Characteristic history
2. Routine urinalysis - glycosuria and ketonuria. In ketoacidotic children, glycosuria and ketonuria

are not enough to establish the diagnosis. A blood glucose > 300 mg% is also necessary to rule out Franconi syndrome and other disease states.
3. Random blood sugar: 180 mg/100 ml (Glucose tolerance test is rarely necessary).

Demonstration of low plasma insulin levels in the face of hyperglycemia has been made in some cases.

Management

Hospitalization is mandatory to closely monitor and evaluate the child's response to the initial treatment when the diagnosis is first established. Also the period of hospital stay can be used to educate the child and his family about the nature of the disease and its implications in the child's new way of life. The primary thrust of therapy is to enable the child and his family to lead a normal or near normal life with minimal psychosocial and physical problems to contend with.

The presence of blood glucose concentration greater than 300 mg/dl, ketonemia and acidosis with a pH of less than 7.3 or serum bicarbonate less than 15 mEq/L establish the diagnosis of diabetic ketoacidosis.

The following plan summarizes the management of children with diabetic ketoacidosis:

1. Initial Management
   a) Insulin therapy (first 24 hours): Regular insulin, roughly a dosage between 0.5 and 2 U/kg depending on the severity of initial manifestations (0.5 U/kg for blood glucose between 300 and 600 mg/dl and 2 U/kg for blood glucose greater than 900 mg/dl and severe ketoacidosis). Administer subcutaneously. In case of vascular collapse give half the calculated dose intravenously. Repeat regular insulin at 2-4-hour intervals if necessary. Choose a dose between 0.5 and 1 U/kg depending on the response to the previous therapy (fall in serum acetone, lowering of blood glucose and ketones in urine). When the blood glucose concentration falls to about 300 mg/dl, administration of insulin can be made every 6-8 hrs at a dose of 0.25-0.5 U/kg.

b) Determination of serum acetone: Make serial dilutions of serum in small test tubes by mixing 1 drop of serum in each tube with 1, 2, 3, 4, 5 to 10 drops of water to give 1:2, 1:3, 1:4, 1:5 to 1:10 dilutions respectively. Test a drop of each dilution with Acetest or Ketostix of Clinitest tablet. Assess the response to therapy by noting the dilution at which the test is positive (purplish color) as the therapy progresses.

c) Many clinicians now prefer the continuous low-dose intravenous infusion of insulin. Briefly, a priming dose of 0.1 U/kg is given initially followed by continuous infusion of 0.1 U/kg/hr. When a blood glucose of 300 mg% is reached, the infusion is continued using 0.05 U/kg/hr in 5% glucose/water or subcutaneous insulin may be used instead. The perceived advantages of this method lie in avoiding insulin shock, and the calling into play of exaggerated metabolic responses to large doses of insulin.

d) Fluids (first 24 hours): Except in very mild cases (children with glycosuria only), IV fluids are necessary (see p. 205 for fluid therapy). Usually after the first 24 hours of IV therapy, clear fluids of high carbohydrate content can be given orally in sufficient amounts. Regular meals can also be given during this period.

2. Later Management (2-3 days after initial treatment)

a) Insulin requirement: Administer one injection of NPH or Lente (intermediate-acting) insulin about 30 minutes before breakfast. The exact requirement varies from individual to individual. Such factors as the duration of the disease and age of the patient influence the need. Usually one-half the total insulin dose of the previous day or a dose between 0.5 and 2 U/kg of body weight will be required per day. Monitor blood glucose to determine if an additional amount of insulin is required.

If the child is noted to develop nocturnal hyperglycemia, divide the daily dose and give approximately one-third to one-fourth of the daily requirement before supper.

Caution: Following the initial control in a new diabetic, the insulin requirement drops precipitously during the remission phase.

b) Diet: Regular diet as eaten by the child's family may be allowed, restricting only concentrated carbohydrate items. Between-meal snacks may be helpful in preventing mild hypoglycemic symptoms. Several factors such as exercise, infection, and growth influence the caloric needs. Hunger should be a useful guide in determining the caloric needs in these situations.

Parent and Child Education

Effective long-term management depends on the degree of emotional acceptance and adjustments that the child and his family can make. Discussion concerning the nature of the disease, the feasibility of leading a normal life, and genetic aspects of the problem would help the family to cope with the problem more easily. Parents and children should be taught to give injections at home. Steps to be taken in case the child develops either intercurrent infection or hypoglycemia—use of crystalline insulin in addition to routinely administered insulin and administration of antibiotics in the former, and ingestion of concentrated carbohydrate such as candy in the latter—should be explained.

Participation in regular school activities should be encouraged. Additional food intake prior to any vigorous activities may be needed to prevent hypoglycemic symptoms.

There is a growing body of evidence showing that long range complications can be minimized by better day-to-day control so that precise insulin administration offers a great deal to the diabetic patient. The advent of pancreatic islet cell transplantation and a simple apparatus allowing automatic administration of insulin by a minipump, worn by the patient, appears to be at hand. This may make insulin administration far simpler, more tolerable, and more precise.

TYPE II OR NONINSULIN-DEPENDENT DIABETES

Children with type II diabetes have intermittent symptoms (polyuria, polydipsia, and polyphagia) and laboratory findings (abnormal glucose tolerance tests) of diabetes mellitus, but ordinarily do not require insulin or become ketotic. Under conditions of strain, e.g., after surgery or during an acute illness, they may, however, become acidotic and require insulin.

The insulin levels of plasma done during glucose tolerance tests are normal and, in some cases, above normal in these children, a finding that differentiates them from children with insulin-dependent overt diabetes mellitus. Approximately 20% of these children eventually develop overt diabetes. Oral hypoglycemic agents such as Orinase or Tolbutamide are of no value in children.

TRANSIENT DIABETES IN THE NEWBORN

Appearing shortly after birth, the syndrome is more common in small for gestational age babies. The etiology is unknown. The characteristic features of the syndrome are weight loss, dehydration with acidosis, failure to thrive and polyuria. Laboratory findings include marked glycosuria and hyperglycemia.

Management consists of administration of fluids parenterally to correct dehydration and insulin for the duration of the diabetic state.

Newborns are very sensitive to insulin and frequent estimation of blood sugar is necessary to avoid hypoglycemia. Approximately 1-3 regular insulin/kg/day in divided doses may be required to control hyperglycemia.

Practical Points

1. An occasional patient presents with a picture of acute appendicitis: abdominal pain, leukocytosis, etc. It is generally a good idea to try several hours of rehydration and insulin therapy before surgery.
2. Screening for diabetes with postprandial blood glucose and glucose tolerance testing usually gives a very low yield even in a population of children at high risk.
3. Diabetic ketoacidosis is defined as glucose > 300 mg%, ketonemia in more than a 1:2 dilution of serum, acidosis (pH < 7.3, HCO_3-15 mEq/L).
4. Nonketotic hyperosmolar coma must be distinguished from ketoacidosis. In this condition blood glucose levels exceed 500 mg% and serum osmolarity is greater than 300 mOsm. In this condition, insulin must be given very slowly to prevent cerebral edema.

HYPERTHYROIDISM (THYROTOXICOSIS)

Increased secretion of thyroid hormone results in hyper-thyroidism. Female children are affected approximately six times more often than male children. The illness may be precipitated by psychic trauma. The disease occurs most often in children reaching adolescence, only rarely affecting children under 10 years of age. There is apparently some genetic basis for the disease, as evidenced by the incidence of the disease in other members of the affected child's family. An autoimmune mechanism with the production of the long-acting thyroid stimulator (LATS) is postulated to ex-plain the pathogenesis of the disease. The manifestations of thyrotoxicosis include:

1. Hyperirritability, hyperexcitability, signs of emotional disturbances.
2. Increased appetite.
3. Tremors, palpitations, restlessness, excessive sweating.
4. Tachycardia, cardiac enlargement, and systolic murmurs, hypertension with widened pulse pressure.
5. Mild to moderate degree of exophthalmos.
6. Variably enlarged thyroid gland.

Laboratory data include:

1. Elevated serum levels of thyroxine (T_4) and triidothyro-nine (T_3)
2. Low levels of thyrotropin hormone (TSH)
3. Abnormal TSH response following the intravenous admin-istration of thyrotropin-releasing hormone (TRH). Norm-ally the level of TSH increases to peak values after the administration of TRH but not in children with thyrotoxi-cosis.

Usually the diagnosis does not present any difficulties. Differential diagnosis includes simple goiter, hyperthyroid phase of Hashimoto's thyroiditis, organic cardiac problems, chorea, and behavior disorders.

MANAGEMENT

Medical management with antithyroid drugs constitutes the first choice of treatment.

In patients who exhibit severe cardiovascular symptoms, propranolol in titrated doses (2-6 mg/kg/day) can be given before starting treatment with the specific antithyroid medications.

The two most commonly used antithyroid drugs are propylthiouracil (the initial dose varies between 300 and 600 mg/day) and methimazole (initial dose varies between 30 and 45 mg/day). Skin rashes and agranulocytosis are some of the side effects associated with these medications. Treatment may be necessary for periods varying between 2 and 4 years. Approximately 75% of the children will show permanent remission. If relapses occur, they generally do so within the first 6 months after therapy is discontinued.

Subtotal surgical thyroidectomy is indicated in children who fail to show permanent remission after adequate therapy with antithyroid drugs or in situations where medical management is not possible for lack of close supervision and adequate cooperation needed for such therapy. The majority of patients undergoing surgery achieve permanent remission. Incidence of hypothyroidism developing after surgery varies from center to center. Use of radioactive iodine for treatment is not recommended in children.

HYPOTHYROIDISM

A deficiency of thyroid hormone results in hypothyroidism. The disorder can result from a variety of causes. The more common ones include developmental defects of the thyroid gland (thyroid dysgenesis), defective synthesis of the thyroid hormone for a variety of reasons, deficiency of iodine which is essential for the production of thyroid hormone, and autoimmune phenomenon (lymphocytic thyroiditis). Defective functioning of the pituitary or hypothalamus can also result in hypothyroidism due to a deficiency in the production of thyroid-stimulating hormone.

Depending on the causative factors, hypothyroidism can be either congenital or acquired. The clinical manifestations in congenital hypothyroidism appear shortly after birth.

These include (1) peculiar facies consisting of coarse facial features with puffiness around the eyes, thick, large protruding tongue, broad flat nose, and hirsutism of the forehead; (2) large abdomen often with an umbilical hernia; (3) respiratory difficulty; (4) feeding problems, often with choking spells; (5) lethargy; (6) constipation; (7) prolongation of physiological jaundice; (8) subnormal temperature; (9) hypotonia; (10) dry and scaly skin. Growth and developmental delay become apparent with advancing age. In acquired hypothyroidism these same manifestations are present but are less pronounced than in infants. It must be remembered that in some cases the manifestations of congenital hypothyroidism may not become evident until sometime after birth.

Laboratory data include:

1. Low levels of T_4 and T_3
2. Elevated levels of thyrotrophic-stimulating hormone (TSH) in primary hypothyroidism
3. Roentgenographic evidence of retardation of osseous growth

Other tests such as thyroid scan, radio iodine studies, and perchlorate discharge tests may be indicated to ascertain the precise etiology of the disorder.

Treatment consists of replacement therapy with thyroid hormone irrespective of the etiology. Preferred treatment for congenital hypothyroidism is now synthetically derived sodium levothyroxine rather than dessicated thyroid. Average effective dose is 5-6 µg/kg which gradually falls to 3-4 µg older children.   Infants with heart involvement or severe hypothyroidism should be started on a quarter of the normal maintenance dose to prevent the rare complication of sudden death. The dose may be raised by quarterly increments q 5 days until maintenance levels are reached. The goal of therapy is to produce normal physical growth and maturation. This may be monitored by T_4, T_3 resin uptake and TSH levels. Normal levels indicate adquate therapy.

Practical Points

1. The potential for mental retardation exists until 2 years of age after which sufficient CNS development has occurred to minimize this.
2. The mean IQ of infants first treated between 3 and 6 months of age is considerably below that of infants treated earlier (70 vs 89). Children treated after 6 months of age are usually retarded.
3. The effects of acquired hypothyroidism after the age of 2 years can usually be reversed with therapy. However, long-standing cases with improper therapy may demonstrate a failure to achieve normal stature.
4. Breast milk has been shown to contain thyroid hormones and breast-fed babies with hypothyroidism have a better prognosis than bottle-fed babies.
5. X-rays demonstrating lack of ossification of the epiphyses of the distal femur, proximal tibia, and the cuboid bone are very helpful.
6. Primary hypothyroidism features a low serum T_4, normal or low serum T_3 resin uptake, and an increased TSH.
7. Newborn screening programs rely on radioimmunoassays of a spot of blood on PKU filter paper of T_4 and/or TSH. A low T_4 and high TSH is indicative of congenital hypothyroidism and definitive serum studies should be carried out.

ADRENOGENITAL SYNDROME

Hyperactivity of the adrenal cortex with hypersecretion of androgenic hormones results in the adrenogenital syndrome. Either congenital adrenal hyperplasia or tumors of the adrenal cortex are responsible for the hyperactivity of the adrenal cortex.

Congenital adrenal hyperplasia results from an autosomal recessive gene in which there is defective biosynthesis of cortisol due to a lack or deficiency of (1) 12-hydroxylase, salt-losing or nonsalt-losing form; (2) 11-beta hydroxylase; (3) 3-beta hydroxy dehydrogenase; and (4) 17-hydroxylase.

Deficient synthesis of cortisol results in increased secretion of corticotropin which in turn produces cortical
hyperplasia. Deficiency of 21-hydroxylase accounts for
nearly 90% of children with this disorder.

CLINICAL MANIFESTATIONS

1. In the male: Premature isosexual development. The
   signs are usually absent at birth. Signs of precocity may
   begin manifesting themselves during the early part of
   the first year. These include enlargement of the penis
   and scrotum and appearance of pubic hair. The testis
   remains small in size.
2. In the female: Ambiguous genitalia at birth. The genitalia resembles that of a male infant with cryptorchidism
   and hypospadias as a result of enlargement of the clitoris
   and varying degrees of labial fusion with a common urogenital opening appearing underneath the enlarged clitoris.
   Shortly after birth, signs of precocious sexual development
   such as appearance of pubic and axillary hair are noted.
   Masculinization progresses as the child grows older.
3. Rapid linear growth in early childhood, advanced bone
   age, premature closure of epiphyses resulting in early
   arrest of growth. (Patients are tall as children but short
   as adults.)
4. Increased development of muscle mass.
5. Salt-losing form. Symptoms include anorexia, vomiting,
   diarrhea, severe dehydration, and electrolyte disturbances
   including hyponatremia and hyperkalemia. These manifestations are mostly seen in children with 21-hydroxylase
   defect and occur in approximately 50% of cases.
6. Hypertension in children with 11-hydroxylase enzyme deficiency. Laboratory data consist of:
   a) Elevated levels of urinary and plasma 17-ketosteroids
   b) Elevated urinary pregnanetriol
   c) Elevated concentration of tetrahydro S (in children
      with 11-hydroxylase defect)
   d) Low levels of blood cortisol in salt-losing forms
   e) Low serum sodium and elevated serum potassium in
      salt losers
   f) Radiological evidence of advanced osseous maturity

g) In females with ambiguous genitalia: Presence of normal chromosomes for female with chromatin-positive pattern and normal female internal genital organs (normal vagina and uterus demonstrated radiologically by injection of contrast media into the urogenital sinus).

MANAGEMENT

Treatment consists of maintaining the affected children on oral hydrocortisone 10-50 mg/day, depending on age, in three divided doses. In addition, children with the salt-losing form must receive supplementary salt intake, and desoxycorticosterone acetate (DOCA) daily intramuscularly or as pellets, subcutaneously. The dose of steroids should be increased during periods of unusual stress such as due to infection or surgery. Clitorectomy or clitoroplasty is usually required to manage the clitoris enlargement.

Virilizing adrenal cortical tumors can be differentiated from congenital adrenal hyperplasia by noting a reduction in the excretion of 17-ketosteroids after the administration of cortisone in children with adrenal hyperplasia. There is no reduction in children with a tumor. Intravenous pyelography usually demonstrates the tumors in most instances. Associated congenital defects are not uncommon in the affected children. Surgical removal of the tumor constitutes the treatment.

Practical Points

1. The chances are one in four that parents having one child with AGS will have another.
2. Since salt-losing crises occur frequently in the first 3-4 weeks of life, any infant suspected of having the disease (ambiguous genitalia) should be carefully monitored at least in the first month of life.
3. Surgical correction of the ambiguous genitalia should be considered before psychosexual misidentification occurs.

CYSTIC FIBROSIS

Cystic fibrosis is an inherited disease affecting the exocrine glands predominantly occurring among white children. The disorder is transmitted as a Mendelian recessive trait. The pathogenesis of the disease is not entirely clear. Abnormally tenacious secretions are elaborated by the exocrine glands which is the underlying defect behind many of the clinical signs and symptoms.

CLINICAL MANIFESTATIONS

Inability of the newborn to gain back the birth weight after the normal initial loss, vomiting, unsatisfactory weight gain in spite of a good appetite, pulmonary symptomatology such as dry cough and wheezing, and intestinal obstruction due to meconium ileus may all characterize the disease in the neonatal period.

Pulmonary manifestations become progressively chronic. Obstruction of bronchi and bronchioles by the tenacious mucus results in their dilatation and consequent damage. As the obstructive process progresses, emphysematous changes take place throughout the lung. Streaky or lobar atelectasis, pulmonary infection, mainly caused by *Staphylococcus aureus* and *Pseudomonas aeruginosa* and abscesses of the lungs, characterize the chronic course. Mediastinal and subcutaneous emphysema, and manifestations of chronic cor pulmonale with clubbing of fingers may result as the pulmonary pathology progresses.

Gastrointestinal manifestations occur as a result of intestinal malabsorption due to a lack of pancreatic enzymes. The steatorrhea is characterized by passage of large, bulky, foul-smelling and greasy stools. The abdomen is distended. Hepatosplenomegaly with cirrhosis of the liver and portal hypertension may be present in a small number of patients.

Other manifestations include involvement of paranasal sinuses, polyps of the nasal mucosa, prolapse of the rectum, glycosuria with an abnormal glucose tolerance test, exudative retinopathy and pulmonary osteoarthropathy associated with chronic pulmonary disease, and edema with hypoproteinemia.

The sweat electrolyte defect that characterizes the disease consists of significantly elevated levels of sodium, chloride and, to a lesser degree, potassium in the sweat of the affected children.

The differential diagnosis includes other causes of intestinal obstruction in the newborn period (see p. 52), various clinical entities associated with steatorrhea such as celiac syndrome and sugar splitting enzyme deficiencies, pulmonary illnesses such as bronchiolitis and pertussis in infancy, asthma, bronchiectasis and pulmonary fibrosis in older children, and other conditions in which children fail to thrive.

Laboratory data include:

1. Elevated sweat sodium and chloride as demonstrated in sweat tests (more than 60 mEq/L is diagnostic). Values between 50 and 60 mEq/L are highly suggestive of the disease.
2. Absent pancreatic enzyme activity (seen in about 95% of affected children). For practical reasons only tryptic activity is studied.
3. Positive malabsorption tests are present.

Practical Points

1. Definitive diagnosis and therapy are best done in a well-established center that exclusively deals with children with cystic fibrosis. If that is impractical, it is recommended that at least a close contact by the family physician should be maintained with such centers for proper guidance in managing these children.
2. Prevention and relief of bronchial obstruction and of pulmonary infection, when it occurs, constitute two of the major goals in the management of children with pulmonary manifestations. Mist tent therapy, postural drainage, and administration of mucolytic agents and expectorant drugs are all part of the therapy in achieving the first goal. Appropriate selection of antibiotics to treat pulmonary infection must be made keeping in mind the common organisms associated with the disease, viz. *S. aureus* and *P. aeruginosa*. Preferably cultures of the sputum and antibiotic sensitivity should be performed. Duration of therapy is dictated by the clinical

response. Aerosol antibiotic therapy may be helpful in some children. Prophylactic use of broad-spectrum antibiotics is not recommended.

3. Therapy for digestive disturbances is directed towards replacing the pancreatic enzymes and maintenance of adequate nutrition. Commercially prepared pancreatic enzymes (Viokase, Cotazyme) administered with meals are usually adequate for pancreatic enzyme replacement. Caloric intake must be larger than normal since there is incomplete absorption of ingested food. Food relatively high in fat content is avoided as it is poorly tolerated. Administration of medium chain triglycerides (MCT) is recommended as they do not depend on pancreatic lipase for absorption. Supplementation of vitamins is recommended. Fat soluble vitamins such as A, D, and E should be administered in a water-miscible form.

4. To compensate for excessive loss of Na and Cl, supplemental salt intake is necessary in hot weather. Ordinarily, such specific therapy is not required.

5. Use of anabolic androgenic steroids to promote growth is of questionable value.

6. Parental education concerning the nature of the illness and the complicated technical aspects of treatment goes a long way in enabling the physician to administer effective comprehensive care to the affected children.

HYDROCEPHALUS

Excessive accumulation of cerebrospinal fluid in the intracranial cavity is termed hydrocephalus. Possible mechanisms that might cause accumulation of excessive fluid are: (1) augmented rate of production of CSF; (2) obstruction to the flow of CSF within the ventricular system or in the subarachnoid space; and (3) impaired resorption of CSF in the subarachnoid spaces.

When the accumulation is greatest in the ventricular system it is termed internal hydrocephalus. When it accumulates primarily in the subarachnoid space it is termed external hydrocephalus. The term communicating hydrocephalus implies that there is free flow of CSF throughout the ventricular system and the cisterns. Hydrocephalus associated with either partial or complete obstruction to such a free flow is defined as obstructive hydrocephalus.

The increases in fluid volume and pressure within the ventricles result in marked enlargement of the ventricular system which in turn results in an increase in head size. Hydrocephalus can be classified into three categories based on etiological considerations:

1. **Congenital Hydrocephalus:** Hydrocephalus resulting from aqueductal stenosis is one well-established example of the congenital form. This is inherited as a sex-linked disorder affecting the male child with the female being the carrier. Hydrocephalus associated with meningomyelocele can also be included in this classification as there is often a familial pattern observed among the affected children.
2. **Idiopathic Hydrocephalus:** Hydrocephalic children in whom no etiological factors can be demonstrated form this group.
3. **Secondary Hydrocephalus:** In these children hydrocephalus results secondarily to a specific primary lesion. The primary lesion may be:
   a) Neoplastic, including those that (1) may cause obstruction to the flow of CSF, e.g., parasellar tumors, leptomeningeal tumors, or (2) increase the amount of CSF secreted, e.g., papilloma of the choroid plexus of the lateral ventricle.
   b) Congenital malformations, that cause obstruction to the flow, e.g., Arnold Chiari type II malformation, Dandy-Walker syndrome.
   c) Posttraumatic and postinflammatory lesions. Infections such as meningitis, toxoplasmosis, and cysticercosis may cause obstruction along the pathway of CSF flow causing hydrocephalus. Similarly, fibrosis of the arachnoid space following an episode of posttraumatic bleeding may impede the flow of CSF at the base of the brain along the extraventricular pathway. Also, some of these clinical entities may alter the cellular mechanism responsible for resorption of CSF thus causing excessive accumulation of the fluid.

CLINICAL FEATURES

1. External signs of increased intracranial pressure: A pulsating, bulging fontanelle with wide separation of sutures.

Loss of firmness along the edges of the frontal and parietal bones. Thinning and pallor of the skin covering the skull with prominently visible and distended veins. Drooping of the eyelids and downward gaze of the eyes with iris only partially visible ("setting sun" sign). Abnormally increasing head size.

2. Other features: High pitched cry, failure to thrive, developmental delays, gait disturbances, and other neurological manifestations. Note: enlarging or enlarged head size is a relatively late manifestation of hydrocephalus, when significant damage to the brain may have already taken place. Other signs of increased intracranial pressure as described above should help identify a child before he has suffered brain damage.

DIAGNOSIS

Diagnosis is easily established by computed tomography. Conditions other than hydrocephalus that can cause abnormal enlargement of the head include megalocephaly and chronic subdural effusion.

MANAGEMENT

Surgical correction of the problem remains the mainstay of treatment and essentially consists of:

1. Rerouting the flow of CSF by way of shunts to an area outside the ventricular and subarachnoid systems for either absorption or excretion. The distal end of the tube in the commonly used ventriculoperitoneal shunt lies in the peritoneal cavity. Infection, occlusion of the shunt system by blood or other tissue fragments, and disconnection of the tubing are some of the complications that may follow the procedures. The infection is usually caused by *S. aureus* and *S. epidermidis,* rarely gram-negative organisms may be responsible.

2. Rerouting of the CSF within the ventricular system itself by passing the point of obstruction, e.g., Torkildsen procedure (ventriculocisternostomy) for aqueductal stenosis. Occasionally medical treatment has been directed towards reducing the rate of production of cerebrospinal fluid by the use of acetazolamide (Diamox) and hypertonic agents.

CEREBRAL PALSY

The term cerebral palsy refers to a varied group of non-progressive disorders due to pathology of the motor control centers of the brain characterized by paralysis, weakness, incoordination, or other aberrations of motor function. Cerebral palsy originates prenatally, during birth, or before the central nervous system has reached relative maturity.

The child with cerebral palsy may have other symptoms secondary to brain damage. There may be mental retardation, seizures, visual, hearing or perceptual problems, speech pathology, and behavioral and emotional disturbances.

TYPES OF CEREBRAL PALSY

Spastic — the stretch reflex is hyperactive and muscle tone is constantly exaggerated.

Athetoid — choreoathetoid movements and rigidity are characteristic. The cortex appears unable to suppress segmental and brain stem reflex activities when movement is initiated.

Ataxic — primarily incoordination due to disturbance of kinesthetic or balance sense or both atonia and hypotonia may be prominent.

Rigidity — the main characteristics are hypertonicity, normal or diminished reflexes, no clonus or stretch reflexes, and the absence of an involuntary motion of resistance to passive motion is continuous. It is referred to as lead-pipe rigidity. If intermittent, it is termed cog-wheel rigidity.

In addition to the typing of cerebral palsy based on neurological characteristics, one can distinguish different forms based on the following sites of anatomic involvement:

Hemiplegia: the limbs on one side are affected

Tetraplegia: all limbs are affected

Diplegia: all limbs are affected but the lower ones more so

Paraplegia: only the lower limbs are affected

Double hemiplegia: upper limbs more severely affected than lower limbs with associated bulbar and higher center involvement

EARLY RECOGNITION

It is important to realize that developmental delay, particularly when it is confined to the motor area, is an early manifestation of cerebral palsy. Testing for spasticity, ataxia, athetoid movements, and rigidity should be then thoroughly carried out in addition to other neurological examinations.

Spastic children are generally detected by testing for resistance on passive movement of a limb. Sudden passive flexion will usually demonstrate a degree of increased resistance. The elbow or fingers, thigh or calf are easily tested. The tendon reflexes are also hyperactive and ankle clonus may be elicited. The degree of spasticity should be assessed for each limb.

The child with a slight degree of hemiplegia may be more readily diagnosed by having him run. The spastic arm will not swing while he runs.

Children with the choreoathetoid form of cerebral palsy may present disorders of posture and muscle tone; the jerky, fast movements of chorea; or the slow, almost purposeful movements of athetosis. The first of these is usually present before 6 months of age while the latter two occur about 1 year of age.

Other manifestations include global mental retardation; feeding problems due to hypotonia of the neck or trunk muscles; and a combination of the several types of cerebral palsy.

Practical Points

1. Cerebral palsy is extremely complex in its diagnosis, treatment, and follow-up care. Because of the complexity, care should be given in a recognized, multidisciplinary treatment center.
2. Diagnosis and evaluation should take into account not only the physical, intellectual and emotional deficits but, equally important, the assets of the child.
3. The goal in treatment should be to capitalize on the assets to offset the deficits and, thereby achieve maximal function.
4. Treatment must be comprehensive in nature and needs to be concerned with the whole child, his family, and his community.

Some of the disciplines that are most likely to be necessary in a comprehensive treatment program are:

1. Physiotherapy started in the first year
2. Surgery for contractures
3. Occupational therapy started to prepare the child to earn a living and care for his daily needs
4. Psychiatry for secondary emotional problems
5. Gymnastics for development of motor coordination
6. Pediatric or family practitioner for counselling, general health care, and the coordination of the health specialists involved
7. Neurology for evaluation and management of neurological damage
8. Psychology for evaluation of intellectual potential
9. Special education for the multiple handicapped

Chapter 17

COMMON DIAGNOSTIC PROBLEMS

FEVER OF UNKNOWN ORIGIN

Few clinical problems in pediatrics are as much of an exercise in differential diagnosis as is the fever of unknown origin (FUO). Almost anything can cause it, including a malingering patient. There are several essential ingredients to the definition of FUO. Fever must be persistent or frequently recurrent and over 101°F rectally or 102°F orally. An obvious cause must be lacking after at least a preliminary evaluation has been made. Fever must persist for at least 10 days before one labels it fever of unknown origin.

In approaching such a problem, two valuable aids are helpful: (1) a list of possible causes ranked according to frequency of occurrence, and (2) an in-depth history and thorough physical examination undertaken with the list of causes in mind.

Table 17-1 lists the illnesses most likely to cause an FUO in a pediatric population. This list is helpful at the patient's bedside so that each possibility may be thoroughly pursued in a systematic manner.

Table 17-1 Causes of FUO

Most Common (Approximately 65% of the Cases)

Infectious Diseases
  Respiratory tract infection
    Pneumonia
    Tracheobronchitis
    Sinusitis
    Tuberculosis
  Renal infection
    Pyelonephritis
  CNS infection
    Meningitis (especially partially treated meningitis)
  Cardiac
    Subacute bacterial endocarditis
  Gastrointestinal
    Salmonella enteritis
    Campylobacter enteritis
  Hepatitis

Collagen Diseases
  Rheumatoid arthritis
  Systemic lupus erythematosus
  Rheumatic fever
  Mixed connective tissue disease

Neoplastic Diseases
  Leukemia
  Lymphoma

Miscellaneous
  Regional enteritis
  Drug fever

Nonorganic Illness
  Factitious fever

Table 17-1   (Cont'd.)

Less Common (10%)

Histoplasmosis
Infectious mononucleosis
Neuroblastoma
Sarcoma
Diabetes insipidus
Salicylate intoxication
Hidden abscess
Osteomyelitis
Sickle cell crisis with infarction
Hemorrhage into a body cavity
Cytomegalic inclusion disease
Toxoplasmosis

Rare

Brucellosis
Immunological deficiencies (AIDS)
Thyroiditis
Malaria
Cholangeitis
Ulcerative colitis
Sarcoidosis
Hyperlipemia
Hypothalamic disorders
Periodic diseases

Practical Points

The list of tests needed to establish the diagnosis may be
extensive. A few general principles are needed.

1. Do no harm.
2. Do the simple tests first. The CBC and smears, cultures,
   ESR, tuberculin skin test, and appropriate x-rays will
   provide valuable diagnostic evidence in many of the cases.

3. Make sure each test is performed well. This is particularly true of x-ray studies where a poor x-ray is accepted as normal all too often.
4. Exploratory laparotomy, occasionally helpful in adults with FUO, is only rarely so in children.

Most often the investigator finds an "atypical typical" illness, viral syndrome or UTI as examples. Despite a thorough-going evaluation, about one-third of the children with FUO will never be diagnosed. The majority of these do well and recover completely. Some continue to have their fever and other symptoms and many adapt in a satisfactory way to an unsatisfactory state of affairs.

Further Practical Points

1. Great care must be taken to be sure that bodily temperatures are accurately determined. It is a good practice for the physician to observe the temperature being taken on more than one occasion.
2. Occasionally, previous antibiotic therapy will mask the signs of a bacterial infection and suppress a positive culture. Cultures must be taken repeatedly and some time after antibiotic therapy has been discontinued.
3. Early morning fever may indicate tuberculosis, collagen diseases, or salmonella infection.
4. Cytomegalic disease and toxoplasmosis tend to cause an absolute lymphocytosis. When lymphocyte elevations are encountered, these illnesses should be ruled out.
5. Communication between attending physicians is essential to properly evaluate these problems. A covering physician poorly informed of the stage of development of the patient's evaluation can negate completely the diagnostic effort. For example, a prescription for antibiotics prior to obtaining adequate cultures.

THE ABDOMINAL MASS

The child who presents with a mass in the abdomen requires at least two things, a speedy workup and an accurate diagnosis. His physician needs a clear picture of all the diagnostic possibilities and a method of sorting them out.

While the differential diagnosis embraces an enormous number of possibilities, the simple scheme presented in Table 17-2 will in itself suggest most of them.

The diagnostic possibilities in a patient with an abdominal mass are a function of the structure involved and the process causing the enlargement. Thus, the liver may enlarge because of an infection (hepatic abscess) or because of engorgement (cardiac failure) or new growth (hepatoma). The kidney may be enlarged because of distention (hydronephrosis) or malformation (horseshoe kidney) or present as a mass because of relocation to an abnormal site (ectopic kidney). Virtually all diagnostic possibilities will be suggested if one keeps the two columns in mind. It is necessary to have an idea of which ones occur most frequently and to proceed in an orderly way. Table 17-3 lists the more frequent causes of abdominal masses. The following steps are helpful in evaluating the mass:

1. History
   a) Familial history of infection and hereditary diseases
   b) Patient's past geographic locations
   c) Onset and duration
   d) Painful or not
   e) Disturbed bowel or urinary function

Table 17-2   Differential Diagnosis of Abdominal Mass

Structure That May Enlarge	Causative Process
Liver	Infection
Kidney	Infestation
Spleen	Distention
Intestine	Engorgement
Lymphatics	New growth
Vascular	Relocation
Muscular	Malformation
Neuroendocrine	

Table 17-3 More Frequent Causes of Abdominal Masses in Childhood

Intestinal
  Constipation with feces in the sigmoid colon. May be due to primary or secondary megacolon, duplication or malrotation of bowel

Hepatomegaly due to:
  Congestive heart failure
  Fatty liver
  Cysts, abscesses, or neoplasms
  Hepatitis
  Drug therapy (steroids)

Hepatosplenomegaly
  Leukemia or lymphomas
  Various anemias
  Various infectious diseases:
    SBE
    Shigella
    Typhoid
    Malaria
    Histoplasmosis
  Reticuloendotheliosis
  Storage diseases (glycogen)
  Rheumatoid arthritis

Renal enlargement
  Wilms' tumor
  Hydronephrosis
  Polycystic kidney
  Malformed kidney

Adrenal or neurological
  Neuroblastoma

Muscular
  Hernias
  Diastasis recti

f) Presence or absence of systemic symptoms and signs
g) Presence or absence of psychological disturbances
(bezoar)
2. Physical Examination
   a) Complete physical evaluation (weight, blood pressure, etc.)
   b) Site of mass
   c) Size, shape, consistency, mobility
   d) Presence or absence of tenderness, fluctuation, or pulsation
   e) Reducibility
   f) Auscultation for bruits
   g) Rectal examination is mandatory
3. Laboratory and x-ray testing will depend on the results of the first two steps.

TESTS AND THEIR PRIMARY USEFULNESS

Test	Primary Usefulness
Hb or hematocrit	Anemia due to neoplasm, infestation or infection
WBC and differential	Infection, infestation, neoplasm
Tuberculin test	Tuberculosis
Urinalysis and BUN	Urinary tract infection, malformation, neoplasm
Urine culture and Gram's stain	Urinary tract infection
Serum bilirubin, flocculation tests	Hepatic infection, neoplasm, engorgement
SGOT, SGPT, alkaline phosphatase	Neoplasms, infection or engorgement associated with tissue destruction
Ultrasound	For mass size, location, and consistency
Abdominal flat plate	For organ size and opacifications
GI series and barium enema	Intestinal masses

Test	Primary Usefulness
Intravenous pyelogram (IVP)	Possible renal mass
Retrograde pyelogram	When nonfunctioning kidney is present
Aortography, angiography, scanning	Mass suspected in a major abdominal organ and vascular malformations
Lymphangiogram	Lymphatic and splenic masses
Bone scan and chest x-ray	Metastatic tumors, tuberculosis, and other infections or infestations
Bone marrow	Lymphatic neoplasms, tuberculosis, reticulocytosis. Culture and sensitivity for infection
Biopsy	Any major abdominal structure may be biopsied

THE RENAL-ADRENAL MASS

Special mention needs to be made of the differential diagnosis of the two most common abdominal malignancies in childhood, the Wilms' tumor and the neuroblastoma. Both of these tumors present as masses in the renal area. The differential also includes any renal-adrenal mass, i.e., polycystic kidney, hydronephrotic kidney, etc. A renal or adrenal mass may be distinguished from other abdominal structures by palpation. Since the kidney is retroperitoneal, it lacks an up and down excursion during the respiratory cycle unlike liver and spleen. In addition, unless the mass is very large or fixed to neighboring structures, ballottement is elicited. Bilateral kidney masses favor Wilms' tumor or lower tract obstruction. A plain abdominal film may resolve some of the doubt by showing the outline of an enlarged kidney. An intravenous or retrograde pyelogram will serve to confirm the clinical impression.

Neuroblastomas arising in the adrenal gland will displace the kidney downward. The appearance of the kidney on the pyelogram will be that of a normal but dislodged one. In Wilms' tumor, the renal calyces and the outline of the kidney shadow will be markedly distorted, and the kidney will usually not be displaced. Another important x-ray finding is the presence of calcification; neuroblastoma commonly contains areas of calcification while Wilms' tumor does not.

Metastatic sites differ in Wilms' and the neuroblastoma. The former involve regional lymph nodes and the lung, the latter various skeletal areas, particularly the orbital cavities of the skull.

Bone marrow aspiration may reveal neuroblastoma cells. The presence of red cells in the urine favors the diagnosis of Wilms' tumor while the finding of catecholamines and their metabolities, particularly vanillylmandelic acid (VMA), favors neuroblastoma.

HEADACHE IN CHILDHOOD

Frequently recurring headaches are not unusual complaints of school-age children. The causes are multiple and tend to vary with the age of the child. The diagnostic process is usually that of eliminating specific causes until one is left with more vaguely defined entities such as recurring migraines. The check list of etiologies include the following:

1. Local scalp disease - infection
2. Sinusitis
3. Allergy, particularly allergic rhinitis with secondary sinusitis
4. Eye disease - congenital glaucoma, poor visual acuity, strabismus
5. Dental problems - root abscess
6. Ear problems - chronic otitis media
7. Cranial nerve disease - central or peripheral; trigeminal neuralgias; herpes zoster
8. Brain tumor or brain abscess
9. Trauma to the head - cerebral concussion, cerebral contusion, subdural hematoma

10. Cavernous sinusitis and cerebrovascular malformation
11. Chronic poisoning, e.g., mercury, plumbism
12. Drug reactions
13. Convulsive disorders
14. Pseudotumor cerebri
15. Hypertensive disease - nephritis, pheochromocytoma
16. Hypoglycemia
17. Fluid and electrolyte abnormalities
18. Migraine
19. Psychogenic headache
20. Muscle contraction headache
21. Stress related imitation of adult coping behavior

A careful history and physical examination should rule out the majority of the listed causes. This examination repeated, as indicated over several weeks, is the safest, most cost-effective means of excluding serious illness.

Most helpful tests include:

1. Fundoscopic exam
2. Visual acuity and eye muscle balance tests
3. Nasal smear for eosinophils
4. Differential WBC count for eosinophils
5. Dental examination including x-rays
6. Sinus and skull x-rays
7. EEG
8. Brain scan
9. Blood glucose and electrolytes
10. Urinalysis
11. Blood pressure
12. Serial physical examinations to include fundi, EOM, and neurologic system

Other tests will, of course, be indicated if the history of physical examination indicates the possibility of a specific disease, e.g., pheochromocytoma, nephritis.

Migraine headaches are common in childhood. They typically present as one-sided headache and nausea or vomiting. A positive family history and transitory neurological phenomena (vertigo, visual aura, etc.) may be elicited. Attacks vary markedly in frequency from once yearly to several a day. Duration of the headache is often short (1-2 hours) but occasionally may last for 1 or 2 days. The majority of children display somnolence after the headache dissipates. An aura is always present.

An occasional abnormal EEG may be observed, but further workup will rule out organic neurological disease. The possibility of a seizure disorder resulting in migraine symptoms is still conjectural but the incidence of migraine headache is higher in patients with seizure disorders. Allergy also may play a role, perhaps as a precipitating factor. The treatment of migraine has classically been with ergotamine preparations. However, the natural history of migraine is to lessen and then cease after puberty. Therefore, therapy is supportive in most instances: simple analgesics such as acetaminophen, rest in a darkened room, and reassurance.

SOME COMMON MUSCLE AND NEUROMUSCULAR DISEASES

HYPOTONIAS

Half the cases of hypotonia are due to spinal cord disease, trauma, viral infections, tumors, arthrogryposis, and Werdnig-Hoffmann's disease. Another 20% are due to central nervous system disease especially severe mental retardation and the congenital cerebral defects, and 15% are due to muscle and connective tissue problems. Of the remaining 15%, 5% are due to various conditions affecting peripheral nerves, the skeletal system, and the neuromuscular junction, while 10% are not definitely diagnosed.

Werdnig-Hoffmann's Disease (Infantile Spinal Muscular Atrophy)

This condition is inherited as an autosomal recessive, and the manifestations begin in the first year and a half of life. An early onset indicates more severe involvement and a more rapidly progressive course. Proximal muscles are more involved, especially the limb girdle and trunk muscles. No sensory or sphincter control changes occur.

Helpful tests include the EMG which shows scattered, peaked waves and fibrillation potentials indicating changes in the anterior horn cells. Muscle biopsy will indicate atrophy of muscle fiber. Death may occur when the bulbar muscles are affected or due to intercurrent pulmonary infection. There is no specific therapy.

Amyotonia Congenita

Probably not a single disease entity. It may be a more benign variant of Werdnig-Hoffmann's disease. Symptoms are similar but less rapidly progressive. Death usually occurs toward middle age.

Congenital Hypotonia

Weakness exists from birth establishing this entity as congenital in nature. There is no familial pattern of inheritance, however. Some children achieve a spontaneous remission of all findings before puberty, whereas others will continue to have residual muscle weakness, particularly involving the smaller muscles of the body. The EMG shows polyphasic, short lasting potentials. Serum enzymes, the muscle biopsy, and nerve conduction are normal.

MIXED HYPOTONIA AND HYPERTONIA

Arthrogryposis

Joint contractures are present from birth. One or more extremities may be involved but the lower extremities are more commonly afflicted. There may be a number of associated malformations and the physician should make a complete search for them, particularly cardiovascular and renal anomalies which are common. Despite contractures of peripheral muscles, there may be a general hypotonia and, thus, arthrogryposis is included as one of the hypotonias.

HYPERTONIAS

Myotonia Congenita

An autosomal dominant disease, affecting males predominantly. Onset is in the prepubertal school-age child. Stiffness when walking is an early sign. Symmetrical involvement of the skeletal muscles is the rule. Increased muscle tone tends to immobilize joints until repeated movements loosen them up. Cold weather and inactivity cause increased stiffness. Exercise, avoiding cold, and procainamide or quinine are helpful.

THERAPY FOR MUSCULAR DEFECTS

Limitation of movement in any joint and contractures require treatment. Appropriate physical therapy is employed, and in recalcitrant cases, surgical correction is necessary. Growth adds an important factor. Contracted joints must be made to keep apace with growth of the limb.

Upper extremities are made as mobile as possible, lower extremities are aligned for the best weight-bearing position possible. Occupational therapy is very valuable in older children.

MUSCULAR DYSTROPHIES

There are several varieties of muscular dystrophy. Landouzy-Dejerine described the fascioscapulohumeral type; Erb described the limb girdle dystrophy; and Duchenne, the more rapidly progressive and severe pseudohypertrophic type. Other varieties include myotonic dystrophy, dystrophic ophthalmoplegia, and Gower's distal dystrophy.

Mode of Inheritance

Duchenne	Sex-linked recessive
Landouzy-Dejerine	Autosomal dominant
Erb	Autosomal recessive

Duchenne's pseudohypertrophic muscular dystrophy is the most common form. Onset is in early childhood during the preschool years. Gait abnormalities, unsteadiness, and lordosis are early signs. Pseudohypertrophy of the calf muscles is usually prominent. Progression of weakness and muscular atrophy varies markedly from patient to patient. As weakness progresses, contractures and deformities increase. Muscle weakness usually proceeds from the proximal to the distal groups. Respiratory and cardiac functions also deteriorate and death is commonly the result of pulmonary infection and cardiorespiratory failure. Many psychological aberrations may also occur as disabilities increase. Eventually, the child is unable to ambulate by himself and wheelchair life is a necessity. Death in the second or third decade is common.

Landouzy-Dejerine's fascioscapulohumeral dystrophy is slowly progressive. Onset is from early childhood to adult life. Early symptoms are difficulty in closing the eyes and an inexpressive face. Drooping of the shoulders and inability to raise the arms also occur early. Deep tendon reflexes are absent or decreased. Later, lower limb weakness begins. Contractures and deformities develop slowly or sometimes not at all. A normal life span is frequently reached.

Erb's limb girdle dystrophy begins in either childhood or early adult life. It is intermediate in rate of progression between Duchenne and Landouzy-Dejerine varieties. The shoulder girdle muscles are demonstrably weak and affect the movement of the upper extremities. Pelvic girdle involvement results in similar disabilities of the lower extremities and takes the name of Leyden and Moebius dystrophy. The course is slowly progressive, leading to atrophy, contracture and deformity, and death in the third to fifth decade.

Helpful Laboratory Tests

1. Electromyography – low amplitude waves of short duration
2. Serum enzymes – creatine phosphokinase and sometimes SGOT and aldolase are elevated
3. Muscle biopsy – fiber atrophy, etc.
4. Nerve conduction is normal. Management is similar to that of other muscular defects

FAILURE TO THRIVE

Failure to thrive is a general term applicable to children in whom growth failure plays a conspicuous role in their disease process. It is either the presenting complaint or one of the more noticeable features. In general, growth failure is an accompaniment to almost any chronic disease state in a growing organism. The causes of growth failure number in the thousands.

In confronting a child who is obviously failing to grow normally for a less than obvious reason, the clinician's dilemma is just how to proceed in a systematic manner. A thorough history, related particularly to major organ systems, will often make the diagnosis or suggest the course of the workup. Apart from an organ-systems approach, familial diseases, prenatal diseases, and the sociopsychoeconomic aspects of the child's life should be explored rigorously. Last, and very important, a complete dietary history must be obtained. Table 17-4 presents a classification of the major causes of failure to thrive.

It is important to establish the types of growth failure that exist: linear, body size, weight, cranial and chest circumference, sitting to total height ratios, limb length measurements. A bone age x-ray is included in the first steps of the workup. Similar measurements should be made in parents and siblings. Next, the pattern of growth failure should be determined. Was growth abnormally retarded before, since, or well after birth? Are all growth measurements affected? The birth weight, length, and head circumference are of special value as are any available series of measurements made after birth. If none exists, plan to take periodic measurements prospectively. Examination of photographs of family members as well as of the patient at different ages is very helpful to diagnose dysmorphism.

It is appropriate to do a few basic screening tests if no clear indication of etiology is suggested. The following are helpful ones:
First Stage

1. CBC and differential
2. ESR
3. PPD
4. Serology

Table 17-4 Classification of Failure to Thrive

General Disease States
  Infection—tuberculosis, urinary tract infections, etc.
  Infestation—tapeworm, hookworm
  Nutritional—poor diet, quality or quantity
  Metabolic—certain inborn errors of metabolism
  Chronic intoxication—lead poisoning
  Psychogenic—anorexia nervosa, poor maternal-infant bonding

Malfunction of Various Organ Systems
  CNS—brain damage, hypothalamic dysfunction
  GI—malabsorptive states, structural GI anomalies, chronic liver disease
  GU—chronic urinary tract infection, renal tubular disease
  Cardiovascular—cyanotic heart disease, chronic heart failure
  Endocrine—hypothyroidism, Cushing's disease
  Hematopoietic—chronic anemias (sickle cell disease, thalassemia)
  Respiratory—cystic fibrosis, chronic asthma, bronchopulmonary dysplasia

Chromosomal or Genetic Illness-Turner's syndrome, Down's syndrome, etc.

Prenatal—rubella syndrome, placental dysfunction

Environmental Factors—poverty, child abuse and neglect

---

5. Urinalysis, including a specific gravity, reducing substance in urine
6. Nose, throat, stool, blood, and urine cultures
7. Blood glucose, BUN, CO_2, NA, Cl, K, Ca, P, serum carotene, TSH, T_3, T_4, liver function tests, pH, stool pH, and reducing substances, Sudan III stain of feces
8. Chest x-ray

9. Visual fields
10. Dietary diary – all food ingested in kind, quality, and quantity is recorded and the nutritional adequacy of the diet is determined.

<u>Later Stage</u>

If the answer is still not suggested by the foregoing procedures, the following should be undertaken:

1. Diet testing – child is placed on an adequate diet and observed as to weight gain, intake and output, etc.
2. Sweat test
3. GI series and Ba enemas (after thyroid studies are completed)
4. IVP and VCU (after thyroid studies are completed)
5. Skeletal survey
6. Twenty-four hour urine for 17-ketosteroids
7. Muscle biopsy
8. ECG
9. Urine concentration test
10. Tests for malabsorption states:
  a) D-xylose uptake
  b) Stool fat
  c) Carbohydrate absorption
  d) Breath hydrogen test for lactose
  e) Malabsorption
11. Buccal smear and karyotyping

Other specific tests suggested by the workup may then be added. The above list is not meant to be exhaustive, it only indicates the more important and helpful tests. Close observation of the patient's behavior, stool and urine habits, relations with mother and other close relatives, and feeding habits is often very helpful.

Practical Points

1. About 75% of children with failure to thrive have a nutritional disturbance. The most common of these is an inadequate diet.
2. Most genetic causes of short stature present without concomitant inanition. This is an important pattern to recognize.

3. Hypopituitary dwarfism can virtually be ruled out if tooth eruption is proceeding normally.
4. Disproportionate body measurements tend to indicate an endocrinopathy as the etiology.
5. Genetic diseases usually cause other major manifestations besides growth failure.
6. Poor hygiene, diaper dermatitis, signs of multiple injury, and an exceptionally cooperative preschool-age child should lead one to think of child abuse.
7. Children living in substandard housing should be screened for lead poisoning.

MUCOCUTANEOUS LYMPH NODE SYNDROME (KAWASAKI DISEASE)

Mucocutaneous lymph node syndrome is a conditon of uncertain etiology first described in Japan, and still more prevalent there, but that is being reported with greater frequency in the United States. It affects younger children causing an inflammatory process of mucous membranes (conjunctivitis, stomatitis), palmar, plantar, and generalized erythema, lymph node enlargement, arthralgia or arthritis, and fever. It may also cause myocarditis, pericarditis, hepatitis, aseptic meningitis, and pyuria. The disease is protracted over several days to 3 weeks or more and occasions a fine desquamation of the skin over the terminal phalanges of fingers and toes. The most serious complication is coronary artery vasculitis which leads to sudden death in 1-2% of cases. This occurs most commonly from 3 to 6 weeks after onset.

The diagnosis is made on clinical findings. ECG and chest x-rays should be obtained but abnormalities may not be detected by these tests. Serum complement may also rise. Salicylate therapy has been used with some degree of success in treating the symptoms associated with the disease. Hospitalization is essential to monitor cardiac functions. Long-term follow-up to detect lingering cardiac illness should be arranged. Consultation with pediatric cardiologists or infectious disease experts is appropriate to provide comprehensive short- and long-term care.

Chapter 18

COMMON ORTHOPEDIC PROBLEMS

There are several orthopedic conditions that are encountered almost daily in any large well-child oriented practice. All practitioners engaged in rendering such care should be familiar with these common conditions.

THE HIP

CONGENITAL HIP DISLOCATION

This congenital defect constitutes an excellent example of the saying "a stitch in time saves nine." Early recognition and simple inexpensive therapy may lead to complete correction, while delay in therapy results in only partial correction, at great cost to the well-being of the child and his family.

The examination of the hips is one of the most important aspects of the well-baby exam in preambulatory infants. Several clinical criteria (Table 18-1) serve to distinguish the subluxated or frankly dislocated hip from the normal.

X-rays of the hip, while of little or no value in early infancy, will be diagnostic in older infants. Care must be taken to have the child in a frog leg position and in proper

Table 18-1   Procedures to Distinguish the Normal From the Dislocated Hip

	Normal Hip	Dislocated Hip
Range of motion	Abduction of femur is normal	Abduction of femur is limited
Ortolani's sign	No negative click on abduction and external-rotation	Frequently positive click on abduction and external-rotation of involved hip
Gluteal fold	Symmetrical	Asymmetrical
Other leg folds	Symmetrical	May be asymmetrical
Length of femur	Equal both sides	Shorter on affected side
Femoral head	Equal position both sides	May be somewhat lower on affected side
Tug test	Femoral head cannot be luxated with a gentle tug	Femoral head may be luxated by gentle tug

alignment in order to be able to interpret the x-ray with any degree of accuracy. If, in a younger infant, the clinical signs of subluxation are present but the x-ray is normal, treatment is best instituted. In this early phase, splinting the femur so that it is held in abduction allows for better development of the acetabulum. Wide diapering with two or three pairs of diapers is generally enough to accomplish the abduction. Overcorrection by maintaining the hips in extreme abduction beyond an angle of 40-45° may compromise the vascular supply to the femoral head with consequent necrosis.

Perfectly acceptable correction can be achieved without extreme abduction, and necrosis of the femoral head avoided.
A Palov harness is the therapy of choice, fitted and maintained by an orthopedist.

It is extremely important to explain the natural history
and excellent prognosis of congenital hip dislocation to the
parents. The parents must also understand the infrequent
occurrence of a late subluxation of the hip in the 9-12-
month-old. The associated parental misconception that an
earlier lesion was missed, resulting in the late hip disorder,
severely complicates management.

SLIPPED LATERAL FEMORAL EPIPHYSIS

This disease presents as pain and a limp in older children.
The patient is usually an obese, prepubertal male. Often
the pain will be referred to the ipsilateral knee. The hip
x-ray is the best way of making the diagnosis but a lateral
view must be included since the frontal view may not adequately demonstrate the lesion. Early diagnosis is essential to complete care. Therapy is surgical, pins being employed to hold the slipping epiphysis in place.

LEGG-CALVE-PERTHES DISEASE

This condition is one of the juvenile osteochondroses. It presents similarly to slipped femoral epiphysis, as pain in the
hip or knee together with a limp. It does occur in younger
children but rarely before the age of 3 years. The active
phase lasts about $1\frac{1}{2}$ years and after an extended period
remineralization takes place. The diagnosis is made with
an x-ray of the hip showing sclerosis and flattening of the
femoral epiphysis. These changes may not be present in
the early phase. In cases of persistent pain and limp, serial
x-ray should be made when the initial ones fail to demonstrate the lesion. Treatment consists of the avoidance of
weight-bearing on the affected hip during the symptomatic
period.

THE KNEE

GENU VALGUM (KNOCK-KNEE)

A primary and secondary form of genu valgum exists. The secondary form represents a sequelae of various processes among which are rheumatoid arthritis and rickets.

The distance between the medial malleoli of the ankles should not exceed 2.5 in. when the child stands at attention with his knees in light approximation. If there is a greater space, the child is said to have genu valgum. Bracing and splinting are helpful in correction.

GENU VARUS (BOWLEGS)

A mild degree is normal in infants. If it is present after the second year of life, correction may be undertaken, particularly if the deformity is progressive. Splinting with a bar that forces the feet apart is adequate in most cases. In severe cases, bracing and surgery are indicated.

THE FEET

PIGEON-TOES

The inward rotation of any part of the thigh or leg may produce pigeon-toes. Inspection will show which segment of the lower extremities is at fault. Examination in a prone position with the knees bent 90° is helpful. If hip rotation is the problem, the thighs will be seen to be rotated. If tibia or knee is the problem, the thigh will not be rotated but the foot will still be turned in. Aligning the two knees so that they are not rotated, one clearly sees internal tibial torsion by the inward pointing foot (or feet). Forefoot adduction or metatarsus varus (an inward pointing deformity of the distal part of the foot) also may produce this appearance. A convex lateral margin of the sole will help distinguish this condition.

Internal tibial torsion is treated by splinting the feet with a bar splint so that they are held in outward rotation. In nonambulatory children, these should be applied constantly. In the ambulatory, they are used at night. The majority of children will correct spontaneously even without splinting. Metatarsus varus is treated by casting the feet serially until the deformity is corrected and the foot aligned properly. If the metatarsus varus is dynamic, massaging the instep in infancy permits final correction of the intoeing as the child begins to walk.

TOEING-OUT

A common and usually benign condition in infancy. When it occurs in older children and is either marked or progressive, it may require surgical correction.

PES CAVUS (FLATFEET)

Infant's feet, due to the fat pad of the arch, invariably will appear to be flat. Significant flatfeet do not exist unless a bony anomaly such as a vertical talus or an accessory navicular, or other foot deformities such as foot pronation or excessively high arches are present. The type of flatfeet caused by a relaxed ligamental structure rarely gives rise to more than cosmetic difficulties.

The classic simple therapy in the benign flatfoot is the Thomas heel and arch supports. The efficacy of this remains doubtful. Careful palpation of the arch should be carried out. If a bony prominence is felt or if dorsiflexion of the ankle is limited, x-rays should be taken to rule out vertical talus and an accessory navicular bone. Correction is surgical in these instances.

THE SPINE

SCOLIOSIS

Scoliosis is a lateral curvature of the spine which develops in the prepubertal child. Sixty to eighty percent of cases occur in girls. It is familial but is frequently found in individuals with a negative family history. This disorder affects up to 4% of children and today approximately 500,000 American adults have a significant scoliotic deformity.

The majority of children who develop scoliosis had a normal spine at birth. The cause is unknown. The affected

spine has an abnormal thoracic convex curve to the right
and a left convex curve in the lumbar spine. The right
shoulder is higher than the left. The patient or mother presents complaining of poorly fitting clothes or that one
shoulder is higher than the other.

Early diagnosis and therapy are very effective in reducing the severity of the progression of this deformity,
eliminating surgery in many cases.

Scoliosis Screening

School scoliosis screening programs provide an excellent
means of early diagnosis and referral. Initial screenings in
the United States are offered in elementary school and
permit medical intervention prior to the onset of symptoms
which would be apparent to family members. Children
noted to have positive findings during screenings are referred to the physician for further evaluation. Orthopedic
management is mandatory for affected individuals as early
as possible.

Scoliosis screening in elementary schools should be performed by trained personnel. The students, dressed in
shorts and no shirts with girls wearing bras or swimsuit tops,
walk toward the examiner while the gait is assessed for a
limp or lurch suggesting unilateral leg pathology. This screens
for a secondary or compensatory scoliosis which can be present with unequal leg length or muscle strength. Once in
front of the examiner, the student turns so that his back is
to the examiner. The child is requested to bend forward
while looking at his toes with both arms loosely dangling
forward. The spine and thorax are inspected from several
angles and palpated to denote any deformity. The presence
of any abnormality is an indication for referral to the patient's primary physician. The student is examined for elevation of one shoulder, asymmetry in the prominence or level
of either scapula, curvature of the spine, hip height inequal-
ity, a rib hump on bending forward or increased distance between the arm and waist.

This type of screening is very sensitive. One in ten 14-
year-old students have detectable scoliosis. In most scoliosis screening programs, 60-70% of those with positive findings and, therefore, referred for further evaluation, have

radiologically confirmed scoliosis. Most detectable scoliosis
does not require treatment. One 5% of children and adolescents require active management.

Preadolescent and adolescent patients with idiopathic
curves of less than 20-25° require regular observation at 6-
month intervals. Less than 50% of these patients will have
increasing curvature of their spines. Only 1 out of 10 will
require therapy. Those individuals with curves between 25
and 40° require treatment with a brace. A Milwaukee brace
is most commonly prescribed. This is worn 23 hours each
day for an average of 3-4 years.

A curve greater than 50° occurs in 1/1000 children and
requires surgical management by placement of a Harrington
distraction rod along the convexity of the curve and fusion
of the affected vertebrae. Surgery partially corrects and
arrests scoliosis progression. Rehabilitation is protracted
and does not correct any associated cardiorespiratory dysfunction. The patient's psychosocial and educational needs
must be provided for during the prolonged hospitalization.

Examination of the spine should be included in all routine
examinations of patients at all ages. Scoliosis is a lifelong
progressive spinal deformity. A negative examination at one
time does not preclude positive findings at a later date.
Parents should be educated with regard to this fact and the
excellent benefits of early intervention. Medical care offered to the scoliosis patient early in the disease results in
an increase in psychological and physical well-being for those
who are prevented from progressing to spinal deformity.

Athletes who require scoliosis brace treatment should be
encouraged to continue their sports. The brace limits performance but does not prohibit athletic participation with
the exception of competitive contact sports and gymnastics.

TRAUMA

Orthopedic trauma is common in pediatrics, especially
during the warmer months of the year with increased out-
door activity. Most frequently, the injury is to soft tissue
without fractures.

The extent of the injury must be defined. Fracture, dislocation, and ligamentous tears can be excluded by the absence of hemorrhage and point tenderness and the presence of

a full range of active motion, with appropriate function. Then first aid is appropriate.

The proper care at the time of injury offers the patient optimal and speedy recovery. The affected site should be immobilized. Cold should be applied, preferably with ice (not in direct contact with the skin) immediately and then for 15 minutes four times daily for 48 hours. Elevation to minimize edema will greatly relieve discomfort. Elevation should be sufficient to offset gravity rather than extreme, i.e., holding the foot above the head.

Proper training with gradually increasing physiologic stress, good nutrition, and matching of the athlete by age, development, and training to the particular type of athletic participation is good preventive medicine. Young athletes are engaging in an educational experience, which should promote a physiologic and psychosocially sound lifestyle at maturity.

OSGOOD–SCHLATTER DISEASE

Athletic, muscular boys are most frequently seen for leg pain and swelling localized to the tibial tuberosity. This discomfort and swelling worsen with exercise. These symptoms and signs are manifestations of an apophysitis of the tibial tuberosity.

The exact etiology of this disorder is uncertain; however, chronic trauma to the tibial tuberosity by quadriceps overuse is generally considered to be the probable cause. X-rays reveal irregular ossification of the tibial tubercle. Examination of the knee and lower extremity joints is normal. Swelling and point tenderness, which may be exquisite, are always present at the tibial tuberosity.

This disorder is self-limited, but very uncomfortable. Reassurance and limitation of activity as dictated by symptoms are all that is necessary in most cases. Appropriate protection of the area to avoid trauma should be advised. Those patients not finding relief with rest, modified athletic participation, and analgesics should be referred for orthopedic management.

Chapter 19

PSYCHOLOGICAL PROBLEMS

FEEDING

Feeding, the most central function in the earliest mother-child care, is frequently the first problem brought to professional attention. One of the earliest problems, colic, which occurs in the first 3 months of life is discussed on p. 66.

Many early feeding problems are a function of normal parental anxiety, particularly in first-born children and can be relatively easily resolved with careful attention and counselling. Others may extend themselves in time and become more complex problems such as obesity or failure to thrive. Eating difficulties will be categorized here as eating too little, eating too much, and inappropriate eating.

EATING TOO LITTLE

In the too little category are the failure to thrive babies. Failure to thrive is most often due to inadequate nutrition which in turn may be related to a temporary acute illness or to a chronic medical problem. A careful medical workup as described in Chapter 17, p. 401, is necessary to rule out organic causes. Other causes may be poverty, inadequate parental knowledge, parental neglect, or other serious problems in the family. These possibilities must be explored by a thorough psychosocial history along with a complete dietary history. Where psychological causes predominate, clear instruction and support from the physician may need to be supplemented with help from agencies such as public health nursing, or by the services of a nutritionist or mental health professional. During the second year of life, eating too little must be seen in the context of the normal marked decrease in appetite. (See p. 66)

In later childhood, particularly adolescence, "too little" is expressed in a collection of symptoms labeled anorexia nervosa. Anorexia is most frequently found in girls (females predominate in a 10:1 ratio over males) between 12 and 21 but is occasionally observed in boys, younger children, and adults. Its severity ranges from self-induced death to mild cases which begin as reactions to situational stress. Primary symptoms are loss of appetite or actual feelings of revulsion toward food followed by severe weight loss, amenorrhea, constipation, weakness, and exhaustion.

Treatment

A combination of close medical supervision (hospitalization may be necessary in very severe cases) and psychotherapy is the treatment of choice. Recent successful modes of psychologic-psychiatric treatment have included family therapy as well as more individualized attention to the child.

Practical Points

1. Early age of onset during the adolescent period is positively related to treatment outcome.
2. An infinite variety of psychological makeup may be found. Although anorexia is predominantly found in neurotic personalities, it is occasionally associated with normal or with psychotic individuals.
3. A history of eating problems including obesity is frequently but not always present.

EATING TOO MUCH—OBESITY

In adults, obesity is related to an increased incidence of such problems as high blood pressure and coronary artery disease; in its more extreme form, it is associated with a shorter life expectancy. Its medical effects in childhood are less well documented, although current research estimates that 85% of obese children become obese adults. The odds against an overweight child becoming normal increase from 4:1 at 12 years of age to 28:1 after adolescence. The age of onset of childhood obesity is unclear. It appears to be a multidetermined condition which is influenced by genetic, prenatal, and environmental events. Maternal overweight, excessive weight gain in pregnancy, and high birth weight often are related to later childhood obesity. There has been recent interest in excessive weight gain in infancy as possibly related to the hypothesis of hypercellular increase in fat cells at an early critical period. Obese 3 and 4 year olds tend to remain obese, at least in later childhood. Obesity is more frequent in female children and adolescents and the frequency is greater in the lower socioeconomic classes.

Juvenile onset obesity is characterized by much greater emotional distress, particularly in the form of body image disturbances in adult life. Obese children, especially adolescents, are frequently the center of family conflict, are teased and ridiculed by peers, and have great difficulty in maturing and achieving independence.

Treatment

Treatment of childhood and adolescent obesity has met with little success. Even where an initial weight loss has been significant, followup has often shown that the weight has been regained. Weight-reducing drugs are not useful and are contraindicated for children and adolescents. Traditional psychotherapy has generally proved ineffective with obesity. It would seem that early prevention is of utmost importance. Nutritional information and weight control need to be started early in infancy. Females in the lower socioeconomic group are at highest risk for obesity and are prime targets for preventative action. The following treatment modes offer the best possibilities:

1. When handled by the physician, emphasis should be given to the active participation of the child in the treatment plan. If she/he is old enough, a record of food and activity should be kept. A diet and activity schedule that fits in with the child or adolescent's life pattern and interests should be attempted. Monitoring and counselling should be provided on a long-term basis.
2. Behavior modification approaches are now used in some weight clinics and have shown promise. This approach also requires a great deal of input from the patient and focuses on changing eating behavior, e.g., eating only in a certain place unaccompanied by any other activity or eating and chewing very slowly. Although this approach has thus far been used primarily with adults, it may be modifiable for use with children and adolescents.
3. Groups such as TOPS or Weight Watchers have been relatively successful in providing the techniques and the psychological support necessary for weight reduction. These resources may be appropriate for adolescents, especially when adolescent groups are available.

INAPPROPRIATE EATING

The eating of inappropriate substances in its most serious aspect (pica) can result in accidental poisoning discussed on p. 244. Pica is generally used to refer to the consistent searching out of inedible substances such as plaster, ashes, etc., rather than to the indiscriminate mouthing of most everything by youngsters less than 1 year of age. The most well-known result of pica is lead poisoning found in children who have routinely ingested plaster or other lead-containing substances. The diagnosis and treatment for lead poisoning are elaborated in the chapter on accidental poisoning. (See p. 244)

The eating of an inappropriate diet which may result in malnutrition without underfeeding may be caused by poverty or other factors making necessary nutrients unavailable or by parental lack of knowledge of nutritional food values. Specific instruction should be given with an awareness of costs and appropriateness with the family's eating patterns. Long-term monitoring and sometimes home followup by a homemaker or visiting nurse may be necessary. "Finicky eaters" are generally not important medically and become of significance only when this becomes the focus and continuing cause of a disturbed parent/child relationship. In the few instances where finicky eating is thought to be important in malnourishment or where parents are especially concerned about a child's eating habits, a reward system such as a specially liked food for trying a new food or for other *positive* eating behavior may be helpful.

ENURESIS

Involuntary passage of urine beyond the age when normal bladder control is attained is termed enuresis. The majority of children gain sufficient bladder control by about 3 years of age and are able to keep themselves dry all day and most of the night. Complete nocturnal bladder control is attained around 4 years of age in most children. Some children continue to have intermittent nocturnal enuresis until about 5-6 years of age. Males are at least twice as commonly afflicted as females. In a small percentage of children, bedwetting recurs after a variable period of complete bladder control.

Enuresis may reflect the normal variation in the growth and development of children. Psychological trauma in early formative years, parental indifference to toilet training the child who is physiologically ready, or conversely, too early attempts at toilet training, small bladder capacity as documented in many enuretics, are all postulated as possible factors in causing enuresis in childhood. Although its significance and pattern are unclear, there is frequently a positive family incidence. Enuresis is also considered by some as a seizure equivalent. No good correlation has been found between enuresis and occurrence of spina bifida occulta. Occasionally urinary tract infection is associated with enuresis. Very rarely enuresis may be a manifestation of lesions of the genitourinary tract. Diabetes mellitus or diabetes insipidus may cause bedwetting in an occasional child.

Diagnostic procedures include:

1. Routine urinalysis and urine culture
2. Careful neurological evaluation including x-ray examination of the spine (defects of the lower part of the spine may or may not be associated with neurological defects) to rule out abnormalities of the sphincter mechanism

3. Careful urological investigation including IVP and VCU studies where abnormalities of urinary tract are suspected
4. Rectal examination

Management includes:

1. Parental education on the nature of the problem will help allay parents' anxiety and prevent them from developing undesirable attitudes towards the problem. Punishment, shaming, etc. only aggravate the situation. Indicating that the child is suffering too and is not wetting to annoy the parents can be helpful.
2. Bladder exercises to increase the bladder capacity have been advocated by some, particularly for those with diurnal enuresis. Bladder stretching exercise consists of increased fluid intake during the day and suppression of the urge to void to the point of discomfort.
3. The most popular medication is imipramine over a varying period of time—usually 8 weeks—in doses between 25 and 75 mg/day. Recurrence of the problem after a course of therapy is not uncommon.
4. Conditioning—Use of an alarm which awakens the child as soon as he begins to void has had reasonably good success.

ENCOPRESIS

The term encopresis is defined as the passage of formed or liquid fecal material into the child's clothing. Three and a half to four years of age is the lower age limit to distinguish encopresis from normal childhood behavior. The observed incidence of encopresis has varied from 1 to 3% of a normal child population to 5 to 7% of a psychiatric population. It has consistently been observed to be five times as common in males as in females.

In contrast to enuresis, fecal incontinence is more common during the day, particularly late afternoon and evening, than at night. Approximately one-third of encopretic children also demonstrate enuresis. Other symptoms associated with encopresis are abdominal pain and large caliber stools. Children frequently report a lack of sensation or perception of the need to have a bowel movement. It has been postulated that bowel distension sensation or sensitivity to its use

may be limited or lost from a chronically stretched colon
and rectum. The frequency of constipation and stool retention as a concomitant of soiling has been unclear. Recent
studies, however, have reported constipation and fecal impaction in 80-95% of encopretic patients. A history of infantile constipation has been reported in many cases. Very
early or coercive bowel training has also been implicated as
a causal factor.

Practical Points

1. Because of the tendency for encopresis to become entrenched and difficult to correct, prevention is of utmost
   importance. Proper management of bowel training, especially for children having difficulty, and immediate
   attention to children having early constipation due to
   such causes as anal fissures and gastroenteritis, are a
   necessity.
2. Soiling is frequently misdiagnosed as diarrhea with anti-
   diarrheal medication compounding the more basic problem of constipation and impaction.
3. Organic conditions such as cerebral palsy or amyotonia
   congenita which affect the abdominal musculature, obstructive lesions such as Hirschsprung's disease, and other
   organic causes must be carefully ruled out.
4. When encopresis has become an entrenched condition,
   treatment directed at the specific symptom should be
   attempted by either the pediatrician or a mental health
   professional. A program described by Wright in Professional Psychology, May 1973, has proven very successful.
   There are basically two aspects to treatment: (1) the use
   of suppositories which gives more control over the time
   of evacuation, and (2) positive reinforcement in the form
   of "earned time" with a parent.

MENTAL RETARDATION

Mental retardation is defined as significantly subaverage
intellectual functioning becoming apparent during the devel-
mental period and characterized by inadequacy of adaptive
behavior. Each of these characteristics is of importance in

the diagnosis, and the exclusion of either adaptive functioning or intelligence test scores can lead to misdiagnosis.
Although 3% of newborn infants are at some time during
childhood diagnosed as mentally retarded it is estimated
that, at any given time, approximately 1% of the population
would be so characterized. This is due to such factors as
the high death rate of infants and children with severe retardation and the assimilation into the normal adult population of the more mildly impaired individuals. The classification system by intellectual potential within the category
of mental retardation is as follows:

Classification	IQ Score Range	Educational Potential
Mild mental retardation	50–70	Educable
Moderate mental retardation	35–50	Trainable
Severe mental retardation	20–35	Trainable
Profound mental retardation	0–20	Totally dependent

Total dependency encompasses most of the profoundly
retarded and assumes the person will need assistance with
basic physical care, is not responsive to his environment, and
will probably require permanent institutionalization. Only 1
or 2% of all retarded children are in this category. Train-
able potential includes the moderate and severe groups and
suggests that the person will become self-sufficient in self-
care and achieve some competence in social and educational
affairs. A sheltered workshop, usefulness in the home, or
possibly, low skill requirement jobs would be most predictive
of economic self-sufficiency.

The educable person will most likely be totally inde-
pendent in self-care, capable of achieving a fourth to sixth
grade academic education (or finish high school in special
programs), and be self-supporting in occupations not requiring abstract thought.

There will be individuals who cross boundaries in one or
more aspects of these classifications.

ETIOLOGY

Causative factors of mental retardation may be biological, sociocultural, psychological or an interaction of the above. In those cases having a demonstrable biological base there are frequently clinical clues of morphological or anatomical stigmata or progressive developmental deterioration. Included are a long list of chromosomal defects, metabolic dysfunctions, progressive central processes, acquired prenatal, perinatal, and postnatal conditions. These should generally be picked up in infancy or early childhood. In addition to the usual medical and social history, particular attention should be paid to developmental information including genetic, pregnancy, stressful labor, and perinatal course.

DIAGNOSIS

Physical examination should be particularly attentive to the following clues: serial cranial measurements or abnormal cranial configuration, subtle neurological abnormalities, specific abnormalities of the face, eyes, ears, liver, and digits. Commonly found behavioral characteristics are as follows:

1. Delayed development in walking, motor coordination, habit training, and speech
2. Inability to follow directions
3. Difficulty in paying attention
4. Problems in attention span
5. Lack of self-direction in play as well as more formal learning
6. Lack of generalization from one situation to another
7. Lack of ability to deal with abstractions—things not physically present

Routine developmental screening is an important aid in diagnosing mental retardation in the preschool years. (See Appendix H) If a child has not passed two screenings, referral for more detailed psychological assessment is called for. Other consultations such as vision or hearing and speech may be helpful.

It should be emphasized that although early diagnosis is important in preventing secondary learning and emotional problems, speedy diagnosis of mental retardation is not necessary or desirable. Frequently the longitudinal picture lends important perspective in the assessment of proper educational planning. Although some parents are aware and semiprepared for a diagnosis of mental retardation, others may be quite stunned and resistant and most will go through periods of denial, anger, and depression before reaching a level of some acceptance and realistic planning. As in other long-term disabilities, a care plan depends on many factors, e.g., strengths, weaknesses, and desires of the child and other family members, and available physical, monetary, and community resources. Residential placement is sometimes necessary, although current thinking tends to be that early childhood care is beneficial to the child and the family when given within the home. Long-term follow-up and counselling for the family and/or child as he/she meets new developmental challenges are frequently needed. Proper psychoeducational assessment should be made to determine if a special educational program is called for. If so, assistance should be given in finding the optimal resources within the community.

HYPERACTIVITY

Hyperactivity had its beginning in the medical and psychological literature as a primary symptom of the minimal brain dysfunction syndrome. However, it will be discussed separately as it is now frequently considered as an entity in itself.

Hyperactivity is an aspect of behavior that is not easy to separate from the normal activity of children and also holds differing significance with age. It is sometimes delineated by the excessive amount of physical activity, sometimes by its very presence, e.g., "he is *never* quiet," and sometimes by its distractibility component, "he just runs from one thing to the next." Hyperactivity becomes of serious importance when it interferes with the child's ability to learn and is destructive of the parent-child relationship.

ETIOLOGY

There are several possible causes of hyperactive behavior, any one or all of which may be present:

1. A deficit in the central nervous system may be present. Although there is occasionally some known insult, there is most frequently no specifiable injury.
2. Anxiety can be a powerful psychological stimulus, expressing itself in excessive physical activity in children.
3. Environmental causes of hyperactivity can be seen where few, harsh, or very inconsistent limits are set by parents or in overcrowded or highly disorganized households.

TREATMENT

One primary treatment modality is psychological where the physician may provide parental counselling around more effective methods of organization and discipline. If severe anxiety is responsible for the hyperactivity, psychological or psychiatric intervention is most likely to be necessary. A vigorously debated method of control is the dietary restriction of food additives and dyes advocated by Feingold. Inasmuch as some current research indicates that high dosages of food dyes do affect activity and learning levels, a reduction in coloring and additives is a possible avenue of treatment. It is difficult for some parents to comply as it makes shopping very time-consuming and expensive. Some authors think that dietary exclusions can make it possible to reduce and sometimes eliminate medication which is a third treatment method. The use of medication for controlling hyperactivity is discussed under attention deficit disorder below.

ATTENTION DEFICIT DISORDER

Attention deficit disorder (ADD) once called minimal brain dysfunction (MBD) refers to a behavior pattern in children which assumes some kind of nonspecific but altered brain function. The concept of inferring dysfunction has developed over a period of 20 to 30 years beginning with the study of behavior and learning deficits in persons with known injury to the brain from illness or insult. Taking into consideration the difficulties and fuzziness of behavioral diagnoses, several surveys have estimated a 5-40% prevalence rate in school-age children. It is found five times more frequently in males.

SYMPTOMS

1. Motor activity: The most frequent abnormalities are hyperactivity and incoordination. The child is described as "driven," "fidgety," unable to sit even for TV. This tends to be a constant rather than a variable feature of his behavior. Delayed developmental milestones or clumsiness are also frequently described. Bicycle riding, tying shoes, and writing are some of the areas where slowness and awkwardness are noticed.
2. Attention and concentration: The ADD child has a very short attention span and is frequently described as unable to complete anything. He runs from one thing to the next, whether it be schoolwork, toys, or leisure activities. He is seemingly distracted by the most innocuous and extraneous stimuli. Memory is also reported as faulty, e.g., "he doesn't hear anything I say." ADD children have been reported to forget things like a visiting friend or a promised trip as well as forgetting the usual parental injunctions and restrictions.
3. Learning disabilities: Although schools are frequently the first to report a learning disability, a preschool child with ADD often has already accumulated learning deficits before getting to school. Learning the alphabet and learning to read are two early school tasks which are particularly difficult. Printing and writing are other frequently mentioned school problems. Psychological evaluation frequently notes perceptual motor dysfunction showing itself in poor reproduction of designs.
4. Other important and frequent symptoms are impulsivity, emotional lability, and poor peer relationships. Parents often report unusual resistance to punishment. Physical punishment goes virtually unnoticed; as an extension of this concept, the children seem rather impervious to pain of any kind and tend to have frequent accidents. Such children may be relatively insensitive to both pleasure and pain so that either positive or negative reinforcers are poorly utilized.

5. Classical neurological signs are most often negative. Soft neurological signs are found in approximately 50% of ADD children.

DIAGNOSIS

1. A most important element in the diagnosis of ADD is a careful developmental history.
2. Observation of the child during his visit and behavioral reports from a teacher or other significant persons are helpful.
3. If the primary physician is familiar with the developmental soft signs frequently found in ADD children, a more formal referral to a child neurologist may not be necessary.
4. Psychological consultation may be helpful in supporting or not supporting a diagnosis of minimal brain dysfunction.
5. The responsiveness of the child to a trial of therapy with stimulant drugs is also thought to be diagnostic.

TREATMENT

1. Medication: The stimulant drugs which have a paradoxical effect are often the treatment of choice for the ADD syndrome. Methylphenidate (Ritalin) and the amphetamines, particularly d-amphetamine, have been the most effective. Phenobarbital is contraindicated. Failures of medication are frequently due to too little medication over too short a time period. A starting dosage of methylphenidate 5 mg po before breakfast and at lunch with gradual increases until therapeutic benefit or toxicity is reached is recommended. It is suggested that 20-100 mg/day of methylphenidate are the lower and upper limits of this medication.

   Anorexia and insomnia are side effects which tend to abate with continued administration. Recent studies suggest some growth curtailment may be another side effect. The literature reports between 40 and 70% effective responses to medication. The results are frequently very specific with activity level decreasing and attention span increasing to a marked degree. The change has been described by some as enhancing learning or growth-producing as opposed to simple abatement of symptoms.

2. Counselling: Counselling the family of a child with ADD has a specific goal of interrupting the negative cycle of parent-child relationships which have taken place. It is important that some specific successes for the parent and child be achieved rather than aiming to change the parents into the counsellor's image of a good parent. A change in the child's behavior with medication is frequently a strong assist toward positive interaction. Information about the child's deficits may relieve guilt and serve as a starting point for his special needs for consistency and environmental structure.

3. Education: The physician or consultants may need to assist parents and schools with decisions about the optimal place and method for his education based on the extent of learning disabilities, the child's age and amount of missed education, the resources available which may range from an innovative teacher in a normal classroom, to a special class for children of normal intelligence with ADD or to special tutoring. Clinics are available that are skilled in assessment and/or treatment of children with ADD.

4. Psychotherapy: Psychotherapy is a secondary treatment which may be helpful to children and/or parents in understanding their feelings about their many negative experiences. It is an ego-centered type of therapy and the encouragement of unlimited behavior is contraindicated for ADD children.

AUTISM

Infantile autism, also referred to as infantile psychosis, was first described in 1943. It is a collection of associated symptoms for which the etiology is unknown. It is seen four or five times more commonly in boys. The symptoms are:

1. Antisocial, aloof and nonresponsive to human contact
2. A strong need for sameness in the environment and obvious distress at change

3. Preoccupation with mechanical objects, e.g., spinning of tops or wheels on a toy car
4. Repetitive body movements such as rocking or wheeling
5. Noncommunicative, frequently no speech
6. No real eye contact and very inconsistent response to sound
7. Pushing away of physical contact
8. Self-preoccupied, excludes others

In retrospect, parents describe symptoms as beginning very early in life, e.g., "he did not like being held even as a small baby." Onset is seen by definition below 5 years of age, and is now more frequently recognized between 1 and 2 years of age. Motor behavior is generally well developed as may be some specific skills, particularly with such things as form boards or puzzles. Autistic children are often referred to as handsome or good-looking children.

TREATMENT

Traditional psychotherapy, behavior modification techniques and special educational techniques have been used separately and in combination for autistic children. The results of traditional psychotherapy have not been remarkable. Intensive educational input in specialized schools as well as at home is perhaps the most accepted treatment at the present time.

LEARNING DISABILITIES

DEFINITIONS

Learning disability is a general term which will be used to describe children who have adequate intelligence but are unable to achieve certain expected skills. It is most commonly brought to the physician's attention during the early school years, particularly from kindergarten through the third grade.

Skill deficiencies may be presented as an inability to master mathematic concepts, inability to read, difficulties in spelling, writing and speech, and perception.

What is sometimes referred to as SLD, specific learning disability or primary learning disability, has frequently been ascribed to irregular or delayed neurological development.

Some authors would assign it as a major type of minimal brain dysfunction while others feel that the evidence for brain dysfunction being a cause is weak. The concept of general maturational lag is another popular explanation.

SYMPTOMS

Some common symptoms of SLD are poorly developed laterality, disturbances of perception and memory (visual, auditory, or somatosensory), difficulty in integrating auditory and visual perception, defects in motor articulation (speech or graphic). Thus, such children frequently cannot distinguish similar letters or the alphabet, cannot reproduce shapes, etc.

Secondary learning disabilities can be related to emotional disturbance, or to poor opportunities for learning. A much larger incidence of secondary learning disabilities are related to socioeconomic class. Children living in economically deprived areas are likely to begin school behind their more fortunate classmates and by the seventh grade are at least 2 or more years retarded in reading.

DIAGNOSIS

Practical Points

1. Attention to performance on preschool developmental screening tests
2. Presence of soft neurological signs
3. Inadequate performance on a screening test such as the Wide Range Achievement Test for children 5 years or older
4. Careful attention to the child's developmental history and school history

If a disability is suspected, referral is indicated or a more detailed psychoeducational evaluation to pinpoint the patient's strengths and limitations and to give some prescriptions and guidelines for an educational program. Early identification is of great importance so that school failure does not result in serious secondary emotional problems.

REMEDIATIONS

1. Specialized methods of teaching reading and writing skills may be obtained either within the school system or from specialized clinics or tutors.
2. The use of stimulant drugs for SLD children is the subject of controversy. There are those who report significant improvement in such areas as the quality of handwriting but most clinicians feel that available data do not support claims of beneficial results and that drugs are contraindicated and may even be deleterious.
3. Counselling for the family regarding the nature of learning disabilities can be helpful; psychotherapy aimed at correcting learning disorders is ineffective.

FEARS

The emotions of fear and anxiety are present throughout life. The causes of fear, however, may vary as the child grows. Some fears are developmental, that is, are acquired simply by reaching a particular stage of development. Some common ones are fears of sudden and unexpected noises (infancy to 6 months), fear of separation and stranger anxiety (second half of the first year), fear of the dark ($2\frac{1}{2}$ years and up), fear of animals (3 years and up). A second kind of fear is a special fear acquired through a traumatic situation, imitation of a parent, or association with an unpleasant situation. Crying, regression, and withdrawal are common symptoms of fear. Guidance is aimed at reassurance to the parents of the normalcy and universality of childhood fears. Most fears can be resolved by slow incremental exposure to the feared situation with strong support from the parents.

SCHOOL PHOBIA

A special case of fear is found in children who are anxious and panicky about going to school and are said to be school phobic. It is a fairly common problem of childhood (reported incidence of 17 cases per 1000 school children each school year). It is more frequently seen in girls than in boys. Prognosis is negatively related to its duration so that prompt treatment is important.

The child's feelings of dread are frequently accompanied by such symptoms as nausea, vomiting, stomach pains, diarrhea, anorexia, or headache. The somatic symptoms disappear following the critical time of "going to school." Extreme resistance, screaming, and temper tantrums may be encountered when the child is pressed to get ready for and start to school. This may continue all the way into the classroom. On very rare occasions there may be an environmental cause such as a bullying gang, being a lone member of a minority group, or having an unacceptable teacher. One hypothesis is that school-phobic children may overvalue themselves and their achievements and when threatened with competitive peers, they withdraw to safer home territory. However, the most frequent and accepted explanation for school phobia is separation anxiety. Separation anxiety is a normal phenomenon but in its extreme form is related to an overly dependent relationship, usually between the mother and child. Both mother and child are too exclusively invested in the relationship with consequent feelings of resentment due to the restrictions and inconveniences to their own freedom. Maternal guilt over the resentment keeps the cycle going.

Treatment

1. Support the child's prompt return to school. The physician can reassure the parent that there are no serious medical problems and stress that the child's successful return to school is of far more importance for his or her well-being. Specific guidelines such as the child should not remain at home unless his temperature is above 100°F are often helpful.
2. A specific program for returning the child to school should be agreed upon with the parent and with appropriate school personnel.
3. If the program is not carried out promptly and the child is unable to return, referral to a child psychiatrist or child psychologist should be made. Good results have been obtained by mental health personnel with behavior modification and with the more traditional psychotherapeutic approaches.

Contributed by Nancy Paddock-Allen, Ph.D.
Clinical Psychologist
118 Mason Lane
North-East, Maryland

Chapter 20

THE ABUSED CHILD

The battered child syndrome represents the most severe form of child abuse. The syndrome lies at one end of a spectrum of insufficient care and protection. The battered child syndrome may be defined as a clinical condition in young children who have received significant physical abuse generally from a parent or guardian. Other forms of chief abuse differing from the battered child syndrome include repeated minor injuries, failure to thrive due to insufficient love or inadequate nutrition, sexual abuse, and emotional and social deprivation.

The incidence of reported cases of child abuse is quite constant throughout urban and rural America. Nearly 1 million cases of child abuse, sexual misuse, and neglect occur in the United States annually. The number of reported cases represents less than 30-35% of the actual number of afflicted children even though child abuse legislation exists in all 50 states. Studies have indicated that 10% of all trauma seen in children brought to emergency rooms is inflicted rather than accidental. Other studies suggest that 30% of all fractures seen in children under 2 years of age are inflicted.

Parents who physically abuse their children come from all walks of life and from all socioeconomic levels. While it

is beyond the scope of this book to discuss in depth the
psychopathology of abusive parents, several practical points
should be expressed.

Practical Points

1. Less than 10% of abusive parents are aggressive psycho-
   paths or delusional schizophrenics. The prognosis for the
   rehabilitation of these families is very poor.
2. Over 90% of abusive parents belong to a wide variety of
   personality types. The vast majority of these parents
   have in common the fact that they are severely deprived
   individuals who, in early infancy, had very little nurturing
   love from their own parents.
3. The parent or parents are isolated individuals who cannot
   trust or use others.
4. The parents have urealistic expectations of their children
   or themselves.
5. The ability to cope with stress is diminished in the individual and the families of abused children.
6. Given the above conditions, some form of crisis, minor or
   major, must occur in order to trigger off the abusive pattern.

Child abuse is most often diagnosed when the child is
found to have some suspicious injury. Another large group is
recognized because they fail to thrive during early infancy.
(See p. 402) An abused child is an emergency, if not medical
or surgical, then certainly one in which the child is urgently
in need of care and protection. Therefore, every suspected
case of child abuse must be admitted to a hospital. If not,
further battering and death may occur.

SEXUAL ABUSE

Sexual misuse is exposure of a child to sexual stimulation
inappropriate for the child's age, level of psychosocial development, and role in the family. This is the best definition
for the physician. It opens a wide variety of sexual activity
to the physician's judgment. This is not vague; on the contrary, it is a realistic appraisal of the subtleties of human

relations. Child pornography is any visual reproduction of the sexual abuse of children. These definitions encourage early therapeutic intervention when psychopathology is suggested by observed family dynamics.

THE MAGNITUDE OF SEXUAL MISUSE

Sexual misuse can be of an acute or chronic nature. It represents 9-14% of all forms of child abuse affecting 200-500 cases per 1 million population. Incest is seen in 1000 patients per 1 million population, and up to 90% of incest is unreported.

The majority of sexual abuse is between parent(s) and child. All socioeconomic groups are affected. The problem is more common in rural and suburban areas than in urban communities. People of all races, religions, ethnic groups, and education levels can be implicated.

Incest is often of a chronic nature when parent and child are involved. The nonparticipating spouse may be aware of the problem and facilitate the ongoing incestuous relationship having given up their sexual role.

An incestuous relationship most often involves a cooperative preadolescent. The socialization of the child at the onset of the deviant relationship disallows an understanding of the perverted nature of the acts. Likewise, rape may occur in any type of male-female relationship, including incest, and may be committed within the context of the family in an episodic or chronic manner. The absence of consent and the violent nature of this sexual act are additional elements to be dealt with. Coercion or force can be a complicating factor in chronic incestuous relationships as well, magnifying the problem.

THE VICTIM

Every report of incest or sexual misuse disclosed by a child or adolescent must be taken seriously. The patient's account must be evaluated with regard to the age of the child, sexualized family interactions, nature of the act, and the quality of the report.

A preschool child who describes sexual activity accurately is unlikely to be fabricating the story. The history should be elicited, not led by the physician. As age increases, the question of truthfulness is more difficult to assess. In the adolescent, fabrication about sexual abuse is more likely.

The child's age markedly influences the presentation of sexual misuse. Infants demonstrate reddened or traumatized genitalia or more generalized symptoms such as sleep disturbances, altered activity level, or poor feeding. Toddlers and school-aged children present with dysuria, stomach ache, or insomnia and are reluctant to verbalize the cause of their complaints. The physical findings of genital laceration, abrasion, or penile or vaginal discharge in a child of any age should make the examiner consider sexual misuse. The history may be insufficient to explain the physical examination, and signs of physical abuse can be absent in the sexually misused child.

Observation of the victim offers clues through specific behavioral characteristics. Extreme shyness and withdrawal or age-inappropriate seductiveness and pseudomaturity suggest sexual misuse. The examiner may easily assume the attitude of seeing the patient in the role of the victim-perpetrator. This concept suggests an active role on the part of the patient. This erroneous characterization of the patient is destructive to proper objective assessment of patient needs and appropriate intervention by the physician. For example, the seductive child may be at greater risk for abuse because of this attribute and should be appropriately protected rather than seen as a willing contributor to the abusing behavior. Seductive behavior may be learned in order to obtain nurturance.

The patient can be an accidental or participating victim. Accidental victims have been molested by a stranger or near stranger in a single forcible encounter, usually with an associated threat of violence. Participating victims are involved in a sexual relationship with a family member over a period of time, ranging from weeks to years.

THE FAMILY

Marital discord is the most common cause of emotional disorders in children, including incestuous relationships. Dysfunctional families are illustrated by three family settings: infrafamilial, chaotic lifestyle, or isolated.

The infrafamilial family pathology remains hidden; however, the family is dysfunctional. The wife is unavailable through illness or work, and the spouses are sexually estranged. An agreement, conscious or unconscious, exists between family members supporting an incestuous relationship. This is preferred to a breakup of the family. In these families, the mother gives up her role to the daughter.

The chaotic lifestyle, multiple-problems family, is well known to support agencies. Multiple social problems are chronic, and the father forms poor interpersonal relationships, viewing all women as sex objects.

In isolated incest, the accidental victim is molested but does not actively encourage the relationship.

DIAGNOSIS AND MANAGEMENT

Diagnosis requires a high index of suspicion and an investment in one's patients that is evident to the patient. Good physician-patient rapport facilitates communication and provides the basis for sound medical care.

The physician caring for a victim of sexual misuse must be prepared to diagnose and treat physical and psychic trauma, sexually transmitted infections, and pregnancy. Should the patient present within 72 hours of the sexual activity, the physician is obliged to collect appropriate medicolegal specimens. The welfare of the patient is always primary; gathering legal documentary evidence is secondary.

The history is obtained in a confidential manner on an individual basis. Sexual behavior is investigated in the context of the standard medical history. If a history of sexual misuse is elicited, further details should be explored with parents and child separately. The necessity to protect the child from future mishandling must be communicated to the parents.

A general physical examination documenting all abnormalities is indicated in all cases. All details should be carefully charted and positive findings as well as significant negatives stated. Special attention ought to be given to the gynecologic examination, breasts, and oral and anal areas for evidence of trauma and infection. Sexual maturity should be assessed using the Tanner maturity rating scale.

Trauma, genital and nongenital, is more frequent with assaults by strangers. Physical findings vary with age. Younger children are usually the victims of fondling alone and have normal physical examinations. Older children are more likely to experience intercourse and, therefore, show signs of penetration.

Separating the labia while depressing the perineum downward allows visualization into the vagina if the hymenal opening is large enough. If this is not possible, vaginoscopy is indicated. Patience and gentleness on the part of the examiner are mandatory. A Hoffman speculum, a veterinary otoscope speculum, laryngoscope, or a Killian nasal speculum may be utilized to see the cervix. An appropriate-size vaginal speculum or otoscopic speculum is adequate for skillful examination.

Cultures for gonorrhea should be routinely taken from the throat, vagina, and rectum in girls. A boy's throat, urethra, and rectum should be cultured. Serologic testing for syphilis is best done on all patients at the time of presentation. Further investigation for infectious disease may then be directed by the physical findings. Future serology and microscopic testing for hepatitis, monilia, chlamydia, trichomoniasis, and syphilis is indicated as individual patient needs dictate. A urinalysis should be obtained, and a pregnancy test should be done if the patient is fertile.

Evidence of sperm must be sought. Sperm or acid phosphatase may be present supporting the patient's history. The absence of semen does not exclude intercourse or sexual assault. Seminal fluid may not be found because of delayed or inadequate collection of specimens, an assailant's ejaculatory incompetence, or douching.

The judicial process requires proof of the assault. Appropriate collection, tagging, and storage of samples, including items such as fingernail scrapings and other evidence, should follow legal protocol. Consultation by or referral to a sexual assault team answers this need in many communities.

The decision to treat at home or to hospitalize the patient must be made on an individual basis. Regardless of choice, privacy and the protection of the patients must be high priorities. After laboratory studies are completed, appropriate antimicrobial therapy should be administered to prevent sexually transmitted diseases.

To prevent pregnancy (Ovral) 2 tablets po every 12 hours administered twice is prescribed at this time, replacing the use of diethylstilbestrol (DES).

Follow-up care can be best managed through a multi-disciplinary team which may include police, courts, and child protective services, as well as physicians and psychologists.

The prognosis for the sexually misused child is ill-defined. Unfortunately, the literature suggests a high correlation with prostitution and psychiatric disorders in later life.

Practical Points

1. The diagnosis of child abuse must be considered in every young child seen because of traumatic injury, particularly if the child is less than one year old.
2. X-rays of the long bones should be carefully reviewed for evidence of recent or past trauma.
3. Be suspicious of child abuse in infants who show evidence of overall poor care.
4. Young children with unexplained dehydration and/or malnutrition should be carefully evaluated for possible abuse.
5. Evidence of repeated skin injury should alert the physician to further evaluation.
6. In injury cases in which an unusual delay has taken place before the child is brought for medical care, child abuse should be considered.
7. Child abuse should be considered in children who are unusually fearful.
8. Consider the diagnosis of child abuse when one or both parents:
   a) Shows loss of self-control or inability to cope with the situation at hand
   b) Presents a bizarre or contradictory history
   c) Shows a lack of concern for the child
   d) Gives evidence of misusing alcohol or drugs
   e) Refuses consent for further diagnostic studies and/or hospitalization
   f) Has unrealistic expectations of the child or of themselves
9. The physician should include, in his anticipatory guidance, information regarding parental stress points and suggestions for coping. The doctor should be alert to verbal and

nonverbal hints asking for parental support and must assume a posture of openness to intervene effectively in a chain of events potentially lending to an abusive situation.

Ask the parent(s):

1. Is your child a difficult baby for you or your spouse to care for?
2. Do you find youself angry at the baby? How often? What do you do when you have these feelings?
3. Does your husband help you? Who does help you if he does not? Who else is available to assist you in his absence?
4. Would you like help? What kind of help? What did you expect parenting to be like? How is it the same or different?

Most often, a careful inquiry demonstrates a need for information and/or support. Appropriate help can be offered through community resources such as a women's support group. Occasionally the pediatrician may need to counsel and educate the father as to the need for a supportive role. In the absence of extended family, much of the education in parenting offered through grandparents must come from the physician's office.

In most cases, it is not difficult to make the correct diagnosis when the child presents with severe injuries. However, the physician, nurse, or social worker, by keeping in mind the above points may pick up earlier and milder cases of abuse, thus preventing future and more serious injury by instituting proper protection for the child, and appropriate management of the family.

TREATMENT OF THE PHYSICALLY ABUSED CHILD AND HIS FAMILY

1. Early or Emergency Care
   a) As mentioned above, all children in whom the diagnosis of child abuse is entertained must be admitted to a hospital for diagnostic workup, protection, and indicated medical or surgical treatment.

b) The parent or parents should not be accused or confronted with the possibility that their child has been physically abused while they are still in the emergency room .

c) At the earliest possible moment, the child and his family should be seen by a pediatrician and a social worker familiar with the complexities of dealing with the physically abused child.

d) As soon as the diagnosis is established, it must be reported to the appropriate agency designated in the community involved.

2. Therapeutic Program for Families of Abused Children
   a) The reporting mechanism should set into motion the Child Protective Services to insure the safety of the child and to initiate rehabilitation of the family (with adequate resources, this can be done in the vast majority of the cases).
   b) Accurate diagnosis of the family psychodynamics must be made while the child is in the hospital or safely out of the home in order to institute appropriate treatment and follow-up care.

3. Innovative family therapeutic services are having dramatic results where available. The newly established National Center for the Prevention of Child Abuse and Neglect in Denver, Colorado, is an outstanding example of multidisciplinary, comprehensive approach to rehabilitation. Services include:
   a) Lay therapists
   b) Families Anonymous
   c) A Crisis Nursery (drop-off service, no questions asked, 24 hr/day, 7 days/week)
   d) A therapeutic day care center

Chapter 21

ADOLESCENT MEDICINE

Adolescent medicine (ephebiatrics) is a recognized inter-
disciplinary health care specialty. The medical care of the
adolescent is directed towards the psychosocial and developmental needs of the patient as well as his physical well-
being. The attainment of each person's full potential is the
responsibility and goal of ephebiatrics. Adolescent medicine
is primarily a specific approach to a challenging age group.
Its practice requires the physician to hear what is not said
and become adept at deciphering the underlying cause for
a complaint.

Practical Points

1. Puberty is a physiologic process through which growth
   occurs and reproductive capability is acquired.
2. Adolescence is a psychosocial process and a transition
   period between childhood and maturity.
3. There are marked cultural differences in the way young
   women and men attain maturity. These differences also
   affect the duration of adolescence.
4. The physician/patient relationship is affected to a great
   degree by individual cultural traits.
5. The patient must be recognized as the unique individual
   he is and will become.

THE MEDICAL HISTORY

The history should be obtained in a conversational manner. Empathy and a trustworthy, understanding attitude must be conveyed to the patient. This is particularly true in evaluating the areas of drugs, alcohol, and sex.

Physician personalities vary, and interviewing styles will reflect these differences. Try to permit the adolescent an opportunity to develop his or her own story. Once a topic is touched upon, appropriate inquiry is made. Should further information be desirable and the patient is not volunteering information, let the item drop and return to it later. This is easily done as related areas of discussion arise or as bodily systems are examined.

The adolescent is forming an opinion of the practitioner as quickly as the physician is assessing the patient's needs. Teenagers are remarkably perceptive and easily grasp role-playing or deception. A physician who is at ease with himself as a person is best able to care for the adolescent patient.

In conducting the patient interview and examination, there are several "B" rules:

Be yourself
Be honest
Be nonjudgmental
Be considerate and sympathetic
Be private
Be comprehensive

CONFIDENTIALITY

Should private matters require parental knowledge, physician support of the adolescent as he informs his parent is a wise approach.

Confidentiality and consent policies must address the unique development status of the adolescent. These young people are increasingly capable of exercising rational choice and informed consent, which demands flexible guidance and support by parents and/or other adults. The law is beginning to recognize that maturity is differentially acquired and that the parent-child relationship exists largely for the protection of the child. Thus, the parent can establish codes of conduct and speak for the child. The traditionally emancipated youth can consent for himself when he is 16 years of age or older, away from home with parental permission, and self-supporting. The doctrine of the mature minor recognizes adult rights, privileges, and responsibilities in those residing at home in advance of the age of maturity. An absence of liability for the physician in treating adolescents on their own consent is gaining greater legal acceptance. In 1973, the American Academy of Pediatrics adopted the Model Act which provided for the consent of minors for health services. The Model Act accepts the concept that receiving health services is a basic right which promotes family harmony and a minor's maturity. Statutes are subject to change and legal precedents dictate court judgments requiring, therefore, that the physician keep abreast of these changes in his own locality.

PHYSICAL EXAMINATION

Physical examination of the adolescent should be done in an informal, relaxed, unhurried manner. Patient and physician needs for modesty and trust differ and must be met on an individual basis. Appropriate privacy should always be available.

The adolescent requires a yearly comprehensive physical examination, which should include the Tanner staging of sexual development (Figure 21-1). The examination of all organ systems must be in detail, emphasizing growth and development. Normal and abnormal physical findings of all systems including the skin, neuroendocrine, musculoskeletal, and reproductive organs should be recorded.

Reproductive growth must be recorded according to acceptable maturity charts because skeletal growth parameters are no longer helpful in adolescents. To define an adolescent stage precisely may require laboratory support with an alkaline phosphatase determination. Active skeletal growth in Tanner stage 3 adolescence will result in an elevated serum alkaline phosphatase which will drop as the growth rate lessens in stages 4 and 5. In the male, the serial complete blood count (CBC) should show a high hemoglobin

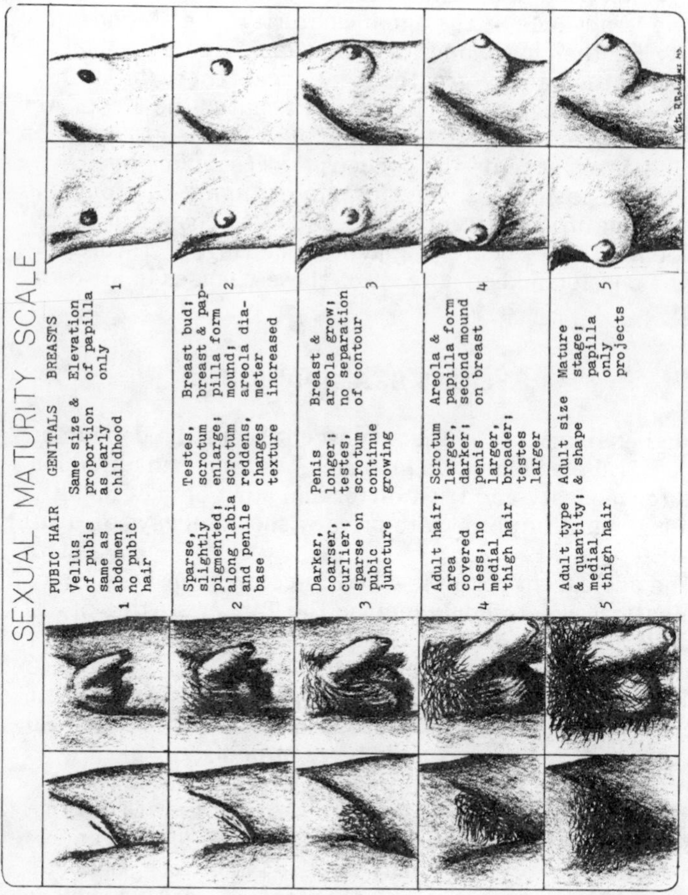

SEXUAL MATURITY SCALE

	PUBIC HAIR	GENITALS	BREASTS
1	Vellus of pubis same as abdomen; no pubic hair	Same size & proportion as early childhood	Elevation of papilla only
2	Sparse, slightly pigmented; along labia and penile base	Testes, scrotum enlarge; scrotum reddens, changes texture	Breast bud; breast & papilla form mound; areola diameter increased
3	Darker, coarser, curlier; sparse on pubic juncture	Penis, longer; testes; scrotum continue growing	Breast & areola grow; no separation of contour
4	Adult hair; area covered less; no medial thigh hair	Scrotum larger, darker; penis larger, broader; testes larger	Areola & papilla form second mound on breast
5	Adult type & quantity; medial thigh hair	Adult size & shape	Mature stage; papilla only projects

Figure 21-1

secondary to rising testosterone levels. A normal value suggests iron deficiency. A female should also have a yearly CBC because of growth, dietary demands, and menstruation.

Adolescence is an appropriate time to screen for predictors of adult disease such as hyperlipidemia and thyroid disorders. Adolescent goiter is a commonplace example. Many of the chronic disorders of adult life can be approached at this time to foster continued sound health habits and prevent illness in later years.

ATHLETICS

The adolescent athlete, when presenting himself or herself for a preparticipation sports examination, requires special attention. The examiner must be aware of the particular hazards of a sport to either sex as well as its physical conditioning requirements. The psychosocial demands must also be weighed. The medical permission to participate in athletics or its denial must be based on valid considerations.

PSYCHOLOGY OF ADOLESCENCE

Adolescents must master four developmental tasks. They must separate from their parents, develop peer relationships outside their family, establish and define their own identity, and decide appropriate hopes and goals for their future.

These tasks are not necessarily approached in chronological sequence. However, the individual must succeed to some degree with self-identity and human relationships to progress further and choose appropriate career goals. Therefore, there is a priority in the importance of each task, with self-identity as paramount.

Adolescent development is divided into three stages: early, middle, and late adolescence. During early adolescence, intense physiologic change occurs. The young adolescent is then most comfortable with peers of the same sex while separating from the parent of identical sex. The question of identity, "Who am I?" is all encompassing at this stage.

In middle adolescence, very strong peer relationships replace forsaken parental ties. Heterosexual relationships form and dating begins. Autonomy is a universal goal of this age group; therefore, adult relationships are strained while they are redefined.

Physiologic growth is completed for the male and female during late adolescence. At this point, a stability is gained with regard to self, and career plans assume a proportionately greater importance. The ability to make commitments and form lasting relationships outside the family is acquired.

The emerging adult continues to require the support and guidance the family and parents can provide. The physician is in a unique position to encourage parenting to support teenage maturation.

The parents should be instructed, as needed, in adolescent development to permit them to better understand their children. Although an adolescent may appear to be an adult, the teenager is limited in his ability to function psychosocially. Parental roles are redefined but are no less essential to the well-being of the adolescent.

Assistance in this parental process is well rewarded in the growth in responsibility on the part of the adolescent. Transient adjustment reactions, acting-out behavior, school problems, acute and chronic disease are all managed more efficiently when parents continue to be invested in their young. Antisocial behavior frequently is a cry for parental attention.

Practical Points

1. Provide time for counselling when scheduling appointments for adolescents.
2. Patient and parents should be seen together as well as separately to adequately assess and address their needs.

PHYSIOLOGY OF ADOLESCENCE

Puberty occurs when the adolescent undergoes the physiologic changes inherent in the ability to reproduce. In North America, the first signs of sexual development begin at age eight in the female and age nine in the male. A reproductive capability is then achieved as the individual approaches an adult stature. Each individual has a unique growth pattern based on the interaction of their genetic sex and its lifelong modification by hormonal and environmental factors. The dynamic interaction of the genetic constitution, the nervous system, and organs and humoral factors influence growth and development and determine biologic sex. The genetic sex (female XX or male XY) is fixed at conception and is transmitted unchanged to all cells of the conception. Thus, the patient's pattern of pubescence is a function of the same-gender parent's stature (mother-daughter or father-son) and the usual age of pubarche in the family for each sex.

Sex-specific characteristics are associated with adolescent maturation of the reproductive system. The male demonstrates a greater height, blood pressure, pulse, hemoglobin, and alkaline phosphotase value than the female. At an earlier age, the female undergoes a growth spurt, and possesses an advanced bone age, more adipose tissue, higher basal body temperature, and earlier psychosocial maturity.

These physiologic processes and the bodily changes affected by them are controlled by the long and short feedback loops of the hypothalamic-pituitary-adrenal-gonadal axis. The hypothalamic-pituitary-adrenal-gonadal axis is active in utero promoting sex-specific organogenesis. In childhood, this axis continues to function for proper growth and development. As the child ages, changing sensitivity of the long and short feedback loops of the axis increases. In the prepubertal child, this axis matures and regulates growth and development of the reproductive system. In adolescence, this axis becomes completely functional as a feedback loop. In the adult, this same neuroendocrine axis ensures homeostasis and full reproductive capability.

Practical Points

1. The average age of menarche is 12.5 years in North America.
2. Menarchal age is occurring earlier at a rate of 3 months per decade over the last century. This is possibly due to an increasingly improved diet.
3. The finding of Tanner stage II development in males before age 11 or age 9 years in the female merits evaluation (look for genetic or acquired endocrine causes).

4. An adolescent girl age 13.5 years or a boy age 15.5 years, who is still Tanner stage I, requires evaluation (bone age and skull films and further studies as indicated).
5. The woman should reach menarche within five years of Tanner stage II breast development.
6. The male should reach stage V genitalia size from stage II within 5 years.
7. Once menarche occurs, the average girl grows 2.5 inches taller.
8. Peak height velocity (PHV) occurs at age 14 in males at stage IV development and averages 10.3 cm/year.
9. Peak height velocity (PHV) occurs at age 12 in females at stage III development and averages 8.4 cm/year.
10. The lymphatic system including the thymus, adenoid-tonsillar tissue, spleen, intestine, appendix, and mesenteric lymph nodes is the only organ system whose growth decelerates during adolescence.

SOMATIC VALUES IN ADOLESCENT MEDICINE

Average Size of Testes in Adolescence

Age	Length and Width (cm)
10	1.8 x 1.1
11	2.0 x 1.4
12	2.3 x 1.8
13	3.0 x 2.3
14	3.4 x 2.5
15	3.6 x 2.6
16	3.8 x 2.7
17	4.0 x 2.8

Average Size of Penis in Adolescence (measured with gentle traction)

Age	Length (cm)	Circumference (cm)
10	6.2	4.5
11	6.5	4.7
12	7.1	5.0

Age	Length (cm)	Circumference (cm)
13	8.7	5.7
14	9.7	6.8
15	11.8	7.6
16	12.5	7.9
17	13.2	8.4

Blood Pressure mmHg (right arm, seated). Age range: 10–15 years

	Female	Male
Systolic	90 – 140 ± 5	88 – 140 ± 5
Diastolic	55 – 90 + 5	55 – 90 ± 5

For blood pressures of 140–160/90–95, serial measurements are needed to define the level accurately. Blood pressures of 160/95 are in the abnormal range.

Practical Points

The patient is much more at ease at the end of the physical examination; the blood pressure may be measured more accurately at that time.

SELECTED LABORATORY VALUES IN THE ADOLESCENT

	Female over 11 years	Male over 11 years
Hemoglobin	11–15 g%	12–16 g%
Average	12.4 g%	12.4 g%
Hematocrit	39–40%	41–43%
Average	40%	42%

Practical Points

1. Anemia in the adolescent female is represented by a hemoglobin of less than 11.5 g. Anemia in the adolescent male is represented by a hemoglobin of less than 13.0 g.

2. A CBC, routine and microscopic urinalysis, and tuberculin testing are probably best obtained yearly in the teenager.
3. A fasting chemistry profile should be performed in early adolescence and, therafter, as indicated, to screen for early manifestations of adult disease, i.e., hypertension or cardiovascular risk factors.

Chapter 22

A PRACTICAL GUIDE TO THE MANAGEMENT
OF DRUG ABUSE

Pediatricians and other health personnel dealing with children and adolescents must be prepared to deal with the drug abuse problem. Certainly, many of the complex aspects of drug abuse by children and young people today are not medical but are sociologic, psychologic, and environmental in nature. Yet the knowledgeable physician often can be an important contributor to the control and prevention of this serious problem. The adverse reactions related to drug abuse are medical in nature and frequently mimic other pathological conditions.

While volumes of information are available concerning drug abuse, it is hard to find a readily available, concise and practical guide for the management of the medical aspects. This brief guide is therefore presented as an attempt to meet this need.

Practical Points

1. Marijuana (Indian hemp, *Cannabis sativa*) — is referred to in street language as "grass," "pot," "tea," or "Mary Jane." The active ingredient is tetrahydrocannabinol (THC) which is a hallucinogen with a sedative effect. Although a few

451

toxic reactions have been reported, the use of **marijuana** does not lead to medical emergencies. A user will often have redness of the conjunctivae but the pupils remain normal or dilated. The patient may be euphoric and is occasionally disoriented as to time and space. Hashish ("hash") is a concentrated form (five times) which produces similar but more severe symptoms than simple marijuana use.

If a child or adolescent is brought to an emergency ward in connection with marijuana, the health personnel must be alert for related problems such as contaminants, other drugs, emotional problems, or other illnesses.

2. Hallucinogens
   a) Phencyclidine (PCP) (Angel Dust) — Originally developed as an anesthetic but now most commonly used as a psychedelic on the street, it is a white powder or colorless solution and may come as tablets. Smoked, inhaled, swallowed, or injected it causes disorganization, stimulation, agressiveness, euphoria, hallucinations, and delusions. Overdose may lead to severe hypertensive states with possible cerebrovascular accidents, miosis, ataxia, drooling, seizures, and respiratory arrest. The schizophrenic-like state it produces on occasion can last for months and can recur even without subsequent use of the drug. It is possible to confirm a suspicion of PCP use by detecting it in urine and blood samples. Many labs can now perform the analysis. The miosis helps distinguish PCP toxicity from that caused by other common hallucinogens (LSD) where midriasis is found.

   Treatment consists of restraint in a quiet room and sedation. Acidification of the urine with 1 or 2% ammonium chloride IV or instilled in the stomach sufficient to lower the pH to 5, together with lasix to induce diuresis, is helpful for overdoses. Diazoxide may be necessary to control hypertension and dilantin may be needed for seizure activity. Intubation is required if there is laryngospasm. Long-term therapy in chronic abusers is difficult. Residential treatment should be considered.
   b) LSD ("Acid") — LSD is a synthetic ergotamine with hallucinogenic properties. The psychedelic experience may last 4-12 hours. Symptoms include an initial

excitement phase followed by depression, headache, mydriasis, tachycardia, nausea, and vomiting. The toxic reaction is referred to as a "bad trip." (See below.)

c) There are a number of other hallucinogens available including DMT, STP (or DOM), mescaline (peyote), psilocybin, morning-glory seeds, and others. They vary in severity and duration of reaction, and toxic effects.

d) "Bad Trips" — For poorly understood reasons, some psychedelic experiences turn out to be harrowing ordeals. If possible, bad trips should be handled by "talking down" the tripper. The use of other drugs should be avoided. Phenothiazines react adversely with anticholinergic contaminants such as atropine and can be dangerous unless one is sure of the nature of the drug taken.

e) The chance that a street drug, regardless of its name, is free of contaminants is very slight. Thus a major problem in treating acute toxic reactions is the identification of the chemical contents of an ingested drug. In a drug related emergency, the physician must be alert to chemical toxicity of any sort. Some of the more common contaminants include atropine, scopolamine, phencyclidine, and strychnine.

3. Amphetamines: Benzedrine ("bennies"), Dexedrine ("dexies"), methedrine-IV ("speed"), "Pep pills," "Ups" — The use of amphetamines varies from the ingestion of small amounts to long periods of ever-increasing dosage using the intravenous route. Signs and symptoms of use of these drugs include excitement, loss of appetite, severe malnutrition, nervousness, dry mouth, hypertension, and tachycardia, mydriasis, and diaphoresis. Acute paranoid psychotic reactions may occur. Hepatitis and septicemia secondary to dirty needles are not infrequent. Treatment of a user includes "talking down," occasional use of Valium (5-10 mg), and appropriate guidance and rehabilitation.

4. Barbiturates ("goof balls," "downs") — In the therapeutic doses, barbiturates depress the actions of nervous tissue, skeletal muscle, and heart muscle. These effects are potentiated by alcohol ingestion. Barbiturates are physically addictive and the chronic user develops extreme tolerance to these drugs.

An overdose of barbiturates causes CNS depression, slow respiratory and heart rates, hypotension, hypoxia, and coma. Pupils are constricted but will react to a bright light. Treatment of overdose includes oxygen and/or assisted breathing, intravenous hydration (for children 3000-4500 ml/m^2 of 5% dextrose in $\frac{1}{4}$ N saline), and alkalinization of the urine. Peritoneal dialysis and hemodialysis have been effective in the management of severe barbiturate poisoning.

Withdrawal from chronically high doses is very dangerous, and must be done in the hospital under closely controlled conditions. Replacement with short-acting barbiturates followed by gradual withdrawal has been the treatment of choice. In the past several years a newer method based on phenobarbital replacement has proven to be very successful.

5. Sniffing — Inhaling one of a variety of solvents is a frequently used method of "getting high," particularly among children. The inhalants used include glue, nail polish, naphtha and carbon tetrachloride (lighter and cleaning fluids), kerosene and gasoline, paint thinners, and deodorant sprays. These agents produce a state similar to alcohol ingestion. Transient euphoria, followed by dullness, loss of coordination and awareness and sleep are common symptoms. When seen in the emergency room the sniffer may demonstrate panic, stupor, or hallucinations. The odors of the inhalant are generally apparent. Management is symptomatic and supportive. Panic may need to be controlled by administration of tranquilizers (thorazine, 1 mg/kg IM).

The chronic use of inhalants can produce liver, kidney, lung, and bone marrow damage. These conditions must be screened for in known cases.

6. Cocaine — "Coke" has a reaction similar to the amphetamines. It has a rapid onset of effect and a short duration of action (15-30 minutes). It may be ingested, inhaled, or injected. The effect of cocaine is to produce an extremely pleasurable state of euphoria. It may cause delusions of grandeur and pleasant hallucinations.

An overdose of cocaine constitutes a medical emergency. The patient is excited and confused. Hyperreflexia, tachycardia, irregular respirations, and mydriasis are

common. Often a chill will be followed by marked hyper-
pyrexia, a very characteristic sign of cocaine overdose.
Terminally, convulsions, coma, and respiratory arrest occur.

Therapy must be rapid and includes lowering of fever,
providing adequate ventilation, and the use of short-acting barbiturates to counteract CNS irritability.

7. Narcotics — While morphine, meperidine, codeine, and
   dilaudid are abused (most often by professionals) the epidemic of narcotic addiction so prevalent in this country
   and throughout the world involves heroin. Street heroin
   ("dope," "H," "horse," "scag," "stuff") is sniffed ("snort-
   ing"), injected subcutaneously ("skin popping"), or taken
   intravenously ("mainlining").

   Signs of heroin usage include drowsiness (nodding),
   anorexia, nausea, urinary retention, decreased sex drive,
   pinpoint pupils, bradycardia and a decreased respiratory
   rate. Needle marks may be apparent but are often well
   hidden.

   If a person becomes addicted to heroin he becomes
   tolerant to the drug and requires ever-increasing amounts.
   Soon his only goal is to get enough heroin for a "fix" every
   4 hours. He must then adopt the lifestyle of the "junkie"
   which in itself is a serious and difficult to reverse social
   state.

   A heroin overdose ("OD") occurs when a person (not
   necessarily an addict) takes more heroin that he can
   tolerate. Generally, this is the result of a larger amount
   of heroin being present in a street "bag." This may be 10
   to 15 times the amount expected. When an "OD" arrives
   at the emergency room he will have pinpoint pupils unless
   hypoxia has produced dilatation. He will have decreased
   respirations, areflexia, and will be cold, pallid, stuporose
   or comatose. Immediate supportive care must be instituted including providing a clean, open airway (endotracheal tube may be necessary) and cardiac massage if
   indicated. Specific therapy consists of Narcan, Nalline,
   or Lorfan. (Also see Chapter 23, p. 496) These medications must be given intravenously in the following dosages:

   a) Narcan or Naloxone (drug of choice because it does
       not cause respiratory depression like other narcotic
       anatagonists).

0.01 mg/kg for children
0.4 mg/dose for adults
May be repeated in 3 minutes.

b) Doses for newborn depressed by maternal narcosis
(1) Nalline
5-10 mg IV to mother
0.1-0.2 mg IV to baby
(0.2 mg/ml is pediatric concentration)
(2) Lorfan
1-2 mg IV to mother
0.005-0.1 mg IV to baby

Withdrawal of heroin from an addict is a complex and difficult procedure. Expertise is of greatest importance. A description of the long-term management of the "junkie" is beyond the scope of this book.

The passively addicted newborn infant of a narcotic addict mother is described in the Newborn section. (See p. 32.)

8. Methadone Poisoning — The average daily dose of methadone given to a narcotic addict on a maintenance program is 60-120 mg. This produces no adverse effects in a tolerant patient but if taken by a child under 6 years of age may cause death within one-half to 3 hours. Emergency treatment is the same as with heroin overdose (see p. 496). The narcotic antagonists may be repeated in 5 and 10 minutes if respirations are improved. If no improvement, the diagnosis should be questioned.

Since the effect of methadone intoxications may last 48 hours and the effect of the antagonists only 2-3 hours, repeated intramuscular doses (50% greater than IV doses) should be given if respiratory function deteriorates. The prolonged CNS depression of methadone and similar products can effect sudden changes in a patient's status. The patient can be speaking to you and lapse into unconsciousness without warning. ICU observation is mandatory. Intravenous infusion of 5% dextrose in $\frac{1}{4}$ N saline should be given continuously to provide adequate hydration and a readily available route for IV medications. Gastric lavage should be used only if the patient is alert. Dialysis and CNS stimulation are contraindicated.

9. Abuse of Multiple Drugs — A mixture of street drugs can be consumed to produce a desired hypnotic effect. Heroin users and non-IV drug abusers appear to consume "hits" consisting of po codeine and glutethimide with increasing frequency. The effect of these two CNS suppressants is addicting and can be lethal. See Table 22-1.

Table 22-1   Tips for the Identification of Drug Abusers

Drugs Used	Physical Symptoms	Look For	Dangers
Glue sniffing	Violence, drunk appearance, dreamy or blank expression	Tubes of glue, glue smears, large paper bags, or handkerchiefs	Lung/brain/liver damage, death through suffocation or choking, anemia
Heroin, morphine, codeine	Stupor, drowsiness, needle marks on body, watery eyes, loss of appetite, blood stain on shirt sleeve, runny nose	Needle or hypodermic syringe, cotton, tourniquet-string, rope, belt, burnt bottle caps or spoons, glassine envelopes	Death from overdose, addiction, liver and other infections due to unsterile needles
Cough medicine containing codeine and opium	Drunk appearance, lack of coordination, confusion, excessive itching	Empty bottle of cough medicine	Addiction

Marijuana ("pot," "grass")	Sleepiness, wandering mind, enlarged pupils, lack of coordination, craving for sweets, increased appetite	Strong odor of burnt leaves, small seeds in pocket lining, cigarette paper, discolored fingers	Inducement to take stronger narcotics. Psychological dependence. Possible physical damage?
Hallucinogens: (LSD, DMT)	Severe hallucinations, feelings of detachment, incoherent speech, cold hands and feet, vomiting, laughing and crying	Cube sugar with discoloration in center, strong body odor, small tube of liquid	Suicidal tendencies, unpredictable behavior, chronic exposure causes brain damage
Stimulants: amphetamines ("pep pills," "ups")	Aggressive behavior, giggling, silliness, rapid speech, confused thinking, no appetite, extreme fatigue, dry mouth, shakiness, insomnia	Pills or capsules of varying colors, chain smoking	Death from overdose, hallucinations, psychosis

Table 22-1 (Cont'd.) Tips for the Identification of Drug Abusers

Drugs Used	Physical Symptoms	Look For	Dangers
Sedatives, barbiturates ("goof balls," "downs")	Drowsiness, stupor, dullness, slurred speech, drunk appearance, vomiting	Pills or capsules of varying colors	Death or unconsciousness from overdose, addiction, convulsions in withdrawal

From NY State Med J: 946, Apr. 15, 1973. (Reproduced by permission of Medical Society of the State of New York.)

Chapter 23

COMMON PEDIATRIC MEDICATIONS

COUGH MEDICATIONS

DEXTROMETHORPHAN

Brand Name: In various combination drugs: Dorcol, Robitussin DM, Triaminicol, Triaminic-DM

    Action: Nonnarcotic cough suppressant
    Strength: Varies from 7.5 mg to 15 mg/5 ml
    Dose of 7.5 mg strength (adjust according to strength
       of preparation): 2-4 years: ¼ tsp q 6-8 hr; 4-12
       years: ½-1 tsp q 6-8 hr; More than 12 years: 1 tsp
       q 6-8 hr
How supplied: 4 oz, 8 oz, 1 pt, 1 gal

GUAIFENESIN
Formerly Glyceryl Guaiacolate

Brand Name: Robitussin, Glycotuss, Hytuss

    Action: Expectorant
    Strength: Tablets: 100 mg; Liquid: 100 mg/5 ml

461

Dose: 1-2 years: 10-15 gtts tid; 2-4 years: $\frac{1}{4}$-$\frac{1}{2}$ tsp
    qid; More than 12 years: 1 tsp qid
How supplied: 2 oz, 4 oz, 1 pt, and 1 gal

POTASSIUM IODIDE

Action: Expectorant
Strength: Saturated solution contains 1 g/ml
Dose: 1 drop per year of age repeated every 8 hr in
    8 oz of juice or milk

ANTIHISTAMINES

CHLORPHENIRAMINE MALEATE

Brand Name: Chlortrimeton, Teldrin

Action: Antihistamine
Strength: Tablets: 4 mg, 8 mg, 12 mg; Syrup: 2
    mg/5 ml; Injection: 10 mg/ml and 100 mg/ml
Dose: 0.35 mg/kg/24 hr divided into 3 or 4 doses
How supplied: Syrup: 1 pt, 1 gal; Injection: 1 ml
    ampules

DIPHENHYDRAMINE

Brand Name: Benadryl

Action: Antihistamine, sedative, antipruritic
Strength: Liquid: 12.5 mg/5 ml; Capsules: 25 mg
    or 50 mg; Ampules: 50 mg; Vials: 10 mg/ml in
    10 ml and 30 ml vials
Dose: 5 mg/kg/24 hr, po, IM or IV in 3 divided
    doses
How supplied: Liquid: 1 pt

PROMETHAZINE

Brand Name: Phenergan, Phenergan Expectorant with or
without Codeine

Action: Antihistamine, sedative, antimotion
    sickness

Strength: Tablets: 12.5 mg; Liquid: 6.25 mg/5 ml;
    Suppository: 25 mg and 50 mg; Vials: 25 mg/
    ml for IM or IV
Dose: 0.5 mg/kg dose. Repeat q 6–8 hr
How supplied: Vials: 10 ml vials or 1 ml tubex;
    Liquid: 4 oz, 1 pt, 1 gal

TRIMEPRAZINE

Brand Name: Temaril

Action: Antipruritic, antihistamine
Strength: Tablets: 2–5 mg, 5 mg; Liquid: 2.5 mg/
    5 ml
Dose: 6 months–2 years: 1.25 mg tid not to ex-
    ceed 5 mg/24 hr; 2–6 years: 2.5 mg tid not to
    exceed 10 mg/24 hr; 6–12 years: 2.5 mg tid
    not to exceed 15 mg/24 hr
How supplied: Liquid: 4 oz

DECONGESTANTS

ACTIFED

Composition: Tablets: Tripolidine HCl 2.5 mg,
    pseudoephedrine HCl 60 mg; Liquid: Equiva-
    lent to ½ a tablet per 5 ml
Dose: 2–6 years, ½ tsp q 6 hr; 7–12 years, 1 tsp q
    6 hr
How supplied: 1 pt

AMBENYL EXPECTORANT

Composition: Liquid: per 5 ml: Codeine sulfate–
    10 mg, Bromodiphenhydramine HCl–3.75 mg,
    Diphenhydramine HCl–8.75 mg, Ammonium
    chloride–80 mg, Potassium guaiacolsulfonate–
    80 mg, menthol–0.5 mg, Alcohol–5%
Dose: 1–4 years: ½ tsp q 6–8 hr; 5–12 years:
    1 tsp q 6–8 hr
How supplied: 4 oz, 16 oz, 1 gal

DIMETAPP ELIXIR

Composition: Tablets: Brompheniramine maleate-
12 mg, Phenylephrine HCl-15 mg, Phenylpropanolamine HCl-15 mg; Liquid: Brompheni-
ramine-4 mg, Phenylephrine HCl-5 mg, Phenylpropanolamine HCl-5 mg, Alcohol-2.3%
Dose: 1-6 months: $\frac{1}{4}$ tsp q 6-8 hr; 6 months-2 years:
$\frac{1}{2}$ tsp q 6-8 hr; 2-4 years: 3/4 tsp q 6-8 hr; 4-12
years: 1 tsp q 6-8 hr
How supplied: 1 pt, 1 gal

TRIAMINIC SYRUP

Composition: Liquid : per 5 ml: Phenylpropanolamine HCl-12.5 mg, Chlorpheniramine ma-
leate-2 mg
Dose: 1-6 years: $\frac{1}{2}$ tsp q 4 hr; 6-12 years: 1 tsp q
4 hr
How supplied: 4 oz, 8 oz, 16 oz

TRIAMINIC EXPECTORANT

Composition: Liquid: per 5 ml: Phenylpropano-
lamine HCl-12.5 mg, Guaifenesin-100 mg,
Alcohol-5%
Dose: 1-6 years: $\frac{1}{2}$ tsp q 4 hr; 6-12 years: 1 tsp q
4 hr
How supplied: 4 oz, 8 oz, 16 oz

TRIAMINIC-DM COUGH FORMULA

Composition: Liquid: per 5 ml: Phenylpropanolamine hydrochloride-12.5 mg, Dextromethorphan hydrobromide-10 mg
Dose: 3 months-2 years: $1\frac{1}{2}$ drops/kg/q 4 hr; 2-6
years: $\frac{1}{2}$ tsp q 4 hr; 6-12 years: 1 tsp q 4 hr
How supplied: 4 oz, 8 oz .

DORCOL PEDIATRIC COUGH SYRUP

Composition: Liquid: per 5 ml: Phenylpropanolamine hydrochloride-6.25 mg, Guaifenesin-50
mg, Dextromethorphan hydrobromide-5 mg,
Alcohol-5%
Dose: 3 months-2 years: 3 drops/kg/q 4 hr; 2-6
years: 1 tsp q 4 hr; 6-12 years: 2 tsp q 4 hr
How supplied: 4 oz, 8 oz

PSEUDOEPHEDRINE

Brand Name: Sudafed

Composition: Syrup 30 mg/5 ml; Tablets: 30, 60 mg
Dose: 5 mg/kg in 3-4 doses

TRIAMINIC ORAL INFANT DROPS

Composition: Each ml contains: Phenylpropanolamine HCl-20 mg, Pheniramine maleate-
10 mg, pyrilamine maleate-10 mg
Dose: 1 drop/2 lb body weight administered 4
times daily
How supplied: 15 ml dropper bottles

ASTHMA MEDICATIONS

AQUEOUS EPINEPHRINE

Action: Bronchodilator
Strength: Dilution 1-1000 (1 mg/ml)
Dose: 0.01 ml/kg may be repeated in 20 min
How supplied: Ampules: 1 ml, 30 ml

BECLOMETHASONE DIPROPIONATE

Brand Name: Vanceril inhaler

Action: Aerosolized corticosteroid

Strength: Each inhaler contains 10 mg of beclomethasone dipropionate and delivers approximately 200 inhalations or 0.05 mg/inhalation
Dose: Children 6-12 years of age: 1-2 inhalations
3-4 times a day, not to exceed 10 inhalations
a day; ≥ 12 years of age: 2 inhalations 3 or
4 times a day not to exceed 20 inhalations a
day
How supplied: Inhaler

CROMOLYN SODIUM

Action: Inhibits bronchoconstriction, nasal
rhinorrhea
Strength: Capules: 20 mg; Nasal solution: 40 mg/
ml
Dose: Asthma: inhale contents of 1 capsule qid
for children over 5 years; Allergic rhinitis:
one spray in each nostril 3-6 times/day for
children ≥ 6 years. Not recommended for
children < 6 years.
How supplied: Spray bottle of 13 ml (520 mg)

EPHEDRINE

Brand Name: Found in Tedral, Quadrinal, etc.

Action: Bronchodilator
Strength: Liquid: Ephedrine sulfate 6 mg/5 ml,
ephedrine hydrochloride 12 mg/5 ml; Tablets:
15, 25, 30, 50 mg; Ampules: 25,50 mg/ml
Dose: 0.5-1 mg/kg/dose po repeat q 4 hr
How supplied: In mixtures of other medications
Tedral, Quadrinal, Marax, etc.

METAPROTERENOL SULFATE

Brand Name: Metaprel

Action: Bronchodilator
Strength: Syrup: 10 mg/5 ml; tablets: 20 mg;
Metered dose inhaler: 0.65 mg/metered
dose (approx)

Dose: Syrup: Children 6-9 years or weight under
60 lb: 1 tsp 3 or 4 times a day; Children over 9
years or weight over 60 lb: 2 tsp 3 or 4 times a
day

OXTRIPHYLLINE

Brand Name: Found in Brondecon

Action: Bronchodilator
Strength: Liquid: 100 mg/5 ml; Tablets: 200 mg
Dose: 12 mg/kg/24 hr po in 4 divided doses
How supplied: Liquid: 8 oz

SUSPHRINE 1-200

Action: Bronchodilator
Strength: 5 mg/ml
Dose: .05-0.1 ml SC q 12 hr prn
How supplied: Bottle: 5 ml; Ampules: 0.5 ml

TERBUTALINE SULFATE

Brand Name: Brethine, Bricanyl Sulfate

Action: Bronchodilator (beta adrenergic receptor
stimulator)
Strength: Tablets: 2.5, 5 mg; Ampules: 1 mg/ml
Dose: Children < 12 years: not recommended.
Children ≥ 12-15 years: 2.5 mg tid not to
exceed 7.5 mg/day. Adolescents and adults:
5 mg tid not to exceed 15 mg/day
How supplied: 1 ml ampules

THEOPHYLLINE

Brand Name: Found in Tedral, Quadrinal, Marax

Action: Bronchodilator
Strength: Liquid: 65 mg/5 cc; Tablets: 130 mg/
tablet
Dose: 15 mg/kg/24 hr po or IV in 4 divided doses
How supplied: In mixtures of other medications,
Tedral, Quadrinal, Marax

THEOPHYLLINE SODIUM GLYCINATE

Brand Name: Asbron G

Action: Bronchodilator
Strength: TSG 300 mg (equivalent to 150 mg of
theophylline), guaifenesin 100 mg in each tablet
or tablespoonful
Dose: Children 6-12: 2-3 tsp 3-4 times a day; 3-6:
1-1½ tsp 3-4 times a day; 1-3: ½-1 tsp 3-4 times
a day

THEOPHYLLINE, SUSTAINED RELEASE

Brand Name: Slo-Phyllin Gyrocaps, Theo-Dur

Action: Bronchodilator
Strength: Slo-Phyllin Gyrocaps: 60, 125, 250 mg;
Theo-Dur tablets: 100, 200, 300 mg
Dose: Slo-Phyllin: 3-5 mg/kg/q 6 hr not to exceed
20 mg/kg/24 hr; Theo-Dur: 8-10 mg/kg q 12 hr

BRONDECON

Oxtriphylline: Liquid: 100 mg/5 ml; Tablets: 200
mg/5 ml
Glyceryl guaiacolate: Liquid: 50 mg/5 ml; Tablets:
100 mg/5 ml
Dose: 12 mg/kg/24 hr in 4 divided doses
How supplied: Liquid 8 oz

ELIXOPHYLLINE

Theophylline: 80 mg/15 ml
Alcohol: 20%
Dose: 13-15 mg/kg/24 hr in 4 divided doses
How supplied: Bottle: 16 oz, 32 oz, 1 gal

ANTIMICROBIALS

AMOXICILLIN

Brand Name: Amoxil, Larotid, Polymox

Action: Broad spectrum antibiotic
Strength: Capules: 250, 500 mg; Liquid: 125 mg/
    5 ml, 250 mg/5 ml; Drops: 50 mg/ml
Dose: 30-40 mg/kg/day po in 3 divided doses
How supplied: Liquid: 80, 100, 150 ml; Drops: 15 ml

AMOXICILLIN/POTASSIUM CLAVULANATE

Brand Name: Augmentin

Action: Broad spectrum antibiotic
Strength: Tablets: 250 mg Amoxicillin + 125 mg
    Clavulinic Acid, 500 mg Amoxicillin + 125 mg
    Clavulinic Acid; Liquid: 125 mg Amoxicillin/5
    ml + 31.25 mg Clavulinic Acid, 250 mg Amoxi-
    cillin/5 ml + 62.50 mg Clavulinic Acid
Dose: Adults and children $\geq$ 40 kg: 250 mg q 8 hr,
    Severe infection: 500 mg q 8 hr. Children
    < 40 kg 20-40 mg/kg/day (based on amoxicillin
    content) q 8 hr
How supplied: Tablets: 250, 500 mg; Liquid: 125
    mg/5 ml, 250 mg/5 ml

AMPICILLIN

Brand Name: Polycillin, Omnipen, Penbritin, Amcill

Action: Broad spectrum antibiotic
Strength: Tablets: 250, 500 mg; Liquid: 125 mg/5
    ml, 250 mg/5 ml
Dose: 50-100 mg/kg/day po in 4 divided doses, 100-
    200 mg/kg/24 hr, IM, IV, q 4-6 hr
How supplied: 60 ml, 80 ml, 150 ml bottles

BENZATHINE PENICILLIN G

Brand Name: L-A Bicillin or C-R Bicillin with Penicillin G

Action: Rheumatic fever prophylaxis
Strength: 1.2 million U/ml
Dose: 1.2 million U IM once monthly
How supplied: Tubex 1.2 million U

BENZATHINE PENICILLIN (600,000 U)
AND PROCAINE PENICILLIN G (600,000 U)

Brand Name: C-R Bicillin

For therapy of nonsevere streptococcal infections

> Dose: 600,000 U IM under 1 year of age, 1,200,000 U
> IM over 1 year of age

CEFACLOR

Brand Name: Ceclor

> Action: Broad spectrum antibiotic
> Strength: Suspension: 125, 250 mg/5 ml; Cap-
> sules: 250, 500 mg
> Dose: 40 mg/kg/day po in 3 divided doses

CEFAMANDOLE NAFATE

Brand Name: Mandol

> Action: Broad spectrum antibiotic
> Strength: 0.5, 1, 2 g vials
> Dose: 50-150 mg/kg/24 hr, IM, IV in 4-6 divided
> doses

CEFOXITIN SODIUM

Brand Name: Mefoxin

> Action: Broad spectrum antibiotic
> Strength: 1, 2, 10 g vials
> Dose: 80-160 mg/kg/24 hr IM, IV in 4-6 divided
> doses

CEPHALOTHIN SODIUM/CEPHALEXIN
MONOHYDRATE

Brand Name: Keflin, Keflex

> Action: Broad spectrum antibiotic

Strength: Liquid: 125 mg/5 ml; Capsules: 250 mg
Dose: (Keflin) 75–125 mg/kg/24 hr IM, IV q 4–6 hr
    in 4 divided doses; (Keflex) 25–50 mg/kg/24 hr
    po in 4 divided doses
How supplied: Liquid: (Keflex) 100 ml; Ampules:
    (Keflin) 1 g/10 ml, 4 g/50 ml

CHLORAMPHENICOL

Brand Name: Chloromycetin

Action: Broad spectrum antibiotic
Strength: Capsules: 50 mg, 100 mg, 250 mg;
    Liquid: 150 mg/5 ml; IV solution: 250 mg/ml;
    in powder: 1000 mg
Dose: 50–100 mg/kg/24 hr in 4 divided doses po,
    IM, or IV; Newborns: 25 mg/kg/24 hr in 4
    divided doses
How supplied: Liquid: 60 ml bottles

CLOXACILLIN

Brand Name: Tegopen

Action: Antipenicillin resistant staphylococcus and
    other gram-positive organisms
Strength: Capsules: 125, 250 mg; Liquid 125 mg/
    5 ml
Dose: 50–300 mg/kg/24 hr po in 4 divided doses
How supplied: 80, 150 ml

COLISTIN

Brand Name: Coly-Mycin S

Action: Anti some gram-negative organisms, *(E.
    Coli)*
Strength: Liquid: 25 mg/5 ml; Vials: 150 mg
Dose: 7.5 mg–10 mg/kg/24 hr po in 3 divided doses;
    1.5–5 mg/kg/24 hr IM in 2–4 divided doses
How supplied: Liquid: 60 ml

ERYTHROMYCIN

Brand Name: Ilosone, Ilotycin, Erythrocin, Pediamycin

Action: Against gram-positive bacteria
Strength: Tablets: 100, 125, 200, 250 mg; Liquid:
200 mg/5 ml; Vials: 250, 300, 500, 1000 mg;
Ampules: 50 mg/ml
Dose: 20–40 mg/kg/24 hr po or IV in 4 divided doses
How supplied: Liquid: 60, 90, 150 ml

ETHAMBUTOL

Brand Name: Myambutol HCl

Action: Antituberculous
Strength: Tablets: 100, 400 mg
Dose: 20 mg/kg/24 hr in a single dose po

ETHIONAMIDE

Action: Antituberculous
Strength: Tablets: 250 mg
Dose: 10–20 mg/kg/24 hr po in 2-3 divided doses not
to exceed 750 mg/day

GENTAMICIN

Brand Name: Garamycin

Action: Broad spectrum, particularly the gram-
negative organisms
Strength: Vials: 40 mg/ml
Dose: Newborn up to 1 week old: 2.5 mg/kg q 12
hr IM or IV: 1 week to 1 month: 2.5 mg/kg q 8
hr IM; Children over 1 month: 2.5 mg/kg/24
hr q 6-8 hr IM or IV
How supplied: 2 ml vials for injection

ISONIAZID

Brand Name: Niadox, Nydrazid

Action: Antituberculous
Strength: Tablets: 50, 100 mg; Capsules: 50, 100
mg; Liquid: 50 mg/5 ml; Ampules: 100 mg/ml
Dose: 15-30 mg/kg/24 hr q 6-8 hr po or IM
How supplied: Liquid: 1 pt; Vials: 10 ml

KANAMYCIN

Brand Name: Kantrex

Action: Broad spectrum antibiotic but mostly used
for gram-negative organisms and staphylococcus
Strength: Capsules: 500 mg; Vials: 37.5 mg/ml, 250
mg/ml, 333 mg/ml
Dose: 50 mg/kg/24 hr in 4 divided doses po; 15
mg/kg/24 hr q 12 hr IM; Newborns: 5-15 mg/
kg/24 hr q 12 hr IM
How supplied: Vials: 2, 3 ml

METHICILLIN SODIUM

Brand Name: Staphcillin

Action: Antipenicillin-resistant staphylococcus
and other gram-positive organisms
Strength: Vials: 1000, 4000, 6000 mg
Dose: 100-400 mg/kg/24 hr in 4 or 6 divided doses,
IM or IV
How supplied: Vials: 1, 4, 6 g

MOXALACTAM

Brand Name: Moxam

Action: Broad spectrum antibiotic
Strength: 1, 2 g vial
Dose: 150-200 mg/kg/24 hr IV in 3-4 divided doses

NAFCILLIN MONOHYDRATE, SODIUM

Brand Name: Nafcil, Unipen

Action: Antipenicillin-resistant staphylococcus
and other gram-positive organisms
Strength: Oral: 250, 500 mg capsules, 250 mg/
5 ml; Parenteral: 0.5, 1, 2 g vial
Dose: 50-100 mg/kg/day po in 4 divided doses,
150 mg/kg/24 hr IM, IV in 4 divided doses

NITROFURANTOIN

Brand Name: Furadantin

Action: Broad spectrum antimicrobial useful in
kidney infections
Strength: Liquid: 25 mg/5 ml; Tablets: 50 mg/100
mg; Vials: 180 mg/20 ml
Dose: 5-10 mg/kg/24 hr in 4 divided doses po, in 2
divided doses IM
How supplied: Liquid: 60 ml, 473 ml; Vials: 20 ml

NYSTATIN

Brand Name: Mycostatin, ointment or cream

Action: Antimonilia
Strength: Tablets: 500,000 U; Liquid: 10,000 U/ml;
Ointment and cream: 100,000 U/g
Dose: (For Thrush) 1 ml q 6 hr for 5 days to 14 days
How supplied: Cream: 15 g; Ointment: 15, 30 g;
Liquid: 24 ml

OXACILLIN

Brand Name: Prostaphlin

Action: Antipenicillin-resistant staphylococcus and
other gram-positive organisms
Strength: Capsules: 125, 250, 500 mg; Liquid: 250
mg/5 ml; Vials: 250 mg, 500 mg, 1000 mg

Dose: 50-200 mg/kg/24 hr in 4 divided doses po
How supplied: Liquid: 100 ml bottles; Vials: 250
mg, 500 mg, 1 g

p-AMINO-SALICYLIC ACID

Brand Name: Rezipas, Pas-C (Pascorbic)

Action: Antituberculous
Strength: Tablets: 300, 500, 1000, 2000 mg; Vials:
100 mg/ml; Liquid: 500 mg/5 ml
Dose: 200 mg/kg/24 hr q 8 hr po

PENICILLIN G
(POTASSIUM OR SODIUM SALTS OF PENICILLIN G)

Brand Name: Pentids, Wycillin

Action: Against gram-positive bacteria
Strength: Tablets: 125 mg (200,000 U), 250 mg,
(400,000 U), 500 mg (800,000 U); Liquid: 125
mg (200,000 U)/5 ml, 250 mg, (400,000U)/5 ml;
Vials: Tubex 1.2 million U/2 ml
Dose: 50,000-250,000 U/kg/24 hr IM or IV in 4 di-
vided doses
How supplied: Liquid: 80, 150 ml

PHENOXYMETHYL PENICILLIN

Brand Name: Pen Vee, V-cillin

Action: Against gram-positive bacteria
Strength: Tablets: 125 mg (200,000 U), 250 mg
(400,000 U), 500 mg (800,000 U); Liquid: 5 ml
125 mg (200,000 U), 250 mg (400,000 U)
Dose: 25,000-50,000 U/ kg/24 hr po in 4 divided
doses
How supplied: Liquid: 40, 80, 150 ml

POLYMYXIN-B SULFATE

Brand Name: Aerosporin

Action: Against gram negative bacteria except
Proteus, especially for *Pseudomonas*
Strength: Tablets: 25, 50 mg; Vials: 50 mg
Dose: Enteric: 20 mg/kg/24 hr in 4 divided doses
po; Systemic: Newborns and prematures: 3-4
mg/kg/24 hr IM or IV in 4 divided doses
How supplied: Liquid: 50 mg vials to be diluted

RIFAMYCIN

Brand Name: Rifampin

Action: Antituberculous and H. Influenza prophylaxis
Strength: Capsules: 300, 600 mg
Dose: 20 mg/kg/24 hr in 2 divided doses po

STREPTOMYCIN SULFATE

Action: Antituberculous and against some gram-
negative organisms
Strength: Powder: 1, 5 g; Vials: 50 mg/ml, 500
mg/ml
Dose: 20-40 mg/kg/24 hr in 1 or 2 daily doses
How supplied: Vials: 50 mg/ml: 2, 10 ml, 400 mg/
ml: 2.5, 12.5 ml

SULFISOXAZOLE

Brand Name: Gantrisin

Action: Broad spectrum antimicrobial
Strength: Tablets: 500 mg; Liquid: 500 mg/5 ml;
Ampules: 400 mg/ml
Dose: 150-200 mg/kg/24 hr in 4 divided doses po, IM
or IV
How supplied: 120 ml, 1 pt

TETRACYCLINE

Brand name: Achromycin (Tetracycline), Terramycin (Oxytetracyline)

Action: Broad spectrum antibiotic
Strength: Tablets: 50, 100, 250 mg; Capsules: 50,
100, 250-mg; Liquid: 125 mg/5 ml; Vials: 100,
250, 500 mg
Dose: 10-20 mg/kg/24 hr in 4 divided doses po, 12
mg/kg/24 hr q 12 hr IM or IV
How supplied: 60 ml, 1 pt

TMP-SMX

Brand Name: Bactrim, Septra (Trimethoprim-Sulfamethoxazole)

Action: Anti some gram-negative organisms
Strength: Tablets: Trimethoprim - 80 mg, Sulfamethoxazole - 400 mg; Liquid: Trimethoprim -
40 mg, Sulfamethoxazole-200 mg/5 ml
Dose: Children over 12 years: 2 tabs q 12 hr; Children
under 12 years of age, 8 mg of Trimethoprim or
40 mg of Sulfamethoxazole kg/24 hr q 12 hr

ANTICONVULSANTS
CARBAMAZEPINE

Brand Name: Tegretol

Action: Anticonvulsant for psychomotor, petit and
grand mal seizures
Strength: 100 mg tablets
Dose: 10-20 mg/kg/24 hr

DIAZEPAM

Brand Name: Valium

Action: Anticonvulsant for status epilepticus, tran-
quilizer
Strength: Tablets: 2, 5, 10 mg; Ampules: 5 mg/1 cc
Dose: 0.1 mg, 1 mg/kg/24 hr IM, IV, po; Not to ex-
ceed 10 mg
How supplied: Ampules: 2 ml; Vials: 10ml

DIPHENYLHYDANTOIN SODIUM

Brand Name: Dilantin

>   Action: Anticonvulsant for grand mal and focal
>   seizures
>   Strength: Tablets: 50 mg; Liquid: 125 mg/5 ml;
>   Vials: 50 mg/ml
>   Dose: 3-8 mg/kg/24 hr in 2 or 3 divided doses po,
>   IM, or IV
>   How supplied: Vials: 100, 250 mg

ETHOSUXIMIDE

Brand Name: Zarontin

>   Action: Anticonvulsant, for petit mal
>   Strength: Capsules: 250 mg
>   Dose: Children less than 6 years old: 250 mg/24 hr
>   po; Over 6 years old: 500 mg/2 hr po in 2 di-
>   vided doses

PARALDEHYDE

Brand Name: Paral

>   Action: Anticonvulsant, sedative for status epilepti-
>   cus
>   Strength: Capsules: 1000 mg; Ampules: 2, 5, 10 ml;
>   Supplement: 1500 mg
>   Dose: Anticonvulsant: 0.3 ml/kg/dose per rectum,
>   0.15 ml/kg/dose IM or IV, not to exceed 8 ml/
>   dose; Sedative: 0.15 ml/kg/dose po or per rec-
>   tum

PARAMETHADIONE, TRIMETHADIONE

Brand Name: Paradione, Tridione

>   Action: Anticonvulsant for petit mal, myoclonic
>   epilepsy, akinetic seizures
>   Strength: Capsules: 150, 300 mg; Liquid (paradione)
>   300 mg/ml, (tridione) 200 mg/5 ml

Dose: Under 2 years: 300 mg/24 hr po; 2-6 years:
600 mg/24 hr po; Over 6 years: 900 mg/24 hr
po in 3-4 divided doses
How supplied: Paramethadione: Liquid: 50 ml;
Trimethadione: Liquid: 1 pt

PHENOBARBITAL

Brand Name: Luminal

Action: Anticonvulsant, sedative against status
epilepticus, psychomotor, grand mal and focal
seizures
Strength: Tablets: 8, 15, 30, 60, 100 mg; Liquid: 20
mg/5 ml; Vials: 65 mg/ml, 160 mg/ml
Dose: Sedative: 3-5 mg/kg/24 hr in 3 divided doses
po, IM; Anticonvulsant: 5-6 mg/kg dose IM or
IV not to exceed 300 mg
How supplied: Liquid: 1 pt; Ampules: 130, 300 mg;
Vials: 10 ml

PRIMIDONE

Brand Name: Mysoline

Action: Anticonvulsant for grand mal, focal, psychomotor seizures
Strength: Tablets: 50, 250 mg; Liquid: 250 mg/5 ml
Dose: Under 6 years: 125 mg bid or tid; Over 8
years: 250 mg bid, tid or qid, not to exceed 2
g/day
How supplied: Liquid: 240 cc

VALPROIC ACID

Brand Name: Depakene

Action: Anticonvulsant for petit mal seizures
Strength: 250 mg capsule; 250 mg/5 ml syrup
Dose: Starting dose 15 mg/kg/24 hr po; Maximum
dose 60 mg/kg/24 hr po in 2-3 divided doses

ANTIDIARRHEALS

DIPHENOXYLATE HCl WITH ATROPINE SULFATE

Brand Name: Lomotil

> Strength: Diphenoxylate HCl: 2.5 mg per tablet or
> Atropine Sulfate: 0.025 mg, 5 ml
> Dose: 3-6 months: 3 mg ($\frac{1}{2}$ tsp tid); 6-12 months:
> 4 mg($\frac{1}{2}$ tsp qid); 1-2 years: 5 mg ($\frac{1}{2}$ tsp 5 times
> a day); 2-5 years: 6 mg (1 tsp tid); 5-8 years:
> 8 mg (1 tsp qid); 8-12 years: 10 mg (1 tsp 5 times
> a day)
> How supplied: 60 ml bottles

DONNATAL

> Strength: Each tablet, capsule or 5 ml contains:
> Hyoscyamine sulfate-0.1037 mg; Atropine sulf-
> ate-0.0194 mg; Phenobarbital-16.2 mg
> Dose: Infants: 15-30 minims tid; Children: $\frac{1}{2}$-1 tsp
> tid or qid
> How supplied: Liquid: 1 pt, 1 gal

KAOLIN AND PECTIN

Brand Name: Kaopectate

> Strength: Kaolin 90 g and Pectin 2 g/30 ml
> Dose: 3-6 years: 1-2 tablespoons after each loose
> bowel movement; 6-12 years: 2-4 tablespoons
> after each loose bowel movement
> How supplied: 180, 300 ml bottles

PAREGORIC

Brand Name: Parepectolin (Paregoric with opium, kaolin
and pectin)

> Strength: Paregoric 1 g (3.7 ml); Opium 15 mg/30 ml;
> Pectin 162 mg/30 ml; Kaolin 5.5 g/30 ml

Dose: 1-3 years: $\frac{1}{2}$ tsp after each loose stool not to
exceed 4 doses in 12 hr; 3 to 6 years: 1-1$\frac{1}{2}$ tsp
after each loose stool not to exceed 4 doses in
12 hr; More than 6 years: 2 tsp after each loose
stool not to exceed 4 doses in 12 hr
How supplied: 4, 8 oz

ANTIHELMINTIC MEDICATIONS

HEXYLRESORCINOL

Action: Against ascaris and trichuris
Strength: Capsules: 100, 200 mg; Solution: 0.1%
solution for retention enema
Dose: Capsules: 15-30 lb: 200 mg in a single dose,
30-60 lb: 500 mg in a single dose, Over 60 lb:
1000 mg in a single dose; Solution: 5-15 lb:
62.5 ml retained for 1 hr, 15-30 lb: 125 ml retained for 1 hr, 30-60 lb: 250 ml retained for 1
hr, Over 60 lb: 500 ml retained for 1 hr

MEBENDAZOLE

Brand Name: Vermox

Action: Against pinworms, ascaris, trichuris, hookworm
Strength: Tablets: 100 mg
Dose: Varies with type of infestation. For pinworm:
1 tablet; For ascaris, trichuris and hookworm:
1 tablet bid for 3 consecutive days

PIPERAZINE CITRATE

Brand Name: Antepar

Action: Against pinworms and ascaris
Strength: Wafers: 500 mg; Liquid: 500 mg/5 ml
Dose: 150 mg/kg in a single dose not to exceed 3 g;
Most effective: a 7-day course of therapy, Up to
15 lb: $\frac{1}{2}$ tsp or wafers once daily, 15-30 lb: 1 tsp

or wafers once daily, 30–60 lb: 2 tsp or wafers
once daily, Over 60 lb: 4 tsp or wafers once
daily
How supplied: Liquid: 1 pt; Wafers: 28/box

PYRANTEL PAMOATE

Brand Name: Antiminth

Action: Against pinworms and ascaris
Strength: Liquid: 50 mg/ml
Dose: 11 mg/kg in a single dose not to exceed 1 g
How supplied: 60 ml bottles

PYRVINIUM PAMOATE

Brand Name: Povan

Action: Antipinworms
Strength: Liquid: 10 mg/ml; Tablets: 50 mg
Dose: 5 mg/kg in a single dose, a second dose is
given in 2 weeks
How supplied: 60 ml bottles

VITAMINS AND IRON

IRON DEXTRAN

Brand Name: Imferon

Strength: 50 mg/ml of elemental iron
Dose: # of ml = 0.3 x wgt in lb x
$$\frac{[100 - (Hb \times 6.8)]}{50}$$

See Table 23-1.

IRON (MOLYBDENIZED FERROUS SULFATE)

Brand Name: Mol-iron drops

Strength: Ferrous sulfate: 125 mg/ml, Molybdenum
sesquioxide: 2 mg/ml, equivalent to 25 mg of
elemental iron

Table 23-1   Dosage Table

Pts wt in lbs	30% 4.4 g/ 100 ml	40% 5.9 g/ 100 ml	50% 7.4 g/ 100 ml	60% 8.9 g/ 100 ml	70% 10.4 g/ 100 ml
10	5	4	3	3	2
20	9	8	6	5	4
30	13	11	9	8	6
40	17	15	12	10	7
50	21	18	15	12	9
60	25	22	18	15	11
70	30	25	21	17	13
80	34	29	24	19	15
90	38	32	27	22	16
100	42	36	30	24	18
110	46	39	33	26	20
120	51	43	36	29	22
130	55	47	39	31	23

How supplied: Ampules, 2 ml and 10 ml

Dose: Prophylactic: less than 6 years: 0.3 ml/day, over 6 years: 0.6 ml/day; Therapeutic: 3 ml/day
How supplied: 15, 50 ml bottles

MULTIVITAMINS

Brand Name: Poly-Vi-Sol

Strength: Viamin A: 3000/U 0.6 ml, Vitamin D: 400 U/0.6 ml, Vitamin C: 60 mg/0.6 ml, Vitamin B_1: 1.0 mg/0.6 ml, Vitamin B_2: 1.2 mg/0.6 ml, Niacinamide: 8 mg/0.6 ml
Maintenance Dose: 0.6 ml/day
How supplied: 15, 30, 50 ml bottles

VITAMINS A, D, C

Brand Name: Tri-Vi-Sol

Strength: Vitamin A: 3000 U/0.6 ml, Vitamin D:
400 U/0.6 ml, Vitamin C: 60 mg/0.6 ml
Maintenance Dose: 0.6 ml/day
How supplied: 15, 30, 50 ml bottles

TOPICAL MEDICATIONS

BACITRACIN 400 U/G, POLYMYXIN 5000 U/G, NEOMYCIN 5 MG/G

Brand Name: Neosporin Ointment, Neopolycin

Action: Antibiotic for superficial skin infections
Dose: Apply tid, qid, or 5 times daily to affected
part
How supplied: 15, 30 g

COAL TAR

Brand Name: Tarbonis

Action: Keratolytic agent for chronic dermatoses:
eczema, seborrhea
Strength: Coal tars 5% in a hydrophilic base
Dose: Apply tid to affected areas
How supplied: 60 g, 1 lb jars

DESITIN OINTMENT

Vitamins A and D, Zinc oxide, Lanolin, Petrola-
tum, Talcum
Action: Soothing agent for dry, irritated skin;
moisture repellant
Dose: Apply 3 or more times daily as needed
How supplied: 30, 60, 125 g

FLURANDRENOLIDE CREAM OR OINTMENT

Brand Name: Cordran

Action: Potent steroid action
Strength: 0.05, 0.025%
Dose: Apply tid to affected area
How supplied: 7.5, 15, 60, 225 g

HYDROCORTISONE CREAM

Brand Name: Cort Dome Cream, Hytone Cream

Action: Antiinflammatory—eczema
Strength: Various strengths: 1/8, 1/4, 1/2, and 1%
Dose: Apply tid to affected area
How supplied: 15, 30, 120 g

HYDROCORTISONE—VIOFORM CREAM

Brand Name: Vioform—Hydrocortisone, Vio-Dydrosone
cream, Doneform-HC

Action: Antibacterial, antifungal, antiinflammatory,
    antipruritic for eczema, tinea
Strength: (Available in various strengths) Average:
    hydrocortisone 1%, iodochlorhydroxyquin 3%
Dose: Apply tid to affected area
How supplied: 5, 15, 20 g

NYSTATIN

Brand Name: Mycostatin cream or ointment

Action: Antimonilial
Strength: 100,000 U/g
Dose: Apply tid to affected area
How supplied: 15, 30 g

NYSTATIN, NEOMYCIN, GRAMICIDIN, TRIAMCINOLONE

Brand Name: Mycolog

> Action: Antimonilial, antibacterial, antiinflammatory
> Strength: Nystatin: 100,000 U/g; Neomycin SO_4: 2.5 mg/g; Gramicidin: 0.25 mg/g; Triamcinolone acetonide: 1 mg/g
> Dose: Apply tid to affected area
> How supplied: 5, 15, 30, 120 g

SALICYLIC ACID 3%, BENZOIC ACID 3%

Brand Name: Whitfield's Ointment

> Action: Antifungal
> Dose: Apply tid to affected part

TOLNAFTATE

Brand Name: Tinactin

> Action: Antifungal agent
> Strength: Cream: 1% Tolnaftate 10 mg/g; Solution: 1% Tolnaftate 10 mg/ml
> Dose: Apply bid for 2-3 weeks
> How supplied: Cream: 15 g tube; Solution: 10 ml bottle

TRIAMCINOLONE ACETONIDE

Brand Name: Kenalog

> Action: Potent steroid action
> Strength: 0.1, 0.025%
> Dose: Apply tid to affected area
> How supplied: 5, 15 g

UNDECYLENIC ACID, ZINC UNDECYLENATE OINTMENT

Brand Name: Desenex

Action: Antifungal agent
Strength: Undecylenic acid 5%; Zinc undecylinate 20%
Dose: Apply bid to affected area
How supplied: 0.9 oz and 1.8 oz tubes, 1 lb jars

EAR MEDICATIONS

CARBAMIDE PEROXIDE

Brand Name: Debrox

Action: Cerumen softener for removal of hardened, impacted ear wax
Strength: Carbamide peroxide 6.5% in glycerol
Dose: 5 drops in affected ear bid for 3-4 days
How supplied: 15 ml bottles

COLISTIN-NEOMYCIN-HYDROCORTISONE DROPS

Brand Name: Coly-Mycins Otic

Action: Antibacterial, antiinflammatory for external otitis
Strength: Colistin: 3 mg/ml; Neomycin: 3.3 mg/ml; Hydrocortisone: 3.5 mg/ml
Dose: 4 drops tid
How supplied: 5, 10 ml bottles

NEOMYCIN EAR DROPS

Brand Name: Otobiotic Otic

Action: Antibiotic for external otitis
Strength: Neomycin: 10 mg/ml; Sodium proprionate: 50 mg/ml
Dose: 4-5 drops tid
How supplied: 15 ml bottles

POLYMYXIN B, NEOMYCIN, HYDROCORTISONE DROPS

Brand Name: Cortisporin Otic Drops

Action: Antibiotic for external otitis
Strength: Polymyxin B: 10,000 U/ml; Neomycin:
  3.5 mg/ml; Hydrocortisone: 10 mg/ml
Dose: 4-5 drops tid
How supplied: 5, 10 ml bottles

EYE SOLUTIONS

CHLORAMPHENICOL

Brand Name: Chloromycetin Ophthalmic Solution 1%

Action: Antibacterial for bacterial conjunctivitis
Strength: Solution: Chloramphenicol: 25 mg/ml;
  Ointment: 10 mg/g
Dose: 2 drops in affected eye tid; ointment, bid
How supplied: Solution: 15 ml; Ointment: 1/8 oz

NEOMYCIN-POLYMYXIN-GRAMICIDIN

Brand Name: Neosporin Ophthalmic Solution

Action: Antibacterial for bacterial conjunctivitis
Strength: Solution: Polymyxin B: 5,000 U/ml,
  Neomycin: 2.5 mg/ml, Gramicidin: 0.025
  mg/ml
Dose: 1-2 drops in affected eye 4-6 times daily
How supplied: 10 ml bottles

SEDATIVES AND TRANQUILIZERS
See also Anticonvulsants

CHLORAL HYDRATE

Brand Name: Noctec

Action: Sedative, hypnotic

Strength: Liquid: 267, 500, 600 mg/5 ml; Capsules:
250, 500, 1000 mg
Dose: Sedative: 10–20 mg/kg/dose q 6–8 hr po;
Hypnotic: 50 mg/kg/dose not to exceed 1 g
How supplied: Liquid: 1 pt, 1 gal

HYDROXYZINE HCl

Brand Name: Atarax

Action: Tranquilizer, muscle relaxant, antispasmodic
Strength: Tablets: 10, 25, 50, 100 mg; Liquid: 10
mg/5 ml; Vials: 25, 50, mg/ml
Dose: 2 mg/kg/24 hr po in 3 divided doses. Not to
exceed 100 mg daily; Preoperative: 1 mg/kg/dose
IM
How supplied: Liquid: 1 pt; Vials: 1, 2, 10 ml

METHYLPHENIDATE HCl

Brand Name: Ritalin

Action: For hyperactivity
Strength: Tablets: 5, 10, 20 mg; Vials: 10 mg/ml
Dose: Initially 5 mg once daily, increase by 5 mg
weekly until desired effect is achieved. Do not
exceed 60 mg/24 hr
How supplied: Vials: 10 ml

SODIUM PENTOBARBITAL

Brand Name: Nembutal

Action: Sedative, hypnotic
Strength: Tablets: 30, 50, 100 mg; Liquid: 20 mg/
5 ml; Ampules: 50 mg/ml; Suppository: 30, 60,
120, 200 mg
Dose: 2–3 mg/kg/dose
How supplied: Liquid: 1 pt, 1 gal; Ampules: 2, 5,
20, 50 ml

ANTIEMETICS
CHLORPROMAZINE HCl

Brand Name: Thorazine

Action: Antiemetic, tranquilizer
Strength: Tablets: 10, 25, 50, 100, 200 mg; Liquid:
10 mg/5 ml; Suppository: 25, 100 mg; Ampules:
25 mg/ml
Dose: 0.5 mg/kg/dose q 6 hr po or IM; 1 mg/kg/dose
q 6 hr per rectum
How supplied: Liquid: 120 ml; Vials: 1, 2, 10 ml

TRIMETHOBENZAMIDE HCl

Brand Name: Tigan

Action: Antiemetic
Strength: Capsules: 100, 250 mg; Suppository: 200
mg; Ampules: 100 mg/ml
Dose: 15-20 mg/kg/24 hr

ANALGESICS AND ANTIPYRETICS

ACETAMINOPHEN

Brand Name: Tylenol, Tempra

Action: Antipyretic, analgesic
Strength: Tablets: 300 mg; Drops: 100 mg/ml;
Liquid: 120 mg/5 ml
Dose: Less than 1 year: 60 mg q 6 hr po; 1-3 years:
120 mg q 6 hr po; 3-6 years: 240 mg q 6 hr po
How supplied: Liquid: 15, 60, 120, 240 ml, 1 pt, 1 gal

ACETYLSALICYLIC ACID

Brand Name: Aspirin

Action: Analgesic, antipyretic
Strength: Tablets: 30, 60 75, 300, 600 mg; Liquid:
150 mg/5 ml; Supplement: 60, 200, 300, 600 mg
Dose: 30-60 mg/kg/24 hr in 6 individual doses po or
pr; For rheumatic fever: 100 mg/kg/24 hr in
4-6 divided doses po, pr

CODEINE PHOSPHATE

Action: Narcotic, analgesic
Strength: Tablets and capsules: 15, 30, 60 mg;
    Ampules: 15, 30, 60 mg
Dose: 0.5-1 mg/kg/dose. May be repeated q 4 hr po
    or sc
How supplied: Ampules: 1, 20 ml

MEPERIDINE HCl

Brand Name: Demerol

Action: Narcotic, analgesic, antispasmodic
Strength: Tablets: 50, 100 mg; Liquid: 10 mg/ml,
    50 mg/ml; Ampules: 50 mg/ml and 100 mg/ml
Dose: 1-1.5 mg/kg/dose q 4 hr po or IM. Do not ex-
    ceed 6 mg/kg/24 hr
How supplied: Liquid: 1 pt; Ampules: 0.5, 1, 1.5,
    2 ml; Vials: 20 ml

MORPHINE SULFATE

Action: Narcotic, analgesic, antispasmodic
Strength: Tablets: 5, 8, 10, 15, 30 mg; Vials: 10, 30
    mg/ml
Dose: 0.2 mg/kg/dose may be repeated q 4-6 hr po
    or IM
How supplied: Ampules: 1 ml; Vials: 20 ml

MISCELLANEOUS MEDICATIONS

ACETAZOLAMIDE

Brand Name: Diamox

Action: Diuretic
Strength: Tablets: 125, 250 mg; Liquid: 250 mg/
    5 ml; Vials: 500 mg
Dose: 10-30 mg/kg/24 hr po in 4 divided doses;
    Salicylate poisoning: 5 mg/kg q 4 hr x 3 IM after
    diuresis is induced

ATROPINE SULFATE

Action: Cholinergic blocking agent
Strength: Tablets: 0.32, 0.4, 0.65, 1.2 mg; Ampules:
0.4 mg/ml
Dose: 0.01 mg/dose po or sc not to exceed 0.4 mg

CALCIUM

Strength: 1 g of CaGluconate = 110 mg Ca; 1 g of
CaLactate = 180 mg Ca; 1 g of CaChloride = 360
mg Ca
Dose: Elemental calcium 2 g/M^2 po, IV in 1-3 divided doses

GLUBIONATE CALCIUM

Brand Name: Neo-Calglucon Syrup

Strength: 1.8 g/5 ml (calcium content 115 mg, providing same amount at 1.2 g calcium gluconate)
Dose: Supplement: Adults and children > 4 years—
1 tbs tid, 1.0 g cal/day, 104% USRDA; Children
< 4 years—2 tsp tid 0.7 g cal/day, 86% USRDA;
Infants—1 tsp 5 times daily (may be taken un-
diluted, mixed with infant's formula or fruit
juice) (Part of need is supplied by diet), 0.6 g
cal/day, 96% USRDA
How supplied: 16 oz bottles

CHLOROTHIAZIDE

Brand Name: Diuril

Action: Diuretic
Strength: Tablets: 250, 500 mg; Liquid: 250 mg/5
ml; Ampules: 500 mg
Dose: 10-40 mg/kg/24 hr divided in 1-4 doses po or
IV
How supplied: Liquid: 237 ml

DIGOXIN

Brand Name: Lanoxin

Action: Cardiotonic
Strength: Tablets: 0.125, 0.25, 0.5 mg; Liquid:
0.05 mg/ml
Total digitalizing dose: Newborns: 0.03-0.04 mg/
kg IM; Less than 2 years: 0.06-0.08 mg/kg/ po,
0.04-0.06 mg/kg IM, IV; More than 2 years: 0.04-
0.06 mg/kg po, 0.02-0.04 mg/kg IM or IV
Digitalization schedule: 1/2 the total digitalizing
dose is given initially, then 1/4 dose q 6-8 hr x
2 with careful clinical and ECG monitoring
Maintenance dose: 1/4 to 1/3 of the total digitalizing dose, divided into 2 doses and given q 12 hr
How supplied: Liquid: 60 ml; Ampules: 2 ml

DIOCTYL SODIUM SULFOSUCCINATE

Brand Name: Colace

Action: Stool softener
Strength: Tablets: 60, 100 mg; Capsules: 20, 50, 60,
100, 240 mg; Liquid: 10 mg/ml, 50 mg/ml;
Suppository: 100 mg
Dose: 5 mg/kg/24 hr in 3-4 divided doses po
How supplied: Liquid: 30, 240 ml, 1 pt

ETHACRYNIC ACID

Brand Name: Edecrin

Action: Diuretic
Strength: Tablets: 25, 50 mg; Vials: 50 mg
Dose: 0.4-1 mg/kg/dose IV; 10-20 mg/kg/24 hr in 4
divided doses po

FLUNISOLIDE NASAL SOLUTION

Brand Name: Nasalide, Nasal Solution 0.025%

Action: Antiinflammatory, antiallergic

Strength: 24 µg/metered spray
Dose: Children > 14 years: 2 sprays (50 µg) in each
nostril bid; Children 6-14 years: 2 sprays (50 µg)
in each nostril bid; or 1 spray (24 µg) in each nostril
tid; Not recommended for children < 6 years
How supplied: 25 ml spray bottles

GRISEOFULVIN (MICROSIZE)

Brand Name: Griseofulvin, Grifulvin [microsized],
Grisactin [microsized], Fulvin U/F [microsized]

Action: Antifungal agent
Strength: Tablets: 125, 250, 500 mg; Liquid: 250
mg/5 ml
Dose:. 20 mg/kg/24 hr in 1-3 divided doses, po; 10
mg/kg/24 hr or 1-3 doses daily po for microsize
griseofulvin
How supplied: Liquid: 125 ml

GRISEOFULVIN (ULTRAMICROSIZE)

Brand Name: Gris-PEG

Action: Antifungal agent
Strength: Tablets: 125 mg (biologically equivalent
to 250 mg of microsize griseofulvin)
Dose: Children: Approximately 5 mg/kg (2.5 mg/lb)
of body weight per day

HEPARIN SODIUM

Action: Anticoagulant
Strength: Tablets: (sublingual): 1800 U; Ampules:
1000, 5000, 10,000, 20,000, 40,000 U (1 U =
.0083 mg)
Dose: Initially: 50 U/kg IV; Maintenance: 100 U/kg
q 4 hr IV titrated so clotting time is between 20
and 30 minutes
How supplied: Ampules: 1 ml; Vials: 2, 4, 5, 10 ml

HYDRALAZINE HCl

Brand Name: Apresoline

Action: Antihypertensive
Strength: Tablets: 10, 25, 50, 100 mg; Ampules:
20 mg/ml
Dose: 0.75 mg/kg/24 hr po in 4 divided doses; 1.7–
3.5 mg/kg/24 hr IM in 4 divided doses; With
Reserpine: 0.15 mg/kg q 12–24 hr
How supplied: Ampules: 1 ml

HYDROCORTISONE SUCCINATE

Brand Name: Solu-Cortef

Action: Systemic steroid
Strength: Vials: 50 mg/ml, 125 mg/ml; Liquid:
2 mg/ml; Tablets: 5, 10, 20 mg
Dose: Gram–negative shock: Initial dose: 50 mg/
kg, then 50–75 mg/kg/24 hr in 4 divided doses
IM
How supplied: Vial: 5 ml; Liquid: 125 ml

IPECAC, SYRUP OF

Action: Emetic
Strength: 0.14% solution
Dose: More than 1 year: 15 ml po, may be repeated
in 20 min
How supplied: Liquid: 30 ml provided without pre-
scription, 1 pt bottles

ISOPROTERENOL HCl

Brand name: Isuprel

Action: Cardiotonic, bronchodilator, peripheral
vasodilator
Strength: Tablets: 5, 10, 15 mg; Liquid: 2.5 mg/
15 ml; Ampules: 200 µg/ml
Dose: 2–10, mg tid, sublingually; 5–15 mg qid per
rectum; 0.1–0.5 mg sc; 0.05–4 µgm/min IV
How supplied: Ampules: 1, 5 ml

MAGNESIUM SULFATE

Action: Cathartic, antihypertensive
Strength: Ampules: 10, 25, 50%, (500 mg/ml)
Dose: Cathartic: 250 mg/kg/dose po; For hyper-
   tension: 0.2 ml/kg/dose IM of 50% solution q
   4-6 hr, up to 100 mg/kg/dose IV
How supplied: Ampules: 2 ml, 10 ml

MANNITOL

Action: Diuresis (osmotic)
Strength: 250 mg/ml (25% solution)
Dose: 1 g/kg IV in 15-30 min q 6 hr
How supplied: Ampules: 50 ml; IV solution: 500,
   1000 ml

NALOXONE HYDROCHLORIDE

Brand Name: Narcan

Action: Neutralizes morphine and derivatives
Strength: Ampules: 0.4 mg/ml
Dose: 0.01 mg/kg for children; 0.4 mg/dose for
   adults
How supplied: Ampules: 1, 2 ml

PREDNISONE

Brand Name: Meticorten, Deltra, Deltasone

Action: Systemic steroid
Strength: Tablets: 1, 2.5, 5 mg
Dose: 1 mg/kg/24 hr

QUINIDINE SULFATE

Action: For cardiac arrhythmias (see cardiology)
Strength: Tablets: 100, 200, 300 mg; Capules: 200
   mg; Vials: 80 mg/ml, 200 mg/ml
Dose: Initial test dose 2 mg/kg po, IM, IV; Therapeutic dose: 30 mg/kg/24 hr divided into 5
   daily doses po, IM, or IV

RESERPINE

Brand Name: Serpasil

Action: Antihypertensive agent
Strength: Tablets: 0.1, 0.25, 1 mg; Liquid: 0.2 mg/
   4 ml; Ampules: 250 g/ml
Dose: Acute hypertension: 0.07 mg/kg IM (maximum dose 2 mg) may be repeated in 12 hr
How supplied: Tablets: 1 mg—bottles of 100,
   0.25 mg—bottles of 100, 500, 1000, 5000,
   0.1 mg—bottles of 100, 500, 1000; Elixir: 0.2
   mg/4 ml tsp—1 pt bottles; Ampules: 2 ml

SODIUM POLYSTYRENE SULFONATE

Brand Name: Kayexalate

Action: Cation exchange resin for potassium removal
Strength: Powder: 450 g
Dose: 1 g of resin exchanges 1 mEq of potassium
   ion. Given as high rectal enema, dissolved in
   sorbital or glucose water. May be repeated q
   6 hr

UREA

Action: Reduce cerebral edema (osmotic diuresis)
Strength: 40 g in 93 ml of 10% invert sugar or in
   210 ml of 10% invert sugar
Dose: 1-1.5 g/kg/dose as 30% solution in 30 min IV
How supplied: Bottles with sterile powder and
   diluent: 40, 90 g

XYLOCAINE HCl

Brand Name: Lidocaine

Action: Cardiotonic, for arrhythmias (see cardi-
   ology), local anesthetic
Strength: Vials: 0.5, 1, 2%
Dose: Arrhythmias: 1 mg/kg IV
How supplied: Ampules: 2, 10 ml; Vials: 20, 50 ml

PERCENTILE CHART FOR MEASUREMENT
OF INFANT BOYS

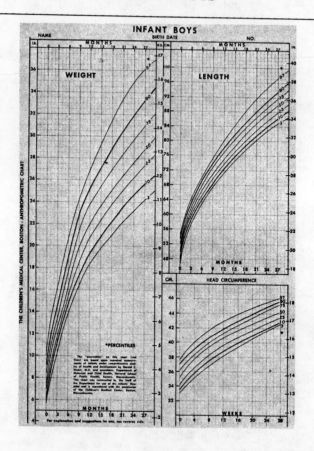

PERCENTILE CHART FOR MEASUREMENT
OF INFANT GIRLS

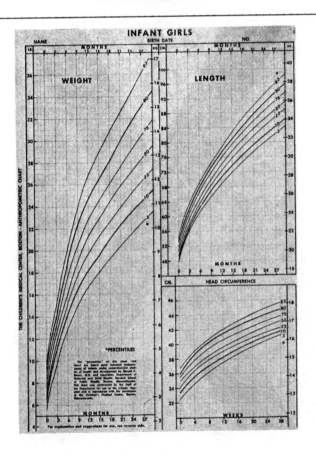

Appendix A-3

PERCENTILE CHART FOR MEASUREMENT OF BOYS

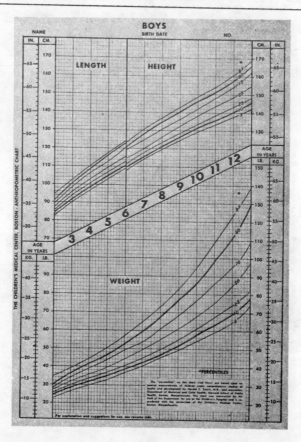

PERCENTILE CHART FOR MEASUREMENT OF GIRLS

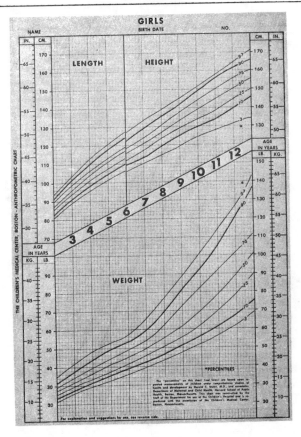

Appendix B-1

HEAD CIRCUMFERENCE FOR BOYS

Name _____

Birth Date _____

Notes:

PATIENT INFORMATION:

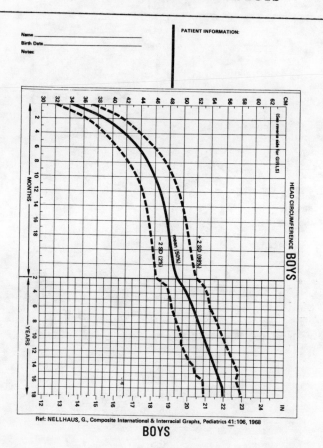

Ref: NELLHAUS, G., Composite International & Interracial Graphs, Pediatrics 41:106, 1968

BOYS

502

HEAD CIRCUMFERENCE FOR GIRLS

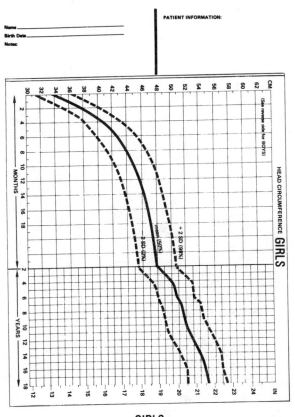

PATIENT INFORMATION:

Name

Birth Date

Notes:

GIRLS

Appendix C

GRID FOR RECORDING THE WEIGHT OF PREMATURE INFANTS

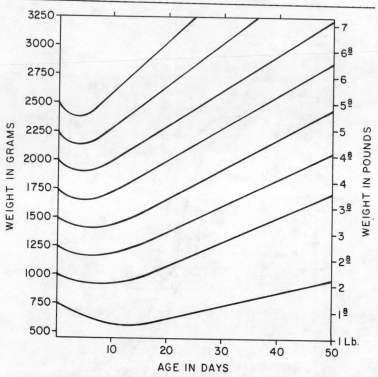

From Dancis J. et al.: J. Pediatrics 30:570, 1948. (Reproduced with permission of C.V. Mosby Co., St. Louis.)

Appendix D

ORGAN GROWTH CURVES*

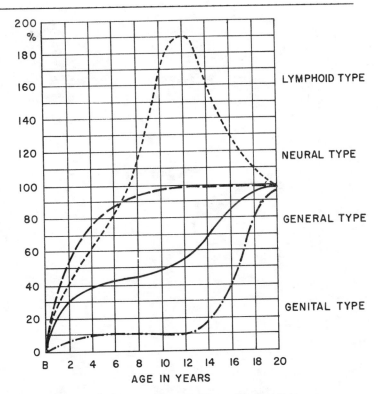

*Organ growth curves, drawn to a common scale by computing their values at successive ages in terms of their total (average) postnatal increments. (From Harris, J.A., et al.: The Measurement of Man, University of Minnesota Press, Minneapolis, 1930. Reproduced with publisher's permission.)

Appendix E-1

PRIMARY OR DECIDUOUS TEETH

| | Calcification | | Eruption | | Shedding | |
	Begins at	Complete at	Maxillary	Mandibular	Maxillary	Mandibular
Central incisors	5th fetal month	18-24 months	6-8 months	5-7 months	7-8 years	6-7 years
Lateral incisors	5th fetal month	18-24 months	8-11 months	7-10 months	8-9 years	7-8 years
Cuspids	6th fetal month	30-36 months	16-20 months	16-20 months	11-12 years	9-11 years
First molars	5th fetal month	24-30 months	10-16 months	10-16 months	10-11 years	10-12 years
Second molars	6th fetal month	36 months	20-30 months	20-30 months	10-12 years	11-13 years

AGE OF ERUPTION OF DECIDUOUS TEETH

Sexes are combined although girls tend to be slightly advanced over boys. Averages are approximate values derived from various studies. From Winkelstein, J.A., Ed.: Harriet Lane Handbook, Year Book Medical Publishers, 1972. (Reproduced with publisher's permission.)

Appendix E-2

SECONDARY OR PERMANENT TEETH

| | Calcification | | Eruption | |
	Begins at	Complete at	Maxillary	Mandibular
Central incisors	3-4 months	9-10 years	7-8 years	6-7 years
Lateral incisors	Max., 10-12 months Mand.,3-4 months	10-11 years	8-9 years	7-8 years
Cuspids	4-5 months	12-15 years	11-12 years	9-11 years
First premolars	18-21 months	12-13 years	10-11 years	10-12 years
Second premolars	24-30 months	12-14 years	10-12 years	11-13 years

Appendix E-2 (Cont'd.) Secondary or Permanent Teeth

First molars	Birth	9–10 years	6–7 years	6–7 years
Second molars	30–36 months	14–16 years	12–13 years	12–13 years
Third molars	Max., 7–9 years Mand., 8–10 years	18–25 years	17–22 years	17–22 years

AGE OF ERUPTION OF SECONDARY OR
PERMANENT TEETH

From Nelson, W.,E.: Textbook of Pediatrics, W.B. Saunders Co., Philadelphia, 1964. (Reproduced with publisher's permission.)

Appendix F

NORMAL BLOOD PRESSURE VALUES AT VARIOUS AGES

Age in Years*	Mean Systolic	Range in 95% of Normal Children	Age in Years*	Mean Diastolic	Range in 95% of Normal Children
$\frac{1}{2}$–1 year	90	±25	$\frac{1}{2}$–1 year	61	±19
1–2 years	96	±27	1–2 years	65	±27
2–3 years	95	±24	2–3 years	61	±24
3–4 years	99	±23	3–4 years	65	±19
4–5 years	99	±21	4–5 years	65	±15
5 years	94	±14	5 years	55	±9
6 years	100	±15	6 years	56	±8
7 years	102	±15	7 years	56	±8
8 years	105	±16	8 years	57	±9
9 years	107	±16	9 years	57	±9
10 years	109	±16	10 years	58	±10
11 years	111	±17	11 years	59	±10
12 years	113	±18	12 years	59	±10
13 years	115	±19	13 years	60	±10
14 years	118	±19	14 years	61	±10
15 years	121	±19	15 years	61	±10

*Data for $\frac{1}{2}$ to 5 years. From Allen–Williams, G.M.: Pulse-rate and blood pressure in infancy and early childhood. Arch Dis Child, 20:125, 1945. Data for 5 to 15 years. From Graham, A.W., Hines,E.A., Jr,and Gage, R.P.: Blood pressure in children between the ages of five and sixteen years. Amer J Dis Child. 69:203. 1945. (Reproduced with publisher's permission.)

WORKING TABLE FOR COMPARISON OF CHRONOLOGIC AND BONE AGES

Age	Measure of Osseous Development
Birth	Distal epiphysis of femur Astragalus, cuboid, calcaneus
1 year	Wrist—capitate, hamate, distal epiphysis of radius Ankle—addition of cuneiform III, distal epiphysis of tibia
2 years	Capitellum of humerus Wrist—no change Ankle—addition of epiphysis of fibula
3 years	Wrist—addition of triangularis Ankle—addition of cuneiform I
4 years	Wrist—addition of lunate Ankle—addition of cuneiform II, navicular Hip—epiphysis of greater trochanter

Age	Measure of Osseous Development
5 years	Wrist—addition of major multangulum, navicular Knee—patella
6 years	Wrist—addition of minor multangulum, epiphysis of ulna Shoulder—union of head and tuberosity of humerus
8 years	Ankle—epiphysis of calcaneus Union of ischium and pubis
10 years	Wrist—pisiform
12 years	External condyle of humerus Union of trochlea and capitellum of humerus
14 years	Union of proximal epiphysis of radius Union of olecranon and ulna
16 years	Union of epiphyses of metacarpals and metatarsals Appearance of crest of ilium
18 years	Union of distal epiphysis of radius and of ulna Union of distal epiphysis of tibia and of fibula

From Lowrey, G.H.: Growth and Development of Children, Year Book Publishers, Chicago, 1973. (Reproduced with publisher's permission.)

Appendix H

COMPOSITE DEVELOPMENTAL INVENTORY
FOR INFANTS AND YOUNG CHILDREN

Equipment needed:

1. Ring, 4-6 inches in diameter suspended on a string, e.g., embroidery hoop covered with red plastic tape
2. Pencils, not sharpened
3. Cup, plastic or aluminum measuring cup
4. Mirror, e.g., circular shaving mirror about 6 inches in diameter
5. Common objects such as a spoon, tongue depressors, large colorful buttons, rubber ball, etc.
6. Rubber stoppers, size "O"
7. Doughnut shaped breakfast cereal bits — "Cheerios"
8. Wooden blocks, about 1 inch on a side
9. Narrow neck bottle just large enough to admit cereal bits
10. Crayons and paper
11. Picture book of common objects
12. Small box of facial tissue wipes

Age level and observations or reports of activity:

1 Month

Briefly follows moving stimulus. With infant supine on the examining table, the ring is brought into

view at a distance of about 12 inches with gentle
   agitation.
Regards examiner's face momentarily. Again, while
   the child is supine the examiner approaches 18–
   24 inches within field of vision and quietly speaks
   to infant.
Hold head erect briefly when supported in upright
   position. When supported under the arms in a
   sitting position the infant is able to hold his head
   erect for a brief period of time.
Avoidance of mildly annoying stimuli. With infant
   supine on the examining table a tissue is lightly
   placed over his face. He will cry perhaps and
   vigorously turn from side to side to dislodge the
   tissue.
Lifts head slightly when prone. For short periods of
   time the infant can lift his head by extension.
Quieted when picked up. Frequently, but not invariably when crying or fussy, the infant will become quieter and less active when picked up.

2 Months

Head erect with bobbing when supported in sitting
   position. Head tends to remain erect but some
   wobbling occurs from this position.
Follows moving person. While supported upright on
   parent's lap will follow examiner at about 36
   inches when quietly spoken to.
Vocalization other than crying. Other sounds produced in addition to crying.
Smiles at times. When spoken to or gently stimulated with smile.

3 Months

Eyes follow moving objects in all planes. In supine
   position, the infant will follow the ring with his
   eyes in all planes.
Searches for sound with eyes. When bell is gently
   struck out of the infant's view he will search for
   the source of the sound with his eyes.

Lifts head and chest when prone.

Vigorous body movements. Either spontaneously or
when stimulated vigorous movements of the
arms and legs may be noted.

Anticipates feeding upon sight of the bottle with
activity change or movements of mouth. A
crying or actively kicking child may become less
active or quieter upon sight of the bottle. For
placid infants a glimpse of the bottle may result
in increased activity.

Cooling or chuckling. Vocalization may be spontaneous or as a result of mild stimuli.

4 Months

Grasps pencil with both hands and holds briefly. When
held near or in contact with one hand both may
reach out to grasp pencil.

Follows moving object when held in sitting position.
Sitting on parent's lap infant will follow ring in
all planes with eyes and by turning head also.

Enjoys play activity. Smiles, chuckles or changes
activity when mildly stimulated and appears to
anticipate play activity.

Rolls from side to side but not completely over.

Initiates smiling and laughs aloud. This may be spontaneously or in response to play activity.

6 Months

Sits with minimal support with stable back and head.
No wobbling of head while sitting and the back
is held relatively straight.

Lifts cup. A cup placed before the infant is grasped
and lifted.

Attempts to attain toy held beyond reach. After a
short period of play with some particular toy, it
is moved just out of reach but still within sight.
The infant may maintain his attention on the toy
and makes an effort to recover it by reaching or
crawling.

Responds to image in mirror. While the infant is
supported in a sitting position, a mirror is slowly
brought within about 12 inches of his face. He
responds by reaching, change in activity and/or
vocalization.

Exploits possibilities of play materials. Several toys
are placed before the infant while he is in a sitting
position. He reaches for one or several objects
and may transfer them to his other hand or mouth
or may bang or shake them.

Rolls over, supine to prone position. The infant is
able to roll over from a supine to a prone position.

Babbles in more than two distinct sounds.

Differentiates strangers from family. When crying
can only be comforted by familiar person or re-
sents attention by strangers and may cry or show
other signs of apprehension.

9 Months

Uses thumb to help grasp tiny objects. Cereal bits
placed before the infant may be raked into a
better position but are picked up with the thumbs
opposed to one or several fingers.

Holds and manipulates two objects at a time. From
several toys placed before the infant at least two
are held and banged or transferred or shaken.

Sits alone and can change positions without falling.
Sits without support and from a prone position
can sit up.

Says "mama" or "dada." This item would apply only
if it is clear that some effort had been made to
use these words in play with the infant.

Plays interpersonal games. Can play such games as
peek-a-boo and pat-a-cake roughly following
the proper actions.

12 Months

Hands toy to examiner when requested to do so.
Some time should be allowed for the child to
become familiar with the examiner before this
is attempted. The child may more easily hand a
toy to the parent.

Puts small objects into a cup and removes them
also. After demonstration the child is able to
drop or place rubber stoppers in cup and remove
them also by pouring or by picking them up.

Will retrieve a hidden toy. A familiar toy placed
under a cup, a box or handkerchief is recovered.
The toy is concealed after the child has played
with it for a short while.

Stands with support and takes steps when supported.
The parent may assist in demonstrating this.
While holding to some object the child can stand
and when his hands are held he can take several
steps also.

Words (two or three) in additon to "mama" and
dada." They may be sounds which are used to
indicate specific objects and are understood by
the parent. They may not be conventional words
but have some resemblance to them.

Gives affection. Will hug or kiss the parent either
spontaneously or at their urging.

Holds cup with assistance for taking fluids. Can
manipulate a small tumbler or cup for drinking
with only moderate spillage.

15 Months

Can stack two blocks one on top of the other. This
is done after a demonstration by the examiner.
It is best to remove other toys at this time.

Can imitate placing a small object in a narrow
necked bottle and if demonstrated can "pour"
object out of bottle. The cereal bits are used
for this and the bottle neck should be just large
enough to admit them easily.

Can scribble by imitation. A blank sheet of paper
is used and soft colored pencil or a crayon is used
for marking.

Walks without support. Unsteadiness may persist
with few falls also.

Climbs onto low chair or stairs. If stairs are negoti-
ated this is usually by creeping at this time.

Uses about five words. Words understood by parents
and have some slight resemblance to the actual
word sound.

Shows interest in picture books. May turn pages of
magazine or picture book and shows some evidence of attention to the pictures presented.
The parent may also be asked to turn pages for
the child to look at.

18 Months

Walks well and runs a bit. Rather steady and can run
without falling too frequently.

Can seat self and climb into chair. May climb onto
chair seat, turn around while standing and then
sit down.

Can walk with pull-toy. Manages pull-toy well and
may take pains to keep toy upright.

Can go up and down stairs. Often creeping or combination of creeping and walking on stairs.

Likes to be read to and interested in books with pictures. This is clearly only applicable when the
parents have made some effort to read to the
child.

Bowel training reasonably well established. During
daytime the child will often but not invariably
indicate to the parent when a bowel movement
is about to occur.

About ten words in vocabulary. Handles spoon fairly
well and feeds self partially. Can manage semi-
solid food, like mashed potatoes, with a spoon
but still unsteady with small bits of solid food.

24 Months

Can deal with a few common household mechanical
devices. Child is able to turn a knob to open
doors or turn a water faucet on.

Can identify a few pictures of common objects by
name. Use a young child's picture book including pictures of such common items as dog, cup,
cat, car, baby, ball, train, chair, bed, etc. It may

be wise to test these pictures on some children
considered normal developmentally to be certain of their clarity. Show the picture and ask,
"What is this," or "What does this look like."
Avoid giving any clues as to the identity of the
picture.

Asks for things by a combination of words and ges-
tures. May ask for specific foods or drink, or
need for toilet or some toy, etc.

Can throw or kick a ball.

Walks up and down stairs alone.

If books are available may sit and "read" little
picture books, turning pages for himself.

Makes sentences of two to three words.

Imitates household tasks. May attempt to sweep, or
imitate kitchen jobs that a parent or older sibling is doing.

Parallel play. Engages in play activities similar to
those of playmate but does not indulge in cooperative or reciprocal play.

Day time bowel and bladder control fairly well established.

If the TV is available in home may spontaneously
identify familiar objects seen on the screen.

30 Months

Can imitate vertical and horizontal strokes on paper.
A crayon is best used for this and the examiner
should demonstrate the movements several times
if necessary.

Can fold a $8\frac{1}{2}$ x 11 inch sheet of paper in half to make
a little book when this is demonstrated.

Can repeat two digits read at the rate of one per second, e.g., four-seven, six-eight, three-two, etc.

Can walk on tiptoes and briefly stand on one foot
when this is demonstrated.

Can relate experiences in simple language. May describe trip to the clinic, or to visit a relative or
to a store. Suitable questions may be inquiries
about how child travelled to the clinic, or whether

or not he helps with shopping at store, or a recent visit to the zoo or a fire house, etc.
If taught the child can tell name and age.
Uses pronouns.
Helps to dress and undress himself by means of a
simple assist, e.g., setting foot partially into
shoe, arms through sleeves, unbuttoning or un-
snapping clothes, etc.
Perceives certain dangerous situations; not likely to
walk into a moving swing, aware of the danger
from cars in the street, etc.

36 Months

Can copy a circle from a sample. Colored pencils or
crayon may be used for this. The drawing is not
to be demonstrated but a previously drawn circle
is merely used as a model.
Can repeat three unrelated digits after the examiner
gives all three at once. One should be correct
out of every three trials.
Can relate things to the action they produce, e.g.,
what barks or meows, flies in the sky, swims,
cuts, etc. Any appropriate answer is acceptable.
When asked by the examiner, the child can give his
last name.
Handles much of dressing, including putting on shoes
but not tying them and fastening accessible buttons.
Goes up and down stairs with one foot on each stair.
Can ride tricycle (if he owns one) using pedals.
Understands sharing and taking turns when playing
with others.

SCORING THE INVENTORY

For general use these scales are not intended to provide a
precise developmental age determination. They are primarily
designed to permit the physician to develop an impression of
how a child compares with a sample of his age mates on certain limited developmental measures. Furthermore, the results of this examination must be interpreted in the light of

all other findings relative to the child. Neurological and sensory abnormalities, hyperactivity and cultural deprivation are a few of the factors which may profoundly affect the developmental estimate. And to repeat what has been said many times before, the marked variability of normal human development must always be considered in judging apparent deviations from the scales.

Before scoring the scales exclude those items which are not applicable such as the identification of objects on TV when the family does not own a set. Eliminate those items requiring reporting by parents when they are unable to supply the information.

For the infrequent user, the scales are best used to indicate the age level at which most items are complete and that level where only a few are accomplished. This will provide a gross estimate of the developmental level. With more experience and increased certainty of uniformity in observing and reporting items, actual counts of items can be used for estimating the developmental age. The basal age level is that at which all items are complete or all but one are positive. The number of items in the next age level is divided into the time interval in months to give estimates between specified ages. When completed items are scattered through several age levels they may all be added to give an estimate of the developmental age. However, since the number of items per time period is not constant at all age levels some interpretations of the total item counts is necessary in order to account for this discrepancy. (From Caldwell, B.M. and Drachman, R.H.: Comparability of the three methods of assessing the developmental level of young infants. Pediatrics 34:51-57, July, 1964. Reproduced with permission of American Academy of Pediatrics.)

Appendix I

DENVER DEVELOPMENTAL SCREENING
TEST (REVISED)*

The Denver Developmental Screening Test (DDST), a device
for detecting developmental delays in infancy and the preschool years, has been standardized on a large cross section
of the Denver population. The test is administered with ease
and speed and lends itself to serial evaluations on the same
test sheet.

TEST MATERIALS

Skein of red wool, box of raisins, rattle with narrow handle,
Abbott aspirin bottle (Abbott-50 children's aluminum), bell,
tennis ball, test form, pencil, eight 1-in. cubical counting
blocks.

GENERAL ADMINISTRATION INSTRUCTIONS

The mother should be told that this is a developmental
screening device to obtain an estimate of the child's level

---

*Prepared by William K. Frankenburg and Josiah B. Dodds,
University of Colorado Medical Center, Denver, Colorado;
reprinted with permission of the authors.

of development. This test relies on observations of what the
child can do and on report by a parent who knows the child.
Direct observation should be used whenever possible. Since
the test requires active participation by the child, every effort should be made to put the child at ease. The child above
6 months of age may be tested while sitting on the mother's
lap. This should be done in such a way that he can comfort-
ably reach the test materials on the table. The test should
be administered before any frightening or painful procedures.
A child will often withdraw if the examiner rushes demands
on the child. One may start by laying out one or two test
items in front of the child while asking the mother whether
he performs some of the personal-social items. It is best to
administer the first few test items well below the child's age
level in order to assure him an initial successful experience.
It is best to remove all test materials from the table, except
the one that is being administered, to avoid distractions.

STEPS IN ADMINISTERING THE TEST

1. Draw a vertical line on the examination sheet through the
   four sectors (Gross Motor, Fine Motor-Adaptive, Language,
   and Personal-Social) to represent the child's chronological
   age. Place the date of the examination at the top of the
   age line. For premature children, subtract the months
   prematurity from the chronological age. After 2 years of
   age it is no longer necessary to compensate for prematurity.
2. The items to be administered are those through which the
   child's chronological age line passes unless there are obvious deviations. In each sector one should establish the
   area where the child passes all of the items and the point
   at which he fails all of the items.
3. In the event that a child refuses to do some of the items
   requested by the examiner, it is suggested that the parent
   administer the item, provided she does so in the prescribed manner.
4. If a child passes an item, a large letter "P" is written on
   the bar at the 50% passing point. "F" designates a failure,
   and "R" designates a refusal.

5. Note how the child adjusted to the examination, that is, his cooperation, attention span, self-confidence, and how he related to his mother, the examiner and the test materials.
6. Ask the parent if the child's performance was typical of his performance at other times.
7. To retest the child on the same form, use a different color pencil for the scoring and age line.
8. Instructions for administering footnoted items are on the back of the test form.

INTERPRETATIONS

The test items are placed in four categories: Gross Motor, Fine Motor-Adaptive, Language, and Personal-Social. each of the test items is designated by a bar which is so located under the age scale as to indicate clearly the ages at which 25%, 50%, 75%, and 90% of the standardization population

| (25%) | (50%) | (75%) | (90%) |

could perform the particular test item. The left end of the bar designates the age at which 25% of the standardization population could perform the item; the hatch mark at the top of the bar, 50%; the left end of the shaded area, 75%; and the right end of the bar the age at which 90% of the standardization population could perform the items.

Failure to pass an item passed by 90% of children should be considered significant. Such a failure may be emphasized by coloring the right end of the bar of the failed item. Several failures in one sector are considered to be developmental delays. These delays may be due to:

1. The unwillingness of the child to use his ability
   a) due to temporary phenomena, such as fatigue, illness, hospitalization, separation from the parent, fear, and so forth,
   b) general unwillingness to do most things that are asked of him—such a condition may be just as detrimental as an inability to perform;

2. An inability to perform the item due to
    a) general retardation,
    b) pathological factors such as deafness or neurological impairment,
    c) familial pattern of slow development in one or more areas. If unexplained developmental delays are noted and are a valid reflection of a child's abilities, he should be rescreened one month later. If the delays persist, he should be further evaluated with more detailed diagnostic studies.

CAUTION

The DDST is not an intelligence test. It is intended as a screening instrument for use in clinical practice to note whether the development of a particular child is within the normal range.

1. Try to get child to smile by smiling, talking or waving to him. Do not touch him.
2. When child is playing with toy, pull it away from him. Pass if he resists.
3. Child does not have to be able to tie shoes or button in the back.
4. Move yarn slowly in an arc from one side to the other, about 6" above child's face. Pass if eyes follow 90° to midline. (Past midline; 180°)
5. Pass if child grasps rattle when it is touched to the backs or tips of fingers.
6. Pass if child continues to look where yarn disappeared or tries to see where it went. Yarn should be dropped quickly from sight from tester's hand without arm movement.
7. Pass if child picks up raisin with any part of thumb and a finger.
8. Pass if child picks up raisin with the ends of thumb and index finger using an overhand approach.

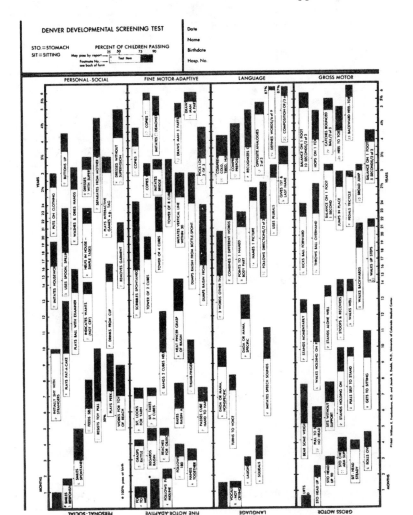

9. Pass any enclosed form. Fail continuous round motions

10. Which line is longer? (Not bigger.) Turn paper upside down and repeat. (3/3 or 5/6)

11. Pass any crossing lines.

12. Have child copy first. If failed, demonstrate

When giving items 9, 11 and 12, do not name the forms. Do not demonstrate 9 and 11.

13. When scoring, each pair (2 arms, 2 legs, etc.) counts as one part.

14. Point to picture and have child name it. (No credit is given for sounds only.)

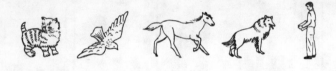

15. Tell child to: Give block to mommie; put block on table; put block on floor. Pass 2 of 3. (Do not help child by pointing, moving head or eyes.)

16. Ask child: What do you do when you are cold? ..hungry? ..tired? Pass 2 of 3.

17. Tell child to: Put block <u>on</u> table; <u>under</u> table; <u>in front of</u> chair; <u>behind</u> chair. Pass 3 of 4. (Do not help child by pointing, moving head or eyes.)

18. Ask child: If fire is hot, ice is? Pass 2 of 3.

19. Ask child: What is a ball? ..lake? ..desk? ..house? ..banana? ..curtain? ..ceiling? ..hedge? ..pavement? Pass if defined in terms of use, shape, what it is made of or general category (such as banana is fruit, not just jellow). Pass 6 of 9.

20. Ask child: What is a spoon made of? ..a shoe made of?
..a door made of? (No other objects may be substituted.)
Pass 3 of 3.

21. When placed on stomach, child lifts chest off table with
support of forearms and/or hands.

22. When child is on back, grasp his hands and pull him to
sitting. Pass if head does not hang back.

23. Child may use wall or rail only, not person. May not
crawl.

24. Child must throw ball overhand 3 feet to within arm's
reach of tester.

25. Child must perform standing broad jump over width of
test sheet. ($8\frac{1}{2}$ in.)

26. Tell child to walk forward, ∞∞∞∞➤   heel within 1
inch of toe. Tester may demonstrate. Child must walk
4 consecutive steps, 2 out of 3 trials.

27. Bounce ball to child who should stand 3 feet away from
tester. Child must catch ball with hands, not arms, 2
out of 3 trials.

28. Tell child to walk backward, ◀∞∞∞∞   to within 1
inch of heel. Tester may demonstrate. Child must walk
4 consecutive steps, 2 out of 3 trials.

Date and behavioral observations (how child feels at time of
test, relation to tester, attention span, verbal behavior, self-
confidence, etc.):

Appendix J

NOMOGRAM FOR ESTIMATION OF SURFACE AREA*

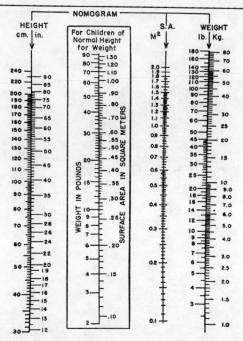

*The surface area is indicated where a straight line connects the height and weight levels intersects the surface area column; or if the patient is roughly of average size, from the weight alone (enclosed area). (Nomogram modified from data of E. Boyd by C.D. West) From Nelson, W.E., Ed.: Textbook of Pediatrics, 9th Ed., W.B. Saunders Co., Philadelphia, 1969. (Reproduced with publisher's permission.)

Appendix K

NORMAL LABORATORY VALUES

A. HEMATOLOGICAL

1. Peripheral blood tests:
   a) Hematocrit: Male: 38–54%
   Female: 36–47%
   Newborn: 53–73%
   b) Hemoglobin: Male: 14–18 g%
   Female: 12–16 g%
   Newborn: 16–22 g%
   3 months: 11.5 g%
   c) WBC count: Newborn: 7000–35,000/cu mm
   1 month: 6000–18,000/ cu mm
   1 year: 6000–15,000/cu mm
   2–12 yrs: 5000–12,000/cu mm
   d) White cell differential:
   Newborn: 45–85% neutrophils
   Less than 6 years: 30–50% neutrophils
   More than 6 years: 40–60% neutrophils
   e) Eosinophils: Absolute Count
   100–600/cu mm, mean = 250/cu mm
   f) Reticulocytes: Newborn: 2.5–6.5%
   greater than 1 year: 0.5–1.0%
   g) Platelet count: 200,000–300,000/cu mm

h) RBC measurements
- **(1)** Diameter: Newborn: 8.5μ
                                            Children: 5.5–8.8μ
- **(2)** Mean corpuscular   Newborn: 106 cuμ
      volume: Children: 80–94 cuμ
- **(3)** Mean corpuscular   Newborn: 38 pg
      Hb: Children: 27–32 pg
- **(4)** Mean corpuscular
      Hb conc.:   33–38%

2. Coagulation tests:
- **a)** Bleeding time   1–3 minutes (Duke)
                                            2–4 minutes (Ivy)
- **b)** Coagulation time   6–12 minutes (Lee-White)
                                            10–30 minutes (Howell)
- **c)** Clot retraction time   2–4 hr
- **d)** Prothrombin time   70–110% of control
- **e)** Sedimentation rate   Male: 0–8 mm/hr (Wintrobe)
                                            Female: 0–15 mm/hr (Wintrobe)
                                            Children: 4–13 mm/hr (Wintrobe)
- **f)** Erythrocyte fragility   0.44–0.35% NaCl
- **g)** Fetal hemoglobin
      Birth: 60–90%
      1 year: 2%

B. BLOOD CHEMISTRIES

1. Serum electrolytes
- **a)** Calcium   4.5–5.7 mEq/L (9–11.5 mg%)
- **b)** Chloride   99–109 mEq/L (348–387 mg%)
- **c)** Magnesium   1.5–2.4 mEq/L (1.8–2.9 mg%)
- **d)** Phosphorus   2.3–3.8 mEq/L (4–6.5 mg%)
- **e)** Potassium   3.6–5.5 mEq/L (14–21.5 mg%)
- **f)** Sodium   135–151 mEq/L (310–356 mg%)

2. Enzymes (serum)
- **a)** Amylase   60–150 U (Somogyi)
- **b)** Lipase   0.2–1.5 U/ml
- **c)** Acid
      phosphatase   0.1–1.0 U (Bodansky)

3. Alkaline phosphatase
   a) Infants: ≤ 14 Bodansky U
   b) Adolescents: ≤ 5 Bodansky U
   c) Adults: 2.0-4.5 Bodansky U
4. Transaminase
   a) SGOT (serum glutamic oxalacetic)
      (1) Newborn (up to first week) 10-120 units
      (2) After first 3 months 10-40 units
   b) SGPT (serum glutamic pyruvic)
      (1) Newborn (up to first week) 10-90 U
      (2) Afterwards 5-45 U
5. LDH (lactic dehydrogenase) 200-600 U/ml
6. Serum proteins
   a) Albumin (serum)
      (1) Newborn: 2.4-5.5 g%
      (2) 1-3 months: 3-4.2 g%
      (3) Afterwards: 3-5 g%
   b) Globulin (serum)
      (1) Newborn: 1.2-4 g%
      (2) 1-3 months: 1-3.3 g%
      (3) Afterwards: 2-4.4 g%
   c) Total protein
      (1) Newborn: 4-6 g%
      (2) 1-3 months: 4.7-7.4 g%
      (3) Afterwards: 6-8.6 g%
   d) Fibrinogen (plasma):   0.22-0.32 g%
   e) Mucoproteins (tyrosine)   1.9-4.5 mg%
   f) Protein electrophoresis

	Mean	Range
(1) Albumin:	58%	45-70%
(2) Alphaglobulin	14%	7-15%
(a) Alpha 1	7.5%	5-10%
(b) Alpha 2	3.5%	2-5%
(3) Betaglobulin	13%	8-14%
(4) Gamma globulin	11%	10-17%
(5) Fibrinogen	4%	2-5%

g) Immunoglobulin levels (serum)

		IGG (mg/ 100 ml)	IGM (mg/ 100 ml)	IGA (mg/ 100 ml)	Total
(1)	9–11 years:	889–1359	46–112	71–191	1080–1588
(2)	12–16 years:	822–1170	39–79	85–211	984–1322
(3)	Adult:	853–1563	72–126	139–261	1104–1810

C. MISCELLANEOUS

1. Bicarbonate or CO_2 combining power	22–30 mEq/L
2. Bilirubin, total (serum)	less than 1 mg%
3. Carbon dioxide content (plasma)	25–33 mEq/L 55–75 vol %
4. pH (serum, arterial) (venous pH is 0.03 lower)	7.35–7.45
5. Carotene (serum)	60–180 mEq%
6. Cholesterol total (serum)	Adolescent: 120–210 mg/ 100 ml Adult: 140–250 mg/100 ml
7. Cholesterol esters (serum)	65–75% of total
8. Cortisol, free (urine)	Adolescent: 5–55 mg/100 ml Adult: 18–90 mg/100 ml Children: 0.3–1.1 mg/100 ml
9. Creatine (serum)	0.17–0.93 mg%
10. Creatinine (serum)	Children: 0.3–1 mg/100 ml Adolescent: 0.5–1.0 mg/ 100 ml Adult male: 0.6–1.2 mg/ 100 ml Adult female: 0.5–1.1 mg/ 100 ml
Creatinine (urine)	Adolescent: 8–30 mg/kg/ 100 ml Adult: 14–26 mg/kg/100 ml
11. Glucose (whole blood)	60–100 mg/100 ml
12. Icteric index	3–8 U
13. Iodine (protein bound) (serum)	4–8 µg/100 ml

14. Iron (serum)   50–180 µg/100 ml
15. Iron binding capacity (serum)   300–360 µg/100 ml
16. Lactic acid (whole blood)   6–20%
17. Lead (whole blood)   0.001–0.04 mg%
18. Lipids
    a) Total (serum or plasma)   400–900 mg%
    b) Phospholipids (serum
       or plasma   Average 225 mg%
                                          Range 125–300 mg%
19. Nonprotein nitrogen (whole
    blood)   25–40 mg%
20. Testosterone (blood)   Adolescent male: 10 mg/
                                          100 ml
                                          Adult male: 0.3–1.0 mg/
                                          100 ml
                                          Adult female: 0–0.1 mg/
                                          100 ml (Average: 0.04)
    Testosterone (urine)   Adolescent male: 47–156
                                          mg/24 hr (Average 70)
                                          Adult male: 0–15 mg/24 hr
                                          (Average < 6)
21. Triglycerides (serum)   Adolescent: 30–150 mg/
                                          100 ml
                                          Adult male: 40–160 mg/
                                          100 ml
                                          Adult female: 35–135 mg/
                                          100 ml
22. Urea (whole blood)   22–40 mg%
23. Urea nitrogen (whole blood)   10–18 mg%
24. Uric acid (serum)   2.5–6.0 mg%
25. Vitamin A   More than 40 µg/%

D. FLOCCULATION TESTS

1. Cephalin flocculation   0–1+
2. Takata ArA test   negative
3. Thymol turbidity   0–4 U
4. Zinc sulfate turbidity   less than 4 U

E. BLOOD GASES

1. pO_2 (arterial, whole blood) 95–100 mmHg
2. pCO_2 (arterial, whole blood) 35–45 mmHg

F. SEROLOGY

1. ASLO titer	less than 50
2. CRP	Negative
3. Heterophile agglutination test	less than 1 to 56
4. Typhoid O or H antigens	less than 1 to 80
5. Paratyphoid A and B antigens	less than 1 to 80

G. URINE

1. pH	–6 (4.8–8.5)
2. Specific gravity (normal range)	1.015–1.025 (Physiological range) 1.003–1.030
3. 17-Hydroxycorticosteroids	2–7 mg/24 hr
4. 17-Ketosteroids	
a) Males	2–25 mg/24 hr
b) Females	1–15 mg/24 hr
c) Children (less than 8 years)	0.8–2.0 mg/24 hr
d) Adolescents	2.0–20.0 mg/24 hr
5. Creatinine	15–25 mg/kg/24 hr
6. Urine volume	Adolescent: 700–1400 mg/ 100 ml
	Adult male: 800–2000 mg/ 100 ml
	Adult female: 800–1600 mg/100 ml
7. Nitrogen	10–15 g/24 hr
8. Protein (albumin)	0.025–0.07 g/24 hr
9. Urea nitrogen	6–17 g/24 hr
10. Ketones	0.3–1.0 g/24 hr
11. Urobilinogen	0–4 µg/24 hr
12. Catecholamines	
a) Epinephrine	less than 10 µg/24 hr
b) Norepinephrine	less than 100 µg/24 hr
c) VMA (Vanillylmandelic acid)	1.8–9 mg/24 hr

H. KIDNEY FUNCTION TESTS

1. Urea clearance standard—
maximum—
     40-65 ml/min
     60-90 ml/min

2. Concentration test
specific gravity   1.025-1.032
after withholding fluids 10
hours or more

3. Dilution test
specific gravity   1.001-1.003
after administering 20-30
ml/kg of water
Maximum—1000 ml in 30-
45 minutes

4. Creatinine clearance
90-130 ml/min/1.73 m^2 of body
surface.
Newborns 40-65 ml/min/1.73 m^2

5. Addis count

a) Children	RBC	1 million/24 hr
	WBC	2 million/24 hr
	Casts	10,000/24 hr
b) Newborn	RBC	600,000/24 hr
	WBC	13 million/24 hr
	Casts	400,000/24 hr

I. CEREBROSPINAL FLUID

1. Amount
  a) Newborn   5 ml
  b) Adults   100-140 ml

2. Appearance, clear, colorless

3. Pressure
  a) Newborn   30-90 mm CSF
  b) Infant   40-150 mm CSF
  c) Child   50-200 mm CSF

4. Specific gravity   1003-1009

5. pH   7.33-7.42

6. Cell count
  a) Newborn   up to 25 WBC and 650
                      RBC/cu mm
  b) Children   up to 10 WBC/cu mm (all
                      lymphocytes)

7. Glucose	40–80 mg% (more than or equal to 50% of the blood sugar)
8. Chlorides	120–130 mEq/L
9. Total protein	
a) Children	5–45 mg%
b) Newborn	5–150 mg%
10. Globulin	4–10 mg%
11. Albumin	16–35 mg%

SUGGESTED READINGS

INFANT AND CHILD HEALTH CARE

GROWTH AND DEVELOPMENT

Barnes, H.V.: Physical growth and development during puberty. *Med Clin North Am* 59:1305, 1975.
Greulich, W.W., and Pyle, S.L.: *Radiographic Atlas of Skeletal Development of the Hand and Wrist,* 2nd ed., Stanford University Press, Stanford, CA, 1959.
Marshall, W.A., and Tanner, J.M.: Variations in the pattern of pubertal changes in girls. *Arch Dis Child* 45:291, 1969.
Marshall, W.A., and Tanner, J.M.: Variations in the pattern of pubertal changes in boys. *Arch Dis Child* 45:13, 1970.
Tanner, J.M.: *Growth at Adolescence,* 2nd ed., Blackwell Scientific Publications, Oxford, 1962.

FEEDING

Committee on Nutrition, American Academy of Pediatrics: Composition of milks. *Pediatrics* 26:1039, 1960.
Committee on Nutrition, American Academy of Pediatrics: *Pediatric Nutrition Handbook,* Chicago, IL, 1979.
Feingold, B.F.: Food additives and child development. *Hosp Pract* 8:11, 1973

Fomon, S.J.: *Infant Nutrition,* 2nd ed., W.B. Saunders, Philadelphia, PA, 1974.

McMillan, J.A., Landau, S.A., and Oski, F.A.: Iron deficiency in breastfed infants and the availability of iron from human milk. *Pediatrics* 58:686, 1976.

NUTRITION

Suskind, R.M., and Varma, R.N.: Assessment of nutritional status of children. In McKay, R.J. Jr. (Ed.): *Peds in Rev* 5:195, 1984.

COMMON COMMUNICABLE DISEASES

CHICKEN POX

Brunell, P.A.: Protection against varicella. *Pediatrics* 59:1, 1977.

EXANTHEM SUBITUM

Letchner, A.: Roseola infantum: A review of 50 cases. *Lancet* 2:1163, 1955.

DIPHTHERIA

Committee on Infectious Diseases, American Academy of Pediatrics: Edition 19. Evanston, IL, 1982.

Pappenheimer, A.M., Jr., and Gill, D.M.: Diphtheria. *Science* 182:353, 1973.

PERTUSSIS

Linnemann, C.C., Jr., Partin, J.C., Perlstein, P.H., et al.: Pertussis: Persistent problems. *J Pediatr* 85:589, 1974.

Nelson, J.D.: The changing epidemiology of pertussis in young infants. *Am J Dis Child* 132:371, 1978.

MEASLES

Krugman, S.: Present status of measles and rubella immunization in the United States: A medical progress report. *J Pediatr* 90:1, 1977.

Moolin, J.F., Jabbour, J.T., Witte, J.T., and Halsey, N.A.:
Epidemiologic studies of measles, measles vaccine, and
subacute sclerosing panencephalitis. *Pediatrics* 59:505,
1977.

MUMPS

Hayden, G.F., Prebulb, S.R., Orenstein, W.A., and Conrad,
J.L.: Current status of mumps and mumps vaccine in the
United States. *Pediatrics* 62:965, 1978.
Sultz, H.A., Hart, B.A., Zielezny, M., and Schlesinger, E.R.:
Is mumps virus an etiologic factor in juvenile diabetes
mellitus? *J Pediatr* 86:654, 1975.

RUBELLA

Cooper, L.Z.: Congenital Rubella in the United States. In
Krugman, S., and Gershon, A.A. (Eds.), *Infections of the
Fetus and Newborn Infant: Progress in Clinical and
Biological Research,* vol. 3, Alan R. Liss, New York,
NY, 1975.
Green, R.H., Balsamo, S.R., Giles, J.P., et al.: Studies of
the natural history and prevention of rubella. *Am J
Dis Child* 110:348, 1965.

COMMON INFECTIONS

PARASITE INFESTATIONS

Amin, N.: Giardiasis. *Postgrad Med J* 66:151-158, 1979.
Belding, D.L.: *Textbook of Parasitology,* 3rd ed., Appleton-
Century-Crofts, New York, NY, 1965.
Katz, M.: Parasitic infections. *J Pediatr* 87:165-178, 1975.
Most, H., and Shookoff, H.B.: *Helminthic Infections.*
Forum on Infections 2:1, 1975, Biomedical Information
Corporation, New York, NY.
Papovich, N.G.: Pinworm infection and its treatment.
Indiana Pharmacist Feb, 1975.
Rajkumar, S., St. John, A., Laude, T.A., Reddy, R.K.,
Rao, A.B., and Rajagopal, V.: Gastrointestinal parasit-
ic infestation in urban population. *NY State J Med*
80(5):763-766, 1980.

COMMON SKIN DISEASES

Hurwitz, S.: *Clinical Pediatric Dermatology.* W.B. Saunders, Philadelphia, PA, 1981.

Laude, T.A., and Russo, R.M.: *Dermatologic Disorders in Black Children and Adolescents.* Medical Examination Publishing Co., New Hyde Park, NY, 1983.

Laude, T.A., Shah, B.R., and Lynfield, Y.: Tinea capitis in Brooklyn. *Am J Dis Child* 136:1047-1050, 1982.

Solomon, L.M.: The management of congenital melanocytic nevi. *Arch Dermatol* 116:1017, 1980.

Solomon, L.M., and Esterly, N.B.: *Neonatal Dermatology.* W.B. Saunders, Philadelphia, PA, 1973.

BRONCHIOLITIS

Wohl, M.E.B., and Chernick, V.: State of the art: Bronchiolitis. *Am Rev Resp Dis* 118:759, 1978.

CROUP

Leipzig, B., Oski, F.A., Cummings, C.W., et al.: A prospective randomized study to determine the efficacy of steroids in the treatment of croup. *J Pediatr* 94:194, 1979.

PNEUMONIA (BACTERIAL)

Cerutl, E., Contrevas, J., and Neira, M.: Staphylococcal pneumonia in childhood: Long-term follow-up including pulmonary function studies. *Am J Dis Child* 122:386, 1971.

Klein, J.O., and Mortimer, E.A.: Use of pneumococcal vaccine in children. *Pediatrics* 61:31, 1978.

BOTULISM

Gunn, R.A., and Terranova, W.A.: Botulism in the United States, 1977. *Rev Infect Dis* 1:722, 1979.

Brown, L.W.: Differential diagnosis of infant botulism. *Rev Infect Dis* 1:625, 1979.

RICKETTSIAL DISEASE

Horsfall, F.L., Jr., and Tamm, I. (Eds.): *Viral and Rickettsial Infections of Man.* J.B. Lippincott, Co., Philadelphia, PA, 1965.

STREP AND SCARLET FEVER

Breese, B.B., Disney, F.A., Tapley, W., et al.: Streptococcal infections in children. *Am J Dis Child* 128:457, 1974.

OSTEOMYELITIS

Waldrogel, F.A., and Vasey, J.: Osteomyelitis: The past decade. *N Engl J Med* 303:360, 1980.

SEPTIC ARTHRITIS

Eyre-Brook, A.L.: Septic arthritis. *J Bone Joint Surg* 42B: 11, 1960.

MYCOPLASMA PNEUMONIA

Fernald, G.W., Collier, A.M., and Clyde, W.A., Jr.: Respiratory infections due to mycoplasma pneumoniae in infants and children. *Pediatrics* 55:327, 1975.

EPIGLOTTITIS

Bates, J.R.: Epiglottitis: Diagnosis and treatment. In Haggerty, R.J. (Ed.): *Peds in Rev* 1:173, 1979.
Faden, H.S.: Treatment of hemophilus influenzae type B epiglottitis. *Pediatrics* 63:402, 1979.
Rapkin, R.H.: The diagnosis of epiglottitis: Simplicity and reliability of radiographs of the neck in differential diagnosis of the croup syndrome. *J Pediatr* 80:96, 1975.

HEPATITIS

Alter, H.J., Purcell, R.H., Feinstone, S.M., et al.: Non A Non B Hepatitis: A Review and Interim Report of an Ongoing Prospective Study. In Vyas, G.N., Cohen, S.N., and Schmid, R. (Eds.): *Viral Hepatitis.* Franklin Institute Press, Philadelphia, PA, 1978.

Krugman, S., and Gocke, D.J.: *Viral Hepatitis.* W.B. Saunders, Philadelphia, PA, 1978.

Krugman, S., Ward, R., and Katz, S.L.: *Infectious Diseases of Children*, 6th ed., C.V. Mosby Co., St. Louis, MO, 1977.

Reesink, H.W., Reesink-Brongers, E.E., Lafeber-Shut, B.J.T., et al.: Prevention of chronic HBsAg positive mothers by hepatitis B immunoglobulin. *Lancet* 2:436, 1979.

GENERAL INFORMATION

Eichenwald, H.F., and McCracken, G.H.: Antimicrobial therapy in infants and children. *J Pediatr* 93:337, 1978.

Feigen, R., and Cherry, J.: *Textbook of Pediatric Infectious Diseases.* W.B. Saunders, Philadelphia, PA, 1981.

Hoekelman, R., Levin, E.B., Shapira, M.B., and Sutherland, S.A.: Potential bacteremia in pediatric practice. *Am J Dis Child* 133:1017, 1979.

McCracken, G.H., Jr., and Nelson, J.D.: *Antimicrobial Therapy for Newborns.* Grune & Stratton, New York, NY, 1977.

INFECTIOUS MONONUCLEOSIS

Henlew, H.: Observations on childhood infections with EBV. *J Infect Dis* 121:303, 1970.

Hoagland, R.J.: *Infectious Mononucleosis.* Grune & Stratton, New York, NY, 1967.

MENINGITIS

Haggerty, R.J., and Ziai, M.: Acute bacterial meningitis. *Adv Pediatr* 13:129, 1964.

Lewin, E.B.: Partially treated meningitis. *Am J Dis Child* 128:145, 1974.

TBC

Lincoln, E.M., and Sewell, E.M.: *Tuberculosis in Children.* McGraw-Hill, New York, NY, 1963.

HERPES SIMPLEX

Wolontis, S., and Jeansson, S.: Correlation of herpes simplex virus types 1 & 2 with clinical features of infection. *J Infect Dis* 135:28, 1977.

H. INFLUENZAE

Jacobsen, J.A., McCormick, J.B., Hayes, P., et al.: Epidemiologic characteristics of infections caused by ampicillin resistant hemophilus influenzae. *Pediatrics* 58: 388, 1976.

COMMON SURGICAL PROBLEMS

INGUINAL HERNIA

Santulli, T.V., and Shaw, A.: Inguinal hernia: Infancy and childhood. *JAMA* 176:110, 1961.

UMBILICAL HERNIA

Halpern, L.J.: Spontaneous healing of umbilical hernia. *JAMA* 182:851, 1962.

MENINGOCELE

Ames, M.D., and Schut, L.: Results of treatment of 171 consecutive myelomeningoceles, 1963-1968. *Pediatrics* 50:466, 1972.

CRYPTORCHIDISM

Allen, T.D.: Cryptorchidism. In McKay, R.J. Jr. (Ed.). *Peds in Rev* 5:317, 1984.

APPENDICITIS

Holgersen, L.O., and Stanley-Brown, E.G.: Acute appendicitis with perforation. *Am J Dis Child* 122:288, 1971.

EMERGENCY CARE

CARBON MONOXIDE TOXICITY

Zarem, H.A., Rattenborg, C.C., and Harmel, M.H.: Carbon monoxide toxicity in human fire victims. *Arch Surg* 107:851, 1973.

DROWNING

Griffin, G.E.: Near drowning: Its pathophysiology and treatment in man. *Milit Med* 131:12, 1966.

CARDIOPULMONARY ARREST

Reece, R.M. (Ed.): *Manual of Emergency Pediatrics,* 2nd ed., W.B. Saunders, Philadelphia, PA, 1978.

SIDS

Beckwith, J.B.: *The Sudden Infant Death Syndrome.* DHEW, Pub. No. (HSA) 75:5137, 1975.

BURNS

Guzzetta, P.C., and Randolph, J.: Burns in children: 1982. In Haggerty, R.J. (Ed.). *Peds in Rev* 4:271, 1983.

ACCIDENTAL POISONING

GENERAL POISONING

Arena, J.M.: *Poisoning, Toxicology, Symptoms, Treatments,* 4th ed., Charles C Thomas, Springfield, IL, 1979.
Goodman, A.G., Goodman, L.S., and Gilman, A.: *The Pharmacological Basis of Therapeutics,* 6th ed., Macmillan, New York, NY, 1980.

ACETAMINOPHEN

Rumack, B.H., Peterson, R.C., Koch, G.G., et al.: Acetaminophen overdosage. *Arch Int Med* 141:380, 1981.

SALICYLATES

Done, A.K.: Aspirin overdosage: Incidence, diagnosis, and management. *Pediatrics* 62:890, 1978, (Suppl.).

HYDROCARBONS

Baldachin, B.J., and Melmed, R.N.: Clinical and therapeutic aspects of kerosene poisoning: A series of 200 cases. *Br Med J* 2:28, 1964.

ALKALI

Haller, J.A., Andrew, H.G., White, J.J., et al.: Pathophysiology and management of acute corrosive burns of the esophagus: Results of treatment of 285 children. *J Pediatr Surg* 6:578, 1971.

IRON

Covey, T.J.: Ferrous sulfate poisoning: A review, case summaries and therapeutic regimen. *J Pediatr* 64:218, 1964.

LEAD

Chisholm, J.J., Jr., and Barltrop, D.: Recognition and management of children with increased lead absorption. *Arch Dis Child* 32:249, 1979.

LONG TERM MANAGEMENT PROBLEMS

HYPERTENSION SCREENING

Goldring, D., Hernandez, A., Choi, S., et al.: Blood pressure in a high school population. Clinical profile of the juvenile hypertensive. *J Pediatr* 95:298, 1979.

Loggie, J.M.H. (Ed.): Symposium on hypertension in childhood and adolescence. *Pediatr Clin North Am* 25(1): Feb 1978.

Report of the task force on blood pressure control in children. *Pediatrics* 59:797, 1977, (Suppl.).

COMMON DIAGNOSTIC PROBLEMS

ABDOMINAL MASS

D'Angio, G.J.: Wilms' Tumor and Neuroblastoma in Children. In McKay, R.J. Jr. (Ed.). *Peds in Rev* 6:10, 1984.

COMMON ORTHOPEDIC PROBLEMS

SCOLIOSIS SCREENING

Berwick, D.M.: Scoliosis Screening. In McKay, R.J. Jr. (Ed.). *Peds in Rev* 5:238, 1984.
Jones, M.C.: Clinical Approach to the Child with Scoliosis. In McKay, R.J. Jr. (Ed.). *Peds in Rev* 6:219, 1985.

ORTHOPEDIC PROBLEMS IN GENERAL

Blockey, N.J.: *Children's Orthopaedics. Practical Problems.* Butterworths, London, 1976.
Lovell, W.W., and Winter, R.B.: *Pediatric Orthopedics.* J.B. Lippincott, Co., Philadelphia, PA, 1972.

CONGENITAL HIP DISLOCATION

Coleman, S.S.: *Congenital Dysplasia and Dislocation of the Hip.* C.V. Mosby Co., St. Louis, MO, 1978.

SLIPPED FEMORAL EPIPHYSIS

Jacobs, B.: Diagnosis and Natural History of Slipped Femoral Capital Epiphysis. In *The American Academy of Orthopedic Surgeons Instructional Course Lectures,* vol. 21. C.V. Mosby Co., St. Louis, MO, 1972.

INDEX

PRODUCT INFORMATION

Tavist®

(clemastine) Syrup 0.5 mg - 5 ml (present as clemastine fumarate 0.67 mg/5 ml)

DESCRIPTION: Each teaspoonful (5 ml) of TAVIST® (clemastine fumarate) Syrup for oral administration contains clemastine 0.5 mg (present as clemastine fumarate 0.67 mg). Other ingredients: alcohol 5.5%, flavors, methylparaben, propylene glycol, propylparaben, purified water, saccharin sodium, sorbitol in a buffered solution. TAVIST (clemastine fumarate) belongs to the benzhydryl ether group of antihistaminic compounds. The chemical name is (+)-(2R)-2-[2-[[(R)-p-Chloro-α-methyl-α-phenylbenzyl]-oxy]-ethyl]-1-methylpyrrolidine fumarate.

Clemastine fumarate occurs as a colorless to faintly yellow, practically odorless, crystalline powder. TAVIST (clemastine fumarate) Syrup has an approximate pH of 6.2.

CLINICAL PHARMACOLOGY: TAVIST (clemastine fumarate) is an antihistamine with anticholinergic (drying) and sedative side effects. Antihistamines competitively antagonize various physiological effects of histamine including increased capillary permeability and dilatation, the formation of edema, the "flare" and "itch" response, and gastrointestinal and respiratory smooth muscle constriction. Within the vascular tree, H_1-receptor antagonists inhibit both the vasoconstrictor and vasodilator effects of histamine. Depending on the dose, H_1-receptor antagonists can produce CNS stimulation or depression. Most antihistamines exhibit central and/or peripheral anticholinergic activity. Antihistamines act by competitively blocking H_1-receptor sites. Antihistamines do not pharmacologically antagonize or chemically inactivate histamine, nor do they prevent the release of histamine.

PHARMACOKINETICS: Antihistamines are well-absorbed following oral administration. Chlorpheniramine maleate, clemastine fumarate, and diphenhydramine hydrochloride achieve peak blood levels within 2-5 hours following oral administration. The absorption of antihistamines is often partially delayed by the use of controlled release dosage forms. In these instances, plasma concentrations from identical doses of the immediate and controlled release dosage forms will not be similar.

Tissue distribution of the antihistamines in humans has not been established.

Antihistamines appear to be metabolized in the liver chiefly via mono- and didemethylation and glucuronide conjugation. Antihistamine metabolites and small amounts of unchanged drug are excreted in the urine. Small amounts of the drugs may also be excreted in breast milk.

In normal human subjects who received histamine injections over a 24-hour period, the antihistaminic activity of TAVIST (clemastine fumarate) reached a peak at 5-7 hours, persisted for 10-12 hours and, in some cases, for as long as 24 hours. Pharmacokinetic studies in man utilizing ^{3}H and ^{14}C labeled compound demonstrates that: TAVIST (clemastine fumarate) is rapidly absorbed from the gastrointestinal tract, peak plasma concentrations are attained in 2-4 hours, and urinary excretion is the major mode of elimination.

INDICATIONS AND USAGE: TAVIST (clemastine fumarate) Syrup is indicated for the relief of symptoms associated with allergic rhinitis such as sneezing, rhinorrhea, pruritus and lacrimation. TAVIST (clemastine fumarate) Syrup is indicated for use in pediatric populations (age 6 years through 12) and adults (see *DOSAGE AND ADMINISTRATION*).

It should be noted that TAVIST (clemastine fumarate) is indicated for the relief of mild uncomplicated allergic skin manifestations of urticaria and angioedema at the 2 mg dosage level only.

CONTRAINDICATIONS: Antihistamines are contraindicated in patients hypersensitive to the drug or to other antihistamines of similar chemical structure (see *PRECAUTIONS—Drug Interactions*).

Antihistamines *should not* be used *in newborn or premature infants.* Because of the higher risk of antihistamines for infants generally and for newborns and prematures in particular, antihistamine therapy is contraindicated *in nursing mothers* (see *PRECAUTIONS—Nursing Mothers*).

WARNINGS: Antihistamines should be used with considerable caution in patients with: narrow angle glaucoma, stenosing peptic ulcer, pyloroduodenal obstruction, symptomatic prostatic hypertrophy, and bladder neck obstruction.

Use with CNS Depressants: TAVIST (clemastine fumarate) has additive effects with alcohol and other CNS depressants (hypnotics, sedatives, tranquilizers, etc.)

Use in Activities Requiring Mental Alertness: Patients should be warned about engaging in activities requiring mental alertness such as driving a car or operating appliances, machinery, etc.

Use in the Elderly (approximately 60 years or older): Antihistamines are more likely to cause dizziness, sedation, and hypotension in elderly patients.

PRECAUTIONS: General: TAVIST (clemastine fumarate) should be used with caution in patients with: history of bronchial asthma, increased intraocular pressure, hyperthyroidism, cardiovascular disease, and hypertension.

Information for Patients:
Patients taking antihistamines should receive the following information and instructions:

1. Antihistamines are prescribed to reduce allergic symptoms.

2. Patients should be questioned regarding a history of glaucoma, peptic ulcer, urinary retention, or pregnancy before starting antihistamine therapy.

3. Patients should be told not to take alcohol, sleeping pills, sedatives, or tranquilizers while taking antihistamines.

4. Antihistamines may cause drowsiness, dizziness, dry mouth, blurred vision, weakness, nausea, headache, or nervousness in some patients.

5. Patients should avoid driving a car or working with hazardous machinery until they assess the effects of this medicine.

6. Patients should be told to store this medicine in a tightly closed container in a dry, cool place away from heat or direct sunlight and out of the reach of children.

Drug Interactions:
Additive CNS depression may occur when antihistamines are administered concomitantly with other CNS depressants including barbiturates, tranquilizers, and alcohol. Patients receiving antihistamines should be advised against the concurrent use of other CNS depressant drugs.

Monoamine oxidase (MAO) inhibitors prolong and intensify the anticholinergic effects of antihistamines.

Carcinogenesis, Mutagenesis, Impairment of Fertility:
Carcinogenesis and Mutagenesis: In a 2-year oral study in the rat at a dose of 84 mg/kg (about 500 times the adult human dose) and an 85-week oral study in the mouse at 206 mg/kg (about 1300 times the adult human dose), clemastine fumarate showed no evidence of carcinogenesis. No mutagenic studies have been conducted with clemastine fumarate.

Impairment of Fertility: Oral doses of clemastine fumarate in the rat produced a decrease in mating ability of the male at 312 times the adult human dose. This effect was not found at 156 times the adult human dose.

Pregnancy:
Pregnancy Category B: Oral reproduction studies performed with clemastine fumarate in rats and rabbits at doses up to 312 and 188 times the adult human doses respectively, have revealed no evidence of teratogenic effects.

There are no adequate and well-controlled studies of TAVIST® (clemastine fumarate) Syrup in pregnant women. Because animal reproduction studies are not always predictive of human response, this drug should be used in pregnancy only if clearly needed.

Nursing Mothers:
Although quantitative determinations of antihistaminic drugs in breast milk have not been reported, qualitative tests have documented the excretion of diphenhydramine, pyrilamine, and tripelennamine in human milk.

Because of the potential for adverse reactions in nursing infants from antihistamines, a decision should be made whether to discontinue nursing or to discontinue the drug.

Pediatric Use:
The safety and efficacy of TAVIST (clemastine fumarate) Syrup has been confirmed in the pediatric population (age 6 years through 12). Safety and dose tolerance studies have confirmed children 6 through 11 years tolerated dosage ranges of 0.75 to 2.25 mg clemastine. In infants and children particularly, antihistamines in overdosage may produce hallucinations, convulsions, and death. Symptoms of antihistamine toxicity in children may include fixed dilated pupils, flushed face, dry mouth, fever, excitation, hallucinations, ataxia, incoordination, athetosis, tonic-clonic convulsions, and postictal depression (see *OVERDOSAGE*).

ADVERSE REACTIONS: The most frequent adverse reactions are underlined:

Nervous System: Sedation, sleepiness, dizziness, disturbed coordination, fatigue, confusion, restlessness, excitation, nervousness, tremor, irritability, insomnia, euphoria, paresthesia, blurred vision, diplopia, vertigo, tinnitus, acute labyrinthitis, hysteria, neuritis, convulsions.

Gastrointestinal System: Epigastric distress, anorexia, nausea, vomiting, diarrhea, constipation.

Respiratory System: Thickening of bronchial secretions, tightness of chest and wheezing, nasal stuffiness.

Cardiovascular System: Hypotension, headache, palpitations, tachycardia, extrasystoles.

Hematologic System: Hemolytic anemia, thrombocytopenia, agranulocytosis.

Genitourinary System: Urinary frequency, difficult urination, urinary retention, early menses.

General: Urticaria, drug rash, anaphylactic shock, photosensitivity, excessive perspiration, chills, dryness of mouth, nose and throat.

OVERDOSAGE: Antihistamine overdosage reactions may vary from central nervous system depression to stimulation. In children, stimulation predominates initially in a syndrome which may include excitement, hallucinations, ataxia, incoordination, muscle twitching, athetosis, hyperthermia, cyanosis convulsions, tremors, and hyperreflexia followed by postictal depression and cardio-respiratory arrest. Convulsions in children may be preceded by mild depression.

Dry mouth, fixed dilated pupils, flushing of the face, and fever are common. In adults, CNS depression, ranging from drowsiness to coma, is more common. The convulsant dose of antihistamines lies near the lethal dose. Convulsions indicate a poor prognosis.

In both children and adults, coma and cardiovascular collapse may occur. Deaths are reported especially in infants and children.

There is no specific therapy for acute overdosage with antihistamines. The latent period from ingestion to appearance of toxic effects is characteristically short (1/2-2 hours). General symptomatic and supportive measures should be instituted promptly and maintained for as long as necessary.

Since overdoses of other classes of drugs (i.e., tricyclic antidepressants) may also present anticholinergic symptomatology, appropriate toxicological analysis should be performed as soon as possible to identify the causative agent.

In the conscious patient, vomiting should be induced even though it may have occurred spontaneously. If vomiting cannot be induced, gastric lavage is indicated. Adequate precautions must be taken to protect against aspiration, especially in infants and children. Charcoal slurry or other suitable agents should be instilled into the stomach after vomiting or lavage. Saline cathartics or milk of magnesia may be of additional benefit.

In the unconscious patient, the airway should be secured with a cuffed endotracheal tube before attempting to evacuate the gastric contents. Intensive supportive and nursing care is indicated, as for any comatose patient.

If breathing is significantly impaired, maintenance of an adequate airway and mechanical support of respiration is the most effective means of providing adequate oxygenation.

Hypotension is an early sign of impending cardiovascular collapse and should be treated vigorously. Although general supportive measures are important, specific treatment with intravenous infusion of a vasopressor titrated to maintain adequate blood pressure may be necessary.

Do not use with CNS stimulants.

Convulsions should be controlled by careful administration of diazepam or a short-acting barbiturate, repeated as necessary. Physostigmine may also be considered for use in controlling centrally mediated convulsions.

Ice packs and cooling sponge baths, not alcohol, can aid in reducing the fever commonly seen in children. A more detailed review of antihistamine toxicology and overdose management is available in Gosselin, R.E., et al., "Clinical Toxicology of Commercial Products."

DOSAGE AND ADMINISTRATION: DOSAGE SHOULD BE INDIVIDUALIZED ACCORDING TO THE NEEDS AND RESPONSE OF THE PATIENT.

Pediatric: Children aged 6 to 12 years:
For Symptoms Of Allergic Rhinitis — The starting dose is 1 teaspoonful (0.5 mg clemastine)

twice daily. Since single doses of up to 2.25 mg clemastine were well tolerated by this age group, dosage may be increased as required, but not to exceed 6 teaspoonsful daily (3 mg clemastine).

For Urticaria and Angioedema — The starting dose is 2 teaspoonsful (1 mg clemastine) twice daily, not to exceed 6 teaspoonsful daily (3 mg clemastine).

Adults and Children 12 Years and Over:
For Symptoms of Allergic Rhinitis — The starting dose is 2 teaspoonsful (1.0 mg clemastine) twice daily. Dosage may be increased as required, but not to exceed 12 teaspoonsful daily (6 mg clemastine).

For Urticaria and Angioedema — The starting dose is 4 teaspoonsful (2 mg clemastine) twice daily, not to exceed 12 teaspoonsful daily (6 mg clemastine).

HOW SUPPLIED: TAVIST (clemastine fumarate) Syrup: clemastine 0.5 mg/5 ml (present as clemastine fumarate 0.67 mg/5 ml). A clear, colorless liquid with a citrus flavor, in 4 fl. oz. bottle (NDC 0078-0222-31).

Store and dispense: Below 77°F (25° C) tight, amber glass bottle. Store in an upright position.

[TAS-Z3   4/1/86]

Tavist-1®

(clemastine fumarate) tablets, USP
1.34 mg

Tavist®

(clemastine fumarate) tablets, USP
2.68 mg

DESCRIPTION: TAVIST (clemastine fumarate) belongs to the benzhydryl ether group of antihistaminic compounds. The chemical name is (+)-2-[-2-[(p-chloro-α-methyl-α-phenyl-benzyl)oxy]ethyl]-1-methyl-pyrrolidine hydrogen fumarate.

1.34 mg and 2.68 mg, Tablets
Active Ingredient: clemastine fumarate, USP
Inactive Ingredients: lactose, povidone, starch, stearic acid, and talc

ACTIONS: TAVIST is an antihistamine with anticholinergic (drying) and sedative side effects. Antihistamines appear to compete with histamine for cell receptor sites on effector cells. The inherently long duration of antihistaminic effects of TAVIST has been demonstrated in wheal and flare studies. In normal human subjects who received histamine injections over a 24-hour period, the antihistaminic activity of TAVIST reached a peak at 5-7 hours, persisted for 10-12 hours and, in some cases, for as long as 24 hours. Pharmacokinetic studies in man utilizing ^{3}H and ^{14}C labeled compound demonstrates that: TAVIST (clemastine fumarate) is rapidly and nearly completely absorbed from the gastrointestinal tract, peak plasma concentrations are attained in 2-4 hours, and urinary excretion is the major mode of elimination.

A3

INDICATIONS: TAVIST-1 Tablets 1.34 mg are indicated for the relief of symptoms associated with allergic rhinitis such as sneezing, rhinorrhea, pruritus and lacrimation.

TAVIST Tablets 2.68 mg are indicated for the relief of symptoms associated with allergic rhinitis such as sneezing, rhinorrhea, pruritus and lacrimation. TAVIST Tablets 2.68 mg are also indicated for the relief of mild, uncomplicated allergic skin manifestations of urticaria and angioedema.

It should be noted that TAVIST (clemastine fumarate) is indicated for the dermatologic indications at the 2.68 mg dosage level only.

CONTRAINDICATIONS: *Use in Nursing Mothers:* Because of the higher risk of antihistamines for infants generally and for newborns and prematures in particular, antihistamine therapy is contraindicated in nursing mothers.

Use in Lower Respiratory Disease: Antihistamines *should not* be used to treat lower respiratory tract symptoms including asthma.

Antihistamines are also contraindicated in the following conditions:

Hypersensitivity to TAVIST (clemastine fumarate) or other antihistamines of similar chemical structure.

Monamine oxidase inhibitor therapy (see Drug Interaction Section).

WARNINGS: Antihistamines should be used with considerable caution in patients with: narrow angle glaucoma, stenosing peptic ulcer, pyloroduodenal obstruction, symptomatic prostatic hypertrophy, and bladder neck obstruction.

Use in Children: Safety and efficacy of TAVIST have not been established in children under the age of 12.

Use in Pregnancy: Experience with this drug in pregnant women is inadequate to determine whether there exists a potential for harm to the developing fetus.

Use with CNS Depressants: TAVIST has additive effects with alcohol and other CNS depressants (hypnotics, sedatives, tranquilizers, etc.).

Use in Activities Requiring Mental Alertness: Patients should be warned about engaging in activities requiring mental alertness such as driving a car or operating appliances, machinery, etc.

Use in the Elderly (approximately 60 years or older): Antihistamines are more likely to cause dizziness, sedation, and hypotension in elderly patients.

PRECAUTIONS: TAVIST (clemastine fumarate) should be used with caution in patients with: history of bronchial asthma, increased intraocular pressure, hyperthyroidism, cardiovascular disease, and hypertension.

Drug Interactions: MAO inhibitors prolong and intensify the anticholinergic (drying) effects of antihistamines.

ADVERSE REACTIONS: Transient drowsiness, the most common adverse reaction associated with TAVIST (clemastine fumarate), occurs relatively frequently and may require discontinuation of therapy in some instances.

Antihistaminic Compounds: It should be noted that the following reactions have occurred with one or more antihistamines and, therefore, should be kept in mind when prescribing drugs belonging to this class, including TAVIST. The most frequent adverse reactions are underlined.

1. *General:* Urticaria, drug rash, anaphylactic shock, photosensitivity, excessive perspiration, chills, dryness of mouth, nose, and throat.

2. *Cardiovascular System:* Hypotension, headache, palpitations, tachycardia, extrasystoles.

3. *Hematologic System:* Hemolytic anemia, thrombocytopenia, agranulocytosis.

4. *Nervous System: Sedation, sleepiness, dizziness, disturbed coordination, fatigue, confusion, restlessness, excitation, nervousness, tremor, irritability, insomnia, euphoria, parasthesias, blurred vision, diplopia, vertigo, tinnitus, acute labyrinthitis, hysteria, neuritis, convulsions.*

5. *GI System:* Epigastric distress, anorexia, nausea, vomiting, diarrhea, constipation.

6. *GU System:* Urinary frequency, difficult urination, urinary retention, early menses.

7. *Respiratory System:* Thickening of bronchial secretions, tightness of chest and wheezing, nasal stuffiness.

OVERDOSAGE: Antihistamine overdosage reactions may vary from central nervous system depression to stimulation. Stimulation is particularly likely in children. Atropine-like signs and symptoms: dry mouth; fixed, dilated pupils; flushing; and gastrointestinal symptoms may also occur.

If vomiting has not occurred spontaneously the conscious patient should be induced to vomit. This is best done by having him drink a glass of water or milk after which he should be made to gag. Precautions against aspiration must be taken, especially in infants and children.

If vomiting is unsuccessful gastric lavage is indicated within 3 hours after ingestion and even later if large amounts of milk or cream were given beforehand. Isotonic and ½ isotonic saline is the lavage solution of choice.

Saline cathartics, such as milk of magnesia, by osmosis draw water into the bowel and therefore, are valuable for their action in rapid dilution of bowel content.

Stimulants should *not* be used.

Vasopressors may be used to treat hypotension.

DOSAGE AND ADMINISTRATION: DOSAGE SHOULD BE INDIVIDUALIZED ACCORDING TO THE NEEDS AND RESPONSE OF THE PATIENT.

TAVIST-1® Tablets 1.34 mg: The recommended starting dose is one tablet twice daily. Dosage may be increased as required, but not to exceed six tablets daily.

TAVIST® Tablets 2.68 mg: The maximum recommended dosage is one tablet three times daily. Many patients respond favorably to a single dose which may be repeated as required, but not to exceed three tablets daily.

HOW SUPPLIED: TAVIST-1 Tablets: 1.34 mg clemastine fumarate. White, oval, compressed, scored tablet, embossed "78-75" on one side, "TAVIST-1" on the other. Packages of 100.

TAVIST Tablets: 2.68 mg clemastine fumarate. White, round compressed tablet, embossed "78-72" and scored on one side, "TAVIST" on the other. Packages of 100.

[TAV-Z3 7/15/86]

Tavist-D®

(clemastine fumarate, USP phenylpropanolamine HCl, USP) Tablets

DESCRIPTION: Each TAVIST-D® (clemastine fumarate/phenylpropanolamine HCl) Tablet contains 1.34 mg clemastine fumarate (equivalent to 1 mg of the free base) and 75 mg phenylpropanolamine hydrochloride. The clemastine fumarate is in the outer shell of the tablet and is immediately released upon dissolution. The tablet's core is a sustained-release matrix which releases the phenylpropanolamine hydrochloride over a 12-hour period at a rate that produces blood levels bioequivalent to those obtained by the administration of 25 mg standard release tablets of phenylpropanolamine hydrochloride every four hours for three doses. Clemastine fumarate belongs to the benzhydryl ether group of antihistaminic compounds. The chemical name is (+)-2-[2-[(p-chloro-α-methyl-α-phenylbenzyl) oxy]ethyl]-1-methylpyrrolidine hydrogen fumarate.

Phenylpropanolamine hydrochloride is a sympathomimetic, orally effective nasal decongestant. Sympathomimetic compounds, whether catecholamines or non-catecholamines, can be regarded as compounds produced by substitution on the -phenylethylamine nucleus common to all these sympathomimetic products, whether their action is on the Alpha receptors of the sympathetic nervous system or on Beta-1 or Beta-2 receptors. The chemical name for phenylpropanolamine hydrochloride is α-(1-Aminoethyl)benzenemethanol hydrochloride.

Active Ingredient: clemastine fumarate, USP phenylpropanolamine HCl, USP

Inactive Ingredients: colloidal silicon dioxide, D&C Yellow #10, dibasic calcium phosphate dihydrate, lactose, magnesium stearate, methylcellulose, polyethylene glycol, povidone, starch, synthetic polymers, and titanium dioxide.

CLINICAL PHARMACOLOGY: Clemastine fumarate is an antihistamine with anticholinergic

(drying) and sedative side effects. Antihistamines appear to compete with histamine for cell receptor sites on effector cells. The inherently long duration of antihistaminic effects of clemastine fumarate has been demonstrated in wheal and flare studies. In normal human subjects who received intradermal histamine injections over a 24-hour period, the antihistaminic activity of clemastine fumarate, as demonstrated by inhibition of the wheal and flare reaction, reached a peak at 5-7 hours, persisted for 10-12 hours and, in some cases, for as long as 24 hours. Pharmacokinetic studies in man utilizing ^{3}H and ^{14}C labeled compound demonstrate that clemastine fumarate is rapidly and nearly completely absorbed from the gastrointestinal tract, peak plasma concentrations are attained in 2-4 hours, and urinary excretion is the major mode of elimination.

Phenylpropanolamine hydrochloride is an Alpha adrenergic stimulator producing nasal decongestion by constriction of arterioles and precapillary arterioles in the nasal mucosa. Phenylpropanolamine hydrochloride is one of the most widely used oral nasal decongestants; it is similar in action to ephedrine, but produces less central nervous system stimulation.

In adult subjects who were given one TAVIST-D (clemastine fumarate/phenylpropanolamine HCl) Tablet, the average peak plasma concentration of phenylpropanolamine was 85.4 ng/ml $\pm$ 13.1 (S.D.) which occurred at about 4.3 hours. In this crossover study these same subjects were given a 25 mg phenylpropanolamine hydrochloride tablet every 4 hours for 3 consecutive doses plus a single dose of a TAVIST-1 Tablet (clemastine fumarate 1.34 mg). The average peak concentration of phenylpropanolamine was found to be 67.6 ng/ml $\pm$ 11.6 (S.D.) which occurred at about 8.2 hours.

In another study, adult subjects received TAVIST-D Tablets every 12 hours for 4 consecutive days. The average peak concentration of phenylpropanolamine was found to be 117.29 ng/ml $\pm$ 14.52 (S.D.) which occurred at about 6.2 hours after the morning dose. In this crossover study these same subjects received a 25 mg phenylpropanolamine hydrochloride tablet every 4 hours for 4 consecutive days. In addition they received a TAVIST-1 Tablet (clemastine fumarate 1.34 mg) every 12 hours for 4 consecutive days. The average peak concentration of phenylpropanolamine was found to be 107.92 ng/ml $\pm$ 15.97 (S.D.) which occurred at about 4.8 hours after the first dose in the morning.

INDICATIONS AND USAGE: TAVIST-D (clemastine fumarate/phenylpropanolamine HCl) Tablets are indicated for the relief of symptoms associated with allergic rhinitis such as sneezing, rhinorrhea, pruritis of the eyes, nose or throat, lacrimation and nasal congestion.

CONTRAINDICATION: TAVIST-D Tablets are contraindicated in patients hypersensitive to any of the components. Antihistamines should not be used in newborn or premature infants or in nursing mothers. Antihistamines should not be used to treat lower respiratory tract symptoms including asthma. Tavist-D Tablets are contraindicated in patients receiving monoamine oxidase inhibitors (see PRECAUTIONS — Drug Interactions) and in patients with severe hypertension or severe coronary artery disease.

WARNINGS: Antihistamines such as clemastine fumarate should be used with considerable caution in patients with: narrow angle glaucoma, stenosing peptic ulcer, pyloroduodenal obstruction, symptomatic prostatic hypertrophy, and bladder neck obstruction. Sympathomimetic drugs such as phenylpropanolamine hydrochloride should be used with caution in hypertension, cardiovascular disease, diabetes mellitus, and uncontrolled hyperthyroidism.

Use with CNS Depressants: Antihistamines have additive effects with alcohol and other CNS depressants (hypnotics, sedatives, tranquilizers, etc.).

Use in Activities Requiring Mental Alertness: Patients should be warned about engaging in activities requiring mental alertness such as driving a car or operating appliances, machinery, etc.

Use in the Elderly (approximately 60 years or older): Antihistamines are more likely to cause dizziness, sedation and hypotension in elderly patients. Overdosages of sympathomimetics in this age group may cause hallucinations, convulsions, CNS depression and death in elderly patients.

Use in Children: Safety and effectiveness of TAVIST-D (clemastine fumarate/phenylpropanolamine HCl) have not been established in children under the age of 12. In infants and children, especially, antihistamines in *overdosage* may cause hallucinations, convulsions or death. As in adults, antihistamines may diminish mental alertness, but they may also produce excitation, particularly in young children.

PRECAUTIONS:
General: TAVIST-D (clemastine fumarate/phenylpropanolamine HCl) Tablets should be used with caution in patients with: History of bronchial asthma, increased intraocular pressure, hyperthyroidism, cardiovascular disease, hypertension, diabetes mellitus, and prostate disease. (See WARNINGS.)

Information for Patients: Patients should be informed of the potential for sedation or drowsiness and warned about driving or operating machinery. The concomitant consumption of alcoholic beverages or other sedative drugs should be avoided.

Due to the inherently long-acting nature of clemastine fumarate and due to the sustained-release of phenylpropanolamine hydrochloride from the tablet's core, TAVIST-D® Tablets provide prolonged symptomatic relief (10-14 hours).

Drug Interactions:
1. Monoamine oxidase inhibitors: MAO inhibitors prolong and intensify the anticholinergic effects of antihistamines and potentiate the pressor effects of sympathomimetics.

2. Alcohol and CNS depressants: These agents potentiate the sedative effects of antihistamines.

3. Certain antihypertensives: Sympathomimetics may reduce the antihypertensive effects of methyldopa, mecamylamine, reserpine and veratrum alkaloids.

Carcinogenesis and Mutagenesis: Carcinogenic studies have not been conducted on the drug combination of clemastine fumarate/phenylpropanolamine hydrochloride. In a two-year oral study in the rat at a dose of 84 mg/Kg (about 1500 times the human dose) and an 85-week oral study in the mouse at 206 mg/Kg (about 3800 times the human dose), clemastine fumarate showed no evidence of carcinogenesis.

No mutagenic studies have been conducted with clemastine fumarate, phenylpropanolamine hydrochloride or the drug combination.

Impairment of Fertility: Oral doses of clemastine fumarate alone in the rat produced a decrease in mating ability of the male at 933 times the human dose. This effect was not found at 466 times the human dose.

Pregnancy — *Pregnancy Category B:* Oral reproduction studies performed with clemastine fumarate alone in rats and rabbits at doses up to 933 and 560 times the human dose, respectively, have revealed no evidence of teratogenic effects. Reproduction studies have not been conducted with phenylpropanolamine hydrochloride alone.

Oral reproduction studies on the drug combination in a ratio of 1 part of clemastine fumarate to 49 parts of phenylpropanolamine hydrochloride in rats and rabbits at doses up to 100 and 67 times the human dose, respectively, have revealed no evidence of teratogenic effects. Adverse reactions attributed to the pharmacological effects of phenylpropanolamine were as follows: Rats — Impaired weight gain and deaths in dams at 33 times the human dose and a slight increase in pre-implantation loss and prenatal deaths, and reduced fetal weights at 100 times the human dose. Rabbits — Increased maternal deaths at 20 times the human dose, and increased maternal deaths and weight loss plus a slight increase in prenatal deaths (within normal limits) at 67 times the human dose.

There are no adequate and well controlled studies of Tavist-D (clemastine fumarate/phenylpropanolamine HCl) Tablets in pregnant women. Because animal reproductive studies are not always predictive of human response, this drug should be used in pregnancy only if clearly needed.

Nursing Mothers: See CONTRAINDICATIONS.

ADVERSE REACTIONS:
Antihistaminic Compounds: It should be noted that the following reactions have occurred with one or more antihistamines and, therefore, should be kept in mind when prescribing drugs belonging to this class, including clemastine fumarate. The most frequent adverse reactions reported with clemastine fumarate are underlined.

1. *General:* Urticaria, drug rash, anaphylactic shock, photosensitivity, excessive perspiration, chills, dryness of mouth, nose and throat.

2. *Cardiovascular System:* Hypotension, headache, palpitations, tachycardia, extrasystoles.

3. *Hematologic System:* Hemolytic anemia, thrombocytopenia, agranulocytosis.

4. *Nervous System:* Sedation, sleepiness, dizziness, disturbed coordination, fatigue, confusion, restlessness, excitation, nervousness, tremor, irritability, insomnia, euphoria, paresthesias, blurred vision, diplopia, vertigo, tinnitus, acute labyrinthitis, hysteria, neuritis, convulsions.

5. *GI System:* Epigastric distress, anorexia, nausea, vomiting, diarrhea, constipation.

6. *GU System:* Urinary frequency, difficult urination, urinary retention, early menses.

7. *Respiratory System:* Thickening of bronchial secretions, tightness of chest and wheezing, nasal stuffiness.

Sympathomimetic Compounds: *Nervous System:* At higher doses may cause drowsiness, dizziness, nervousness, or sleeplessness, and especially in children may cause excitability. Phenylpropanolamine hydrochloride may cause elevated blood pressure and tachyarrhythmias, especially in hyperthyroid patients.

OVERDOSAGE: Antihistamine overdosage reactions may vary from central nervous system depression to stimulation. Stimulation is particularly likely in children. Atropine-like signs and symptoms: dry mouth; fixed, dilated pupils; flushing; and gastrointestinal symptoms may also occur.

Overdosage of the phenylpropanolamine hydrochloride may produce tachycardia, pupillary dilatation, excitation and arrhythmias.

If vomiting has not occurred spontaneously the conscious patient should be induced to vomit. This is best done by having the patient drink a glass of water or milk along with an appropriate amount of Syrup of Ipecac. Precautions against aspiration must be taken, especially in infants and children.

If vomiting is unsuccessful in 20 minutes, gastric lavage is indicated within 3 hours after ingestion and even later if large amounts of milk or cream were given beforehand. Isotonic and ½ isotonic saline is the lavage solution of choice.

Saline cathartics, such as milk of magnesia, by osmosis draw water into the bowel and therefore are valuable for their action in rapid dilution of bowel content.

Stimulants should *not* be used.

Activated charcoal has been demonstrated to interfere with phenylpropanolamine absorption.

The value of dialysis has not been established.

The concentration of phenylpropanolamine hydrochloride or clemastine fumarate in biological fluids associated with toxicity is not known.

The amount of TAVIST-D in single doses associated with significant signs of overdose or death is not known.

The oral LD_{50} for a mixture containing 50 mg phenylpropanolamine hydrochloride and 1.34 mg clemastine fumarate is 1277 mg/Kg in mice, 602 mg/Kg in rats and 634 mg/Kg in rabbits.

DOSAGE AND ADMINISTRATION: Adults and children twelve years and over:
One tablet swallowed whole every twelve hours.

HOW SUPPLIED: TAVIST-D (clemastine fumarate/phenylpropanolamine HCl) Tablets: containing 1.34 mg clemastine fumarate (equivalent to 1 mg of the free base) and 75 mg phenylpropanolamine hydrochloride. White, round, film-coated multiple compressed tablet, embossed "TAVIST-D" on one side and "78-221" on the other. Packages of 100 (NDC 0078-0221-05). TAVIST-D Tablets should be stored and dispensed below 86°F in a tight, light-resistant container.

[TAD-Z4   4/15/86]

Triaminic® Cold Syrup

DESCRIPTION: Each teaspoonful (5 ml) of TRIAMINIC Cold Syrup contains: phenylpropanolamine hydrochloride 12.5 mg and chlorpheniramine maleate 2 mg in a nonalcoholic vehicle. Other ingredients: benzoic acid, edetate disodium, flavors, purified water, sodium hydroxide, sorbitol, sucrose, Yellow 6.

INDICATIONS: Temporarily relieves runny nose, nasal congestion and sneezing due to colds and allergies. Also relieves itching nose or throat and itchy, watery eyes associated with allergies.

WARNINGS: Unless directed by a doctor, do not take this product if you have heart disease, high blood pressure, thyroid disease, diabetes, asthma, glaucoma, difficulty in breathing, enlargement of the prostate gland or are taking a prescription drug for high blood pressure or depression. Do not exceed recommended dosage or take for more than 7 days. If symptoms persist or are accompanied by fever, consult a doctor. May cause excitability especially in children. May cause drowsiness. Avoid drinking alcohol, driving or operating machinery while taking this product. As with any drug, if you are pregnant or nursing a baby seek the advice of a health professional before using this product. Keep this and all drugs out of the reach of children. In case of accidental overdose, seek professional assistance or contact a Poison Control Center immediately.

DOSAGE AND ADMINISTRATION: Adults and children 12 and over — 2 teaspoonfuls every 4 hours. Children 6 to under 12 years — 1 teaspoonful every 4 hours. Unless directed by physician, do not exceed 6 doses in 24 hours. Consult physician for dosage under 6 years of age.

PROFESSIONAL LABELING: The suggested dosage for pediatric patients is:

3-12 months	1 drop/Kg of body weight every 4 hours
12-24 months	3 drops/Kg of body weight every 4 hours
2-6 years	½ teaspoonful every 4 hours

HOW SUPPLIED: TRIAMINIC Cold Syrup (orange), in 4 fl oz and 8 fl oz plastic bottles with tamper-evident band around child-resistant cap.

Triaminic®
Expectorant

DESCRIPTION: Each teaspoonful (5 ml) of TRIAMINIC Expectorant contains: phenylpropanolamine hydrochloride 12.5 mg and guaifenesin 100 mg. Other ingredients: alcohol (5%), benzoic acid, edetate disodium, flavors, purified water, saccharin, saccharin sodium, sodium hydroxide, sorbitol, sucrose, Yellow 6, Yellow 10. ·

INDICATIONS: Helps loosen phlegm and bronchial secretions of a dry cough. Helps rid bronchial passageways of phlegm and relieve dry, irritated throat. Temporarily relieves nasal congestion due to colds, allergies and sinusitis.

WARNINGS: Unless directed by a doctor, do not take this product if you have heart disease, high blood pressure, thyroid disease, diabetes, enlargement of the prostate gland or are taking a prescription drug for high blood pressure or depression. Do not exceed recommended dosage or take for more than 7 days. If symptoms persist, are accompanied by fever, rash or persistent headache or if cough recurs, consult a doctor. As with any drug, if you are pregnant or nursing a baby, seek advice from a health professional before using this product. Keep this and all drugs out of the reach of children. In case of accidental overdose, seek professional assistance or contact a Poison Control Center immediately.

DOSAGE AND ADMINISTRATION: Adults and children 12 and over — 2 teaspoonfuls every 4 hours. Children 6 to under 12 years — 1 teaspoonful every 4 hours. Children 2 to under 6 years — ½ teaspoonful every 4 hours. Unless directed by physician, do not exceed 6 doses in 24 hours or give to children under 2 years of age.

PROFESSIONAL LABELING: The suggested dosage for pediatric patients is:
3-12 months 2 drops/Kg of body weight every 4 hours
12-24 months 3 drops/Kg of body weight every 4 hours

HOW SUPPLIED: TRIAMINIC Expectorant (yellow), in 4 fl oz and 8 fl oz plastic bottles with tamper-evident band around child-resistant cap.

Triaminic-DM®
Cough Formula

DESCRIPTION: Each teaspoonful (5 ml) of TRIAMINIC-DM Cough Formula contains: phenylpropanolamine hydrochloride 12.5 mg and dextromethorphan hydrobromide 10 mg in a nonalcoholic vehicle. Other ingredients: benzoic acid, Blue 1, flavors, propylene glycol, purified water, Red 40, sodium chloride, sorbitol, sucrose.

INDICATIONS: Temporarily relieves coughs due to minor throat and bronchial irritation. Temporarily relieves nasal congestion due to colds, allergies and sinusitis.

WARNINGS: Unless directed by a doctor, **DO NOT** take this product: **1)** if cough is accompanied by excessive secretions, **2)** for persistent cough such as occurs with smoking, asthma or emphysema, or **3)** if you have heart disease, high blood pressure, thyroid disease, diabetes, enlargement of the prostate gland or are taking a prescription drug for high blood pressure or depression. Do not exceed recommended dosage or take for more than 7 days. If symptoms persist, are accompanied by fever, rash or persistent headache or if cough recurs, consult a doctor. As with any drug, if you are pregnant or nursing a baby, seek advice from a health professional before using this product. Keep this and all drugs out of reach of children. In case of accidental overdose, seek professional assistance or contact a Poison Control Center immediately.

DOSAGE AND ADMINISTRATION: Adults and children 12 and over — 2 teaspoonfuls every 4 hours. Children 6 to under 12 years — 1 teaspoonful every 4 hours. Children 2 to under 6 years — ½ teaspoonful every 4 hours. Unless directed by physician, do not exceed 6 doses in 24 hours or give to children under 2 years of age.

PROFESSIONAL LABELING: The suggested dosage for pediatric patients is:
3-12 months 1 drop/Kg of body weight every 4 hours
12-24 months 3 drops/Kg of body weight every 4 hours

HOW SUPPLIED: TRIAMINIC-DM Cough Formula (dark red), in 4 fl oz and 8 fl oz plastic bottles with tamper-evident band around child-resistant cap.

Triaminicol®
Multi-Symptom
Cold Syrup

DESCRIPTION: Each teaspoonful (5 ml) of TRIAMINICOL Multi-Symptom Cold Syrup contains: phenylpropanolamine hydrochloride 12.5 mg, chlorpheniramine maleate 2 mg, dextromethorphan hydrobromide 10 mg in a palatable non-alcoholic vehicle. Other ingredients: benzoic acid, flavors, propylene glycol, purified water, Red 40, saccharin sodium, sodium chloride, sorbitol, sucrose.

INDICATIONS: Temporarily relieves coughs due to minor sore throat and bronchial irritation. Temporarily relieves runny nose, nasal congestion and sneezing due to colds and allergies. Also relieves itching nose or throat and itchy, watery eyes associated with allergies.

WARNINGS: Unless directed by a doctor, **DO NOT** take this product: **1)** if cough is accompanied by excessive secretions, **2)** for persistent cough such as occurs with smoking, asthma or emphysema, or **3)** if you have heart disease, high blood pressure, thyroid disease, diabetes, asthma, glaucoma, difficulty in breathing, enlargement of the prostate gland or are taking a prescription drug for high blood pressure or depression. Do not exceed recommended dosage or take for more than 7 days. If symptoms persist, are accompanied by fever, rash or persistent headache or if cough recurs, consult a doctor. May cause excitability especially in children. May cause drowsiness. Avoid drinking alcohol, driving or operating machinery while taking this product. As with any drug, if you are pregnant or nursing a baby, seek the advice of a health professional before using this product. Keep this and all drugs out of the reach of children. In case of accidental overdose, seek professional assistance or contact a Poison Control Center immediately.

DOSAGE AND ADMINISTRATION: Adults and children 12 and over — 2 teaspoonfuls every 4 hours. Children 6 to under 12 years — 1 teaspoonful every 4 hours. Unless directed by physician, do not exceed 6 doses in 24 hours or give to children under 6 years of age.

PROFESSIONAL LABELING: The suggested dosage for pediatric patients is:
3-12 months   1 drop/Kg of body weight every 4 hours
12-24 months   3 drops/Kg of body weight every 4 hours
2-6 years   ½ teaspoonful every 4 hours

HOW SUPPLIED: TRIAMINICOL Multi-Symptom Cold Syrup (red), in 4 fl oz and 8 fl oz plastic bottles with tamper-evident band around child-resistant cap.

Triaminic® Oral Infant Drops

DESCRIPTION: Each ml of TRIAMINIC Oral Infant Drops contains: phenylpropanolamine hydrochloride 20 mg, pheniramine maleate 10 mg, and pyrilamine maleate 10 mg. Other ingredients: benzoic acid, flavor, glycerin, purified water, Red 33, saccharin sodium, sorbitol, sucrose, Yellow 6.

This product combines the nasal decongestant properties of phenylpropanolamine hydrochloride with the antihistaminic activities of pheniramine maleate and pyrilamine maleate.

Phenylpropanolamine hydrochloride, a sympathomimetic drug, is structurally related to ephedrine and amphetamine. Pheniramine maleate is an antihistamine of the alkylamine class while pyrilamine maleate belongs to the ethylenediamine class.

CLINICAL PHARMACOLOGY: Phenylpropanolamine presumably acts on α-adrenergic receptors in the mucosa of the respiratory tract producing vasoconstriction which results in shrinkage of swollen mucous membranes, reduction of tissue hyperemia, edema and nasal congestion, and an increase in nasal airway patency. Antihistamines competitively act as H, receptor antagonists of histamine. They exhibit anticholinergic (drying) and sedative side effects. There are several classes of antihistamines which vary with respect to potency, dosage and the relative incidence of side effects. Antihistamines inhibit the effects of histamine on capillary permeability and on vascular, bronchial and many other types of smooth muscle.

INDICATIONS AND USAGE: For relief from such symptoms as nasal congestion and post nasal drip associated with colds, allergies, sinusitis and rhinitis. Also for relief of symptoms associated with allergic rhinitis such as sneezing, rhinorrhea, pruritus and lacrimation.

CONTRAINDICATIONS: TRIAMINIC Oral Infant Drops are contraindicated in patients exhibiting hypersensitivity to any of the ingredients. Antihistamines are contraindicated in patients receiving monoamine oxidase inhibitors since these agents may prolong and intensify the anticholinergic and CNS depressant effects of antihistamines (See Drug Interactions). Antihistamines should not be used to treat lower respiratory tract symptoms or be given to premature or newborn infants. Sympathomimetic agents such as phenylpropanolamine are contraindicated in patients with severe hypertension, severe coronary artery disease and in those taking monoamine oxidase inhibitors.

WARNINGS: Sympathomimetic agents should be used with caution in patients with hypertension, hyperthyroidism, diabetes melitus and cardiovascular disease. Antihistamines should be used with caution in patients with narrow angle glaucoma, stenosing peptic ulcer, pyloroduodenal obstruction, symptomatic prostatic hypertrophy, bladder neck obstruction or chronic pulmonary disease.

PRECAUTIONS: General: see WARNINGS.
Information For Patients:
Mothers should be informed of the potential for sedation or drowsiness. When prescribing antihistamine preparations, patients should be cautioned against mechanical activity requiring alertness.

Drug Interactions:
1. Monoamine oxidase inhibitors: MAO inhibitors prolong and intensify the anticholinergic effects of antihistamines and potentiate the pressor effects of sympathomimetics.

2. Alcohol and CNS depressants: These agents potentiate the sedative effects of antihistamines.

3. Certain antihypertensives: Sympathomimetics may reduce the antihypertensive effects of methyldopa, mecamylamine, reserpine and veratrum alkaloids.

Carcinogenesis, Mutagenesis, Impairment Of Fertility: No data are available on the long-term potential for carcinogenicity, mutagenicity or impairment of fertility in animals or humans.

Pediatric Use: TRIAMINIC Oral Infant Drops have been formulated to provide safe and effective symptomatic relief for infants and small children. Precise dosage (on a body weight basis) is facilitated through the use of the plastic squeeze bottle with attached dropper tip (see DOSAGE AND ADMINISTRATION). It is important to note the variability of response infants and small children exhibit to antihistamines and sympathomimetics. As in adults, the combination of an antihistamine and sympathomimetic can elicit either mild stimulation or mild sedation in children. In the young child, mild stimulation is the response most frequently seen. In infants and children, overdosage of antihistamines may cause hallucinations, convulsions or death.

ADVERSE REACTIONS: The most frequent adverse reactions are underlined.

1. *General:* urticaria, drug rash, anaphylactic shock, photosensitivity, excessive perspiration, chills, dryness of mouth, nose and throat.

2. *Cardiovascular System:* hypotension, headache, palpitations, tachycardia, extrasystoles.

3. *Hematologic System:* hemolytic anemia, thrombocytopenia, agranulocytosis.

4. *Nervous System:* Sedation, sleepiness, dizziness, disturbed coordination, fatigue, confusion, restlessness, excitation, nervousness, tremor, irritability, insomnia, euphoria, paresthesias, blurred vision, diplopia, vertigo, tinnitus, acute labyrinthitis, hysteria, neuritis, convulsions, CNS depression, hallucinations.

5. *GI System:* epigastric distress, anorexia, nausea, vomiting, diarrhea, constipation.

6. *GU System:* urinary frequency, difficult urination, urinary retention.

7. *Respiratory System:* thickening of bronchial secretions, tightness of chest and wheezing nasal stuffiness.

OVERDOSAGE: TRIAMINIC product overdosage reactions may vary from central nervous system depression to stimulation. Stimulation is particularly likely in children. Atropine-like signs and symptoms—dry mouth, fixed, dilated pupils; flushing—and gastrointestinal symptoms may also occur.

If vomiting has not occurred spontaneously, the conscious patient should be induced to vomit. This is best done by having the patient drink a glass of water or milk after which they should be made to gag. Precautions against aspiration must be taken, especially in infants and children.

If vomiting is unsuccessful, gastric lavage is indicated within 3 hours after ingestion, and even later if large amounts of milk or cream were given beforehand. Isotonic and ½ isotonic saline is the lavage solution of choice.

Saline cathartics, such as milk of magnesia, draw water by osmosis into the bowel and therefore are valuable for their action in rapid dilution of bowel content.

Stimulants should not be used. Vasopressors may be used to treat hypotension.

DOSAGE AND ADMINISTRATION: 1 drop per 2 pounds of body weight administered orally 4 times daily. The prescribed number of drops may be put directly into child's mouth or on a spoon for administration.

HOW SUPPLIED: TRIAMINIC Oral Infant Drops, in 15 ml plastic squeeze bottles which deliver approximately 24 drops per ml. Store TRIAMINIC Oral Infant Drops at room temperature.